HEALTH CARE FOR SINGLE HOMELESS PEOPLE

HEALTH CARE FOR SINGLE HOMELESS PEOPLE

SANDRA WILLIAMS and ISOBEL ALLEN

Policy Studies Institute

PSI Publications are obtainable from all good bookshops, or by visiting the Institute at 100 Park Village East, London NW1 3SR (01-387 2171).

Sales Representation: Pinter Publishers Ltd.

Individual and Bookshop orders to: Marston Book Services Ltd, PO Box 87, Oxford, OX4 1LB.

A CIP catalogue record of this book is available from the British Library

PSI Research Report 699

ISBN 0 85374 381 9

Laserset by Policy Studies Institute

Printed by BPCC Wheaton's Ltd, Exeter

Acknowledgements

This study was initiated and funded by the Department of Health and Social Security (now the Department of Health). Several members of staff at the Department gave their support and guidance at various stages of the research. Particular thanks are due to Hugh Jones, Doreen Rothman and Lynne Fosh.

The study was designed and directed by Isobel Allen. Sandra Williams was the principal researcher on the project. She was responsible for managing the project and wrote the majority of the report.

Many thanks are due to the interviewers who spent a lot of their time in day centres, night shelters and hostels talking to homeless people, as well as in the field interviewing a range of providers of health care. This study made great demands on their emotional stamina as well as their interviewing skills. The interviewers were Sheila Chetham, Ian Christie, Jenny Green, Jenny Jacoby and Annette Walling.

We are also grateful to Annette Walling for her organisational skills and determination in keeping track of all the contact sheet information about use and users of the pilot schemes. Coding was carried out by Ian Christie, Rosemary Markham and Annette Walling. Karen MacKinnon was responsible for the computing and preparation of tables and her help was much appreciated during the computer analysis of the data. Karin Erskine provided valuable help and guidance on typesetting and presentation.

Marie-Anne Doggett prepared the comprehensive review of the literature on primary health care for single homeless people which is presented at the end of this report. This brings together, for the first time, a vast amount of published and unpublished literature addressing the issue of health care for homeless people

We are grateful to all the health care professionals, voluntary workers and wardens of centres used by homeless people who spared the time to be interviewed by us. In particular, we should like to thank the team members of both pilot schemes for their co-operation during the monitoring period. We recognise that it cannot have been easy starting a new service with a new team while under the close scrutiny of researchers and constrained by a limited time scale. Finally, we owe an enormous amount to the homeless people themselves who talked to us about their use and opinions of health care services. They often have difficulty making their voices heard. We have reported their views and experiences and in so doing we hope to have shed light on some of the misconceptions about homeless people and the realities of providing health care services to them.

Contents

List of Tables

Chapter 4

Appendix 1

Appendix 3

1 Introduction

Aims of the study

This study looks at primary health care for homeless people and, in particular, at two pilot schemes in Inner London which were funded by the Department of Health and Social Security and became operational in 1986. The schemes were located in Tower Hamlets and in Camden and were managed respectively by the City and East London and the Camden and Islington Family Practitioner Committees (FPCs). Through the use of multidisciplinary health care teams they were intended to provide primary health care to homeless people within the locality of their responsible FPCs.

The schemes had a number of objectives: to identify and contact as many homeless people as practicable within the locality of the FPCs, gain their confidence, diagnose and treat their morbidity, and wherever possible, secure their admission to the list of a general medical practitioner. It was also hoped that the problems of alcohol dependence and homelessness would be tackled, with a view to rehabilitation where possible.

The Policy Studies Institute (PSI) was asked by the Department to evaluate the two pilot schemes. The main aims of the research were to assess the schemes in the light of their objectives and to comment on their appropriateness as a model of care for the homeless. It was envisaged that this would be essentially a descriptive study, looking at the organisation and functioning of the health care teams in each of the two project areas, referral patterns into and out of the schemes, and the incidence of morbidity of homeless people using the schemes. In addition, it examined the views of professionals and voluntary workers,

1

as well as the users themselves, on the delivery of primary health care to the homeless. It was also hoped that it would be possible to develop measures of 'outcome' to assess the impact of the schemes on the health and well-being of the consumers - the homeless people.

For the purposes of the study, a homeless person was defined as one who had no fixed abode or who was dwelling in a hostel which was used primarily by homeless people. The study concentrates on the health care experiences of *single* homeless people because it was this group who used the pilot schemes. The Department's expectation that the scheme in Tower Hamlets would be used primarily by single homeless people while the scheme in Camden would in addition deal with homeless families living in hotels and hostels was not borne out in practice. Our frequent use of the phrase single homeless people should not mislead the reader into thinking that we assume that those who are single and homeless constitute a homogeneous group. On the contrary, our research indicates a great diversity of individuals and personal circumstances.

Background to the research

The 'problem': primary health care for homeless people
It is commonly believed that registration with GPs and utilisation of health care services is low among single homeless people compared with the general population. The implications of non-registration are twofold: that homeless people have difficulty in obtaining primary care when they need it; and that without a GP, they also have difficulty in getting hospital care and, on discharge, on-going after-care. However, there is so little systematic evidence about the access of single homeless people to services, based on indicators such as their registration with GPs, the attitudes of health care professionals towards them or their use and misuse of hospital casualty departments, that comparisons with the general population are difficult and uncertain. In the absence of systematic evidence, much of the debate about health care for homeless people has been based upon anecdotal information and stereotypical images of the behaviour and appearance of homeless people.

Studies which have investigated the health needs of single homeless people are discussed in detail in the literature review which is appended to this report. The review is deliberately broad. From the vast literature on both homelessness and primary care services in London it highlights material on the provision of primary health care to single homeless people and gives background information about the population characteristics of Tower Hamlets and Camden, the two areas where the pilot schemes were set up. It also gives details of a number of other special projects which have been set up elsewhere to provide primary health care for homeless people.

The few studies which have looked specifically at the problems of health and homelessness have tended to concentrate on the morbidity characteristics associated with single homelessness and only recently has attention been focused on the related concept, that those in greatest need are often those who *use* services less effectively (McCarthy, 1980). A crucial problem which affects the expression of demand for services by homeless people has been identified as one of access to primary care facilities (SHIL Sub Group, 1987).

There are generally thought to be two main factors affecting this: patient inability or unwillingness to use GP services; and GP reluctance to take on the homeless. In particular, registration difficulties and the attitudes of staff are believed to discourage homeless people from using available primary care services. GPs are commonly thought to be reluctant to register homeless people because they regard them as 'transitory' patients who are likely to create an excessive workload, and whose appearance or behaviour might be off-putting to other patients. They are more likely to treat them on the basis of temporary resident registrations or to use the claims form for immediately necessary treatment, than to take them on their lists on a permanent basis. Homeless people therefore miss out on the advantages of permanent registration, which relate mainly to continuity of care and the fact that the medical history notes of a patient are only sent on to GPs with whom the patient is permanently registered.

A lack of motivation on the part of homeless people themselves has also been identified as a reason for their low take-up of mainstream primary health care services. It has been argued that many single homeless people feel they have no need of medical care, have low expectations regarding their health, are embarrassed about their appearance or are wary of going to a GP's surgery as a result of previous unhappy experiences with primary care services.

Those who have identified the main problem as one of access to primary care facilities argue that the main factor influencing their take-up by homeless people is the manner in which they are delivered, and not simply their availability (Shanks, 1983). Much of the debate about improving the provision of health care for homeless people has centred around the issue of service delivery; in particular, whether homeless people can and should be integrated into mainstream primary health care services, or whether they need a separate and special service.

The Department's response

The DHSS has for some time been concerned about the delivery of primary health care services to the homeless and has encouraged the efforts made by some Family Practitioner Committees and GPs to find locally acceptable solutions to the problem. In 1975, in an attempt to improve the situation in areas of persistent difficulty, the Department issued Guidance to FPCs on the need to develop special medical care arrangements for the homeless and rootless. Provision was made with the Medical Practices Committee to enable restricted Principals to be admitted to FPC lists of Principals in General Practice specifically for this purpose. There is no evidence that this policy has been widely implemented.

In 1981 the problem of health care for the homeless was identified in the Acheson Report - the report of a study group on Primary Care in Inner London, chaired by Professor Acheson (DHSS, May 1981a). This recommended the use of the Secretary of State's powers under Section 56 of the 1977 NHS Act to meet the needs of this particular group. Section 56 provides that the Secretary of State may authorise an FPC to make, or may himself make, 'other arrangements' for the provision of general medical services where 'any considerable number of persons are not receiving satisfactory services'. However, largely because it was evident that this recommendation was not generally supported by the medical profession, the Department did not act upon it at that time.

At the beginning of 1985 the problem was highlighted again, this time by the work of a nursing sister who, describing herself as a 'nurse practitioner', was providing health care for homeless men in East London. The Pharmaceutical Society of Great Britain took action to prevent her continuing to supply 'prescription only' medicine to patients without involving a medical practitioner. This left an identifiable gap in the service, since it was estimated that she had regularly treated 1,000-1,200 patients.

The public interest which this case aroused again called into question the adequacy of primary health care for homeless people in general and for the single homeless in particular. The Department asked all FPCs, as part of the 1985/6 planning exercise, to report on the extent to which the health care needs of homeless people in their locality were being met. At the same time it was considering whether it was now appropriate to exercise the Section 56 powers in the locality of those FPCs where there were sufficiently large numbers of homeless people to warrant such special arrangements.

Establishment of pilot primary health care schemes
It was decided to establish the two pilot schemes for primary health care in Inner London so that the issues could be examined in detail. The funding for the schemes was to come from the £9 million or so set aside by the government, originally over three years from 1983, to fund initiatives for improving primary health care in inner cities. The schemes were funded to run provisionally for three years.

The Department envisaged that the service provided under the pilot schemes would be delivered on an 'outreach' basis, in that in each area a primary health care team would visit and treat homeless people at the places where they congregated, such as day centres, hostels and night shelters. It was expected that this approach would mean close co-operation by the FPCs managing the schemes with health and local authorities and voluntary workers. The FPCs were to employ 'salaried' doctors instead of using local GPs, which was a major departure from the way general practice is organised and which involved securing the necessary professional agreements. It was intended that the doctor would provide short-term treatment and would, wherever possible, secure the admission of patients to GPs' lists in the usual way.

Given the need apparently demonstrated in East London by the work of the 'nurse practitioner', it was decided to locate one of the pilot schemes in the area covered by City and East London FPC. This became known as the East London Homeless Health Project (HHELP). A doctor was already working with homeless people in this area. His funding, which also came from the money set aside by the government for improving primary health care in the inner cities, was re-directed to the pilot scheme and he was employed in March 1986 as the scheme's salaried doctor. He was joined by an alcohol counsellor, a social worker, a community psychiatric nurse and a project co-ordinator. The team was located in its own premises, but was not generally available for consultation there.

It was decided to set up the second pilot project within the locality of Camden and Islington FPC, another area which was known to attract substantial numbers of homeless people. This scheme had a differently constituted team of a salaried doctor, a nurse and a project administrator. It also had its own premises but, as in East London, team members did not treat patients there.

A steering group was appointed to advise on the operation and development of both schemes and PSI was asked to conduct the evaluation.

Design of the study and method
Although it was envisaged that this study would highlight many of the problems relating to the provision of primary health care for homeless people generally, it was designed primarily to be a descriptive study and an assessment of the two pilot schemes. In undertaking the research, we took the view that it was clearly important to assess the views of both providers and consumers of the services, as well as those of others involved in the provision of health and social services to homeless people. In this way, the study breaks new ground in the debate on health care for single homeless people and introduces the voice of the consumer. We adopted two main methods of research to collect evidence for the study:

(i) We designed a system of monitoring the activity, organisation, referral patterns and functioning of the pilot health care teams managed by the two FPCs. We worked closely with both teams to establish a medical record system which could be used by them for practical purposes but also by us for our research and monitoring purposes. It provided a description of the day-to-day work of the two projects and gave detailed information over a twelve month monitoring period (1 January 1987 - 31 December 1987) on numbers, age and sex of clients, their presenting problems, referrals into and out of the schemes, and outcome in so far as this could be defined as the 'terminating actions' to consultations.

(ii) We conducted personal interviews, using semi-structured questionnaires, with:

(a) samples of users and non-users of the services offered by the two pilot health care teams;

(b) all members of the health care teams employed in the two pilot schemes and the Chairmen and Administrators of their managing FPCs;

(c) samples of professionals concerned with the statutory provision of health or social services to homeless people in the two localities and, where appropriate, their managers;

(d) representatives and workers in voluntary agencies offering health care, counselling or social services to homeless people;

(e) wardens of the centres for homeless people where the project doctors established regular clinics.

Interviews with homeless people

Personal interviews were held with a total of 190 homeless people, of whom 50 per cent had used the projects' services and the rest had not. Ninety of these interviews were with individuals attending centres in East London where the project doctor had established regular clinics (45 of them users); and 100 interviews were with people using the centres in Camden where regular clinics were set up (50 of them users). These interviews had to be done on a quota sampling basis because it was impossible to find a sampling frame which would have enabled us to select a random sample of users and non-users. Many of the homeless people attending the centres where the clinics were held were highly mobile and we could not predict who would use the project teams' services on a specific day. A detailed account of the sampling procedure and response rates is given in Appendix 1.

We explored a number of issues in our interviews with clients and potential clients of the services. We wanted to know about their use of GP services and, in particular, whether or not they thought they were registered with a GP. We probed their attitudes towards their GP if they had one and, where appropriate, tried to get some indication of the criteria they used to assess the care received from their GP. We also asked them about their use of other sources of primary health care: for example, doctors at other hostels or day centres and hospital accident and emergency departments. In each project area we explored their attitudes towards the services provided under the pilot schemes. We wanted to know what they liked or disliked about the way the services were organised and delivered and how they thought these services compared with other sources of health care. We were interested to know the extent to which they were aware of the 'team' nature of the scheme and their attitudes towards the primary health care team. The extent to which they wanted to be on a GP's list or whether they preferred to use the special service was a key issue in our interviewing.

Interviews with team members and the FPCs

All team members were interviewed at the beginning, mid-point and end of the monitoring period, which was the calendar year 1987. We collected information about their roles in the project and their patterns of work. We also explored their views about the existing provision of health care for homeless people generally, and more specifically about the pilot scheme for which they worked. We asked them to discuss the objectives of the scheme, its strengths and weaknesses and whether or not they thought homeless people in their locality needed special and separate primary health care services. The purpose of the interim interview was to record any new features developing during the year, either in the structure and functioning of the pilot scheme, or in a team member's views and understanding of the scheme. The purpose of the final interview was to record any such changes or developments and to give team members the opportunity to comment on the achievements of the pilot scheme in their area and to make suggestions about its future. We explored similar issues in our interviews with the Chairmen and Administrators of the managing FPCs.

Interviews with professionals and voluntary workers

Individual interviews were also carried out with a random sample of 76 professionals concerned with the statutory provision of health or social services to homeless people in the locality of each pilot scheme. These included GPs, district nurses, community psychiatric nurses and social workers. Wherever possible, we also interviewed the managers to whom they were professionally accountable. We also interviewed 15 professionals either working in or taking referrals from the accident and emergency departments of two large London teaching hospitals, one in East London and one in the vicinity of the Camden project. These included six senior house officers, six nurses and three social workers. Detailed information about the sampling procedure is contained in Appendix 1. To get some indication of the views of the voluntary sector, we also interviewed representatives from 14 voluntary agencies offering health care, counselling or social services to homeless people in one or other of the two project areas.

We wanted to establish how much they knew about the pilot schemes, how they had acquired information about the schemes and the extent and nature of their liaison with the project teams. We asked them for their assessment of the strengths and weaknesses of the pilot schemes and for the criteria they considered important in estimating the success of the schemes. Key issues were the extent to which they thought homeless people needed special and separate services, and their views on the feasibility of integrating homeless people into the present provision of primary health care. We also sought their views on whether or not the pilot schemes demonstrated an appropriate model of care which could be usefully transferred to other areas known to have substantial numbers of homeless people with unmet health care needs.

Interviews with wardens

We also interviewed the wardens of the centres where the project doctors set up regular clinics during the monitoring period; this included five centres in East London and three centres in Camden. We interviewed each warden twice: at the beginning of the monitoring period and again at the end.

The purpose of the first interview was to collect background information about each of the centres and their clientele, and to establish whether they had offered any medical services before they participated in the pilot scheme. The main purpose of the final interview was to collect their views on the achievements of the pilot scheme in their area and what they thought should happen to the scheme after the initial period of funding expired. Again, we wanted to hear their views on the feasibility of integrating homeless people into mainstream services.

Structure and presentation of the report

This report is divided into three sections. Section 1 (Chapters 2-4) covers how the pilot schemes worked and how they were used. This section contains a great deal of factual detail about the schemes and some readers might prefer to go straight to Section 2 (Chapter 5-8), which is concerned with what people thought about the schemes. Section 3 (Chapters 9-11) draws together the findings of Sections 1 and 2 and assesses the schemes in the light of their objectives.

Section 1

Chapter 2 describes the setting up of the pilot schemes, their structure, and the work roles and patterns developed by team members in each area. More detailed information about the staffing arrangements and the centres visited by the project teams can be found in Appendix 2 and Appendix 3. Chapter 3 gives a profile of all those people who used the schemes during the calendar year 1987. Chapter 4 provides a detailed account of how they used the schemes.

Section 2

Chapters 5-8 deal with the various perceptions of the pilot schemes and primary health care provision more generally for homeless people, as seen by: (i) the homeless people for whom the schemes were designed; (ii) the project team members and the FPCs managing the schemes; (iii) the wardens of the centres participating in the schemes; (iv) health care professionals and voluntary representatives working in the two areas.

In these chapters we have made extensive use of verbatim quotes from respondents to illustrate points made and, wherever possible, to illuminate tables. The quotations are always selected rigorously in proportion to the numbers of respondents making such comments. Much of the richness and poignancy of the data we collected would have been lost if we had not presented the views of the consumers and providers in this way.

Section 3

A discussion of our main findings is presented in Chapter 9, followed by our conclusions and recommendations in Chapter 10. A summary of the report is given in Chapter 11.

2 The Pilot Schemes

Many of the lessons to be learned from the pilot schemes concern their structure and management and the dynamics of multidisciplinary teams. This chapter summarises these aspects of the schemes. It shows how and where team members worked on a day-to-day basis and points to the ways in which their work roles evolved during the monitoring period. Fuller details about staffing arrangements and team management are given in Appendix 2.

The date when each project actually started is not clear-cut because in neither area were team members all appointed at the same time. The appointment of the salaried doctor to each team gives some indication of when they became operational, although in Camden there were delays in finding locations for holding clinics. In City and East London the doctor joined the project in March 1986, although he had been providing a service to homeless people in the area before this; in Camden the appointment of the doctor was made in June 1986. The monitoring period in which we collected information about uses and users of the schemes covered the calendar year 1987.

The two projects shared a similar model of service delivery, but they were set up and staffed in different ways. First we summarise the elements common to the structure and organisation of both schemes. Then we look at the individual schemes.

Common features of the schemes

The pilot schemes were both managed by the local Family Practitioner Committee (FPC): the scheme in Tower Hamlets by the City and East London FPC and the scheme in Camden by the Camden and Islington

FPC. Each project consisted of a multidisciplinary team of workers who were employed to provide primary health care to homeless people within the locality of their responsible FPC. The size and composition of the two teams were quite different. Team members were employed by different authorities, and there were no clear lines of accountability and no clear definition of responsibility. The projects shared a joint Steering Group which included representatives from both statutory and voluntary agencies.

The key difference from general practice in the way that general medical services were provided was that the FPCs employed *salaried doctors* to work for the schemes instead of using local GPs (see Appendix 2). These doctors did not provide 24 hour cover and they had no mechanism for registering patients. They were able to prescribe drugs in the same way as ordinary GPs because, where necessary, arrangements were made for them to be included on their respective FPC's list of general medical practitioners.

The distinctive feature of service delivery under the schemes was that team members were employed to do *outreach work*. They took their services to places where homeless people congregated, instead of expecting users to come to their base. Descriptions of the centres visited by team members during the monitoring period are given in Appendix 4. These centres included day centres, night shelters and hostels. Most were run by voluntary bodies, but some were the responsibility of local statutory authorities.

The fact that both schemes were channelled through particular day centres, night shelters and hostels meant that for the most part they were available only to people who attended these centres. By implication, those homeless people who did not make use of these traditional street agencies or hostels were unlikely to come into contact with the pilot schemes. But not all users of the schemes were regular attenders. Some people would hear about the services on the streets and would go to one of the centres specifically to see the doctor and not to use the general facilities.

Each of the centres where regular surgeries were established had its own set of circumstances and reasons for participating in the schemes, but it was not always clear why these centres and not others were involved. In some cases the centres approached the project teams for help, or were contacted by team members because their users or residents were known to be in great need of medical services, but in other cases the arrangement was more fortuitous. The project teams rarely started from a base-line of no health care provision at the centres they visited but, with few exceptions, existing medical or nursing services were provided on an ad hoc basis by volunteers and were not part of mainstream provision.

The *pattern* of outreach work was similar in both schemes. The salaried doctors established regular clinics in several centres and occasionally provided services elsewhere. Most of the patients they saw had referred themselves, but some had been directed to the medical service by centre staff, by other team members and occasionally by local GPs or staff in accident and emergency departments. Other team members also established regular sessions, but not necessarily in the same centres as the project doctor. They also took referrals from a number of other local centres, where their services were available on a more ad hoc basis. The *nature* and *extent* of outreach services varied between the two projects, partly because of differences between the size and composition of the teams, and partly because of the way team members defined and approached their brief.

Inevitably some of the patients seen by team members needed to be referred to hospital or elsewhere for further investigations or for services that the teams could not provide, and this referral activity is discussed in Chapter 3. Generally speaking, the project doctors appeared to refer as little as possible to hospital consultants and to direct access diagnostic facilities, one reason for this being doubt on their part as to whether many homeless people would actually go.

The quality of the service provided by team members in both project sites depended to some extent on the facilities available to them in individual centres, and these varied considerably. At the beginning of the monitoring period the project doctor in East London told us that only one of the centres he visited had amenities which were adequate for the service he wanted to provide. These included: a separate room, with hot and cold running water, which could be used as a medical room; a couch for examinations; adequate heating; lockable storage space for medical records; and a medicine cabinet, although this was never used to store dangerous drugs. Similarly, only one of centres in Camden was able to offer good facilities for delivering a health service. The majority of centres lacked some of the normal amenities that were necessary for team members, and in particular the doctor, to provide a good standard of service. Many were also unable to provide privacy for patients while they were waiting to see the doctor.

City and East London pilot scheme

Structure and management

The team
The composition of the team in East London was the result of discussions between the DHSS, the FPC and the doctor who was subsequently employed on the project. The East London team did not have their full complement of members during the monitoring period and in their view this affected both the way they functioned as a team and the range of services they provided.

At the beginning of the monitoring period, in January 1987, the team consisted of a salaried doctor, an alcohol counsellor, a community psychiatric nurse (CPN) and a project co-ordinator. The appointment of the social worker was delayed and he was not in post until March 1987. In the same month the project doctor left to go into general practice and his replacement did not arrive until April. The CPN left in May and was not replaced until May 1988, so that for the rest of the monitoring period the team was without this expertise in mental health care. Towards the end of 1987 the project co-ordinator began to reduce his input into the project before he left for another post.

In addition to these changes to the core team, an American professor of internal medicine on an eight-month sabbatical in England joined the team temporarily in September 1987. It is difficult to assess with any accuracy what impact the attachment of this doctor had on the team. In service terms, he provided an additional input of medical cover for a limited period. He eased the professional isolation of the project doctor and he attended team meetings, but to what extent he influenced the thinking and direction of the team is hard to establish.

The fact that not all team members were appointed at the same time and that there were several changes of personnel not only affected the way the team worked and the service they provided. It also meant that the team we were evaluating at the end of the monitoring period was substantially different from the team we had started out with.

The managers

The City and East London FPC were charged with overall management of the scheme and they appointed a small sub-committee to manage the project on their behalf and to provide clinical back-up for the salaried doctor. However, as the DHSS channelled funding for the scheme through a number of other authorities and agencies, the FPC were the employing authority for the salaried doctor and the project co-ordinator only. The CPN was employed by Tower Hamlets Health Authority, the social worker was employed by Tower Hamlets Social Services Department and the alcohol counsellor was appointed by the Tower Hamlets Inter-Agency Group for Alcohol Services - Inform(AL).

Premises and facilities

The City and East London team were based in office premises in Whitechapel, which were provided at a peppercorn rent by Tower Hamlets local authority. In contrast to the Camden project, the East London team did not have a computer for information storage and retrieval until *after* the monitoring period for the evaluation had finished. Whereas the Camden team were able to computerise their medical record system, the team in East London had to set up and work with a manual medical record system (See Chapter 5).

Outreach approach in practice

Locations for regular surgeries

During the monitoring period the first project doctor employed by the East London scheme held regular surgeries in five centres. His successor took over and continued these surgeries. Two of the centres were residential establishments and both doctors were reluctant to take them on because they thought they should have been covered by local GPs. They eventually agreed to hold surgeries in these centres because both had been unsuccessful in attracting the services of local GPs.

The five centres concerned were:

(i) *Cable Street Day Centre*, a day centre providing a service to single people over the age of 16 with housing needs. The vast majority of users of this centre were men and fell almost equally into three different groups: hostel dwellers; those of no fixed abode; and those who were housed. This centre also acquired the services of a part-time nurse, paid for by the health authority, shortly after the project doctor had set up his surgery there. The timing of her appointment meant that staff as well as users often confused her with the project team. In view of the impracticability of attempting to distinguish her contribution from that of the pilot scheme, we considered her as a team member for the purposes of collecting information about clients' use of and responses to the service as a whole. In assessing the service as a model of provision, it must be borne in mind that this nurse was an extra resource. This centre had a tradition of medical care provided by a nursing sister who described herself as a 'nurse practitioner'. When her services were closed down the centre asked the project doctor to step in. He began visiting in May 1985, before his funding was transferred to the pilot scheme. He continued to hold three surgeries a week at this centre after he was appointed to the scheme and these were taken over by his successor in April 1987.

(ii) *St. Botolph's Crypt Centre*, a centre in Aldgate open to homeless men and women during the day and the evening. (For the purposes of assessing the pilot scheme we were concerned with the evening centre only because this was when the project team's services were available). The wardens estimated that around 30 per cent of users of the evening centre were hostel dwellers, 45 per cent were of no fixed abode and perhaps 25 per cent were housed. Again the majority of users were men. The centre was in great need of medical services and the project doctor started visiting in May 1985, again *before* his funding was transferred to the pilot scheme. On joining the project he continued holding two evening surgeries there a week and these were taken over by his successor in April 1987.

(iii) *Providence Row Refuge*, a hostel with 45 beds providing accommodation usually for a period of 6 weeks only. Approximately a third of the hostel population were women. Hostel staff approached the project team for help and the project doctor started a regular weekly surgery in March 1986. This was taken over by his successor in April 1987.

(iv) *Tower Hamlets Mission*, a day centre on the Mile End Road. Most of the people using this centre were men; around 40 per cent were hostel dwellers, 35 per cent were of no fixed abode and the rest had their own accommodation of some sort. Centre staff had asked for their Mission to be included in the pilot scheme and the first project doctor started twice-weekly surgeries there in October 1986. These surgeries were taken over by his successor in April 1987, but were withdrawn towards the end of 1987.

(v) *Booth House Detoxification Unit*, located in the basement of a large Salvation Army hostel for men and offering treatment for male alcoholics who were suffering from the effects of severe alcohol abuse. The first project doctor started a regular weekly surgery at the unit in October 1986, shortly after the unit had lost the services of a local GP who had provided a weekly service. The second project doctor took over the weekly session in April 1987.

Outreach work by other team members
The other team members had a more flexible work schedule than the project doctors. In some instances they undertook regular sessions with groups or individuals, but in each case this was usually for a limited period of time. Frequently they visited the centres on a more ad hoc basis, responding to the needs of staff or clients. Four of the centres which called upon the services of the *alcohol counsellor* were the same as those visited by the project doctor. She did not visit the detoxification unit on a regular basis to see clients because the unit already had the expertise to deal with alcohol abuse. She visited a number of centres in addition to those where the project doctor had established surgeries, including another popular day centre and a large long-stay hostel for men. The *social worker* wanted to avoid duplicating work at centres where staff already provided social work services and this eliminated a

number of centres where the project doctor had already set up regular surgeries. He also identified a gap in the services offered at several places not visited by the project doctor and began to build up social work support there and, where appropriate, a resettlement service.

Both the alcohol counsellor and the social worker occasionally had people referred to them who did not use any of the centres involved in the pilot scheme. The location for seeing the client would then depend on where was mutually convenient. For the alcohol counsellor there were three main venues: the project team's office base; one of the centres involved in the scheme; or at Inform(AL), the local alcohol agency where she also worked part-time. The social worker operated on a similar basis, but where clients had just been resettled into their own accommodation he would visit them at home to give them support and life-skills training.

Teamwork

Individual roles and work patterns

The success of any team is heavily dependent on the contributions and personalities of its members. With these pilot schemes team members had to be imaginative and adaptable in the way they approached their work. They had to find a way of developing an outreach service which was attractive to users of the centres and acceptable to the staff running them. They also had to undertake a considerable amount of administrative work involved with setting up and running the schemes.

(i)   First project doctor
At the beginning of the pilot scheme there was a great deal of work to be done just setting up the project and the doctor took the lead in this. In an average week he spent as much, if not more, time at the office base sorting out the project's infrastructure, as he did holding surgeries in the centres. For example, he was engaged in acquiring furniture and equipment for the project's base, finding sites for surgeries, organising the arrangements for clinical back-up in terms of necessary supplies and the procedures for prescribing drugs, and making the running in negotiations for employing the alcohol counsellor and the social worker.

Approximately 19-20 hours of his working week were taken up with holding regular surgeries in the five centres. He found that patients were often fairly inarticulate and he estimated that with a new patient it would often take about ten minutes to get information about their medical history and their reason for consulting, and a further ten minutes to sort out a diagnosis and treatment. Whereas in general practice he might see between 15 and 20 patients during a two hour surgery, in the centres he would be able to see only about ten patients in the same amount of time. Patients came to see him for a variety of complex social reasons and not necessarily because they had a medical problem. He thought this was linked to the stereotypical view of a doctor as a source of authority and said 'Patients come to me because of my magic title, "doctor"'.

Although one of the aims of the pilot scheme was to encourage patients to register with a local GP, he saw no point in doing so unless he thought the person was interested in registering and there was a good chance that a local GP would take them on. He met other health care professionals in a variety of contexts: through his participation in various local commmittees or advisory groups; as a result of his attachment to the Department of General Practice at St. Bartholomew's Hospital; and because he talked about the health care problems of homeless people on a number of induction courses for new staff, including one for casualty officers at the London Hospital.

(ii)   Second project doctor

The second project doctor also took the lead on administrative and organisation matters, but by the time he joined the project in April 1987 the majority of the infrastructure was in place and he carried less of an administrative burden. Like his predecessor, much of what he did at the administrative base was paperwork associated with patients he had seen in the centres. He typed his own letters about patients or administrative matters, did much of his own filing and was constantly on the telephone chasing appointments or trying to obtain or confirm information about patients. He compared this aspect of the project with the way a good general practice in Inner London would function and pointed out that in ordinary general practice at least half of these tasks would be delegated to a receptionist. It was not clear why more of them could not have been delegated to the project co-ordinator.

Like his predecessor, he found that consultations with the client group encountered in the centres took longer than in general practice. He also did not routinely recommend homeless patients to register with a local GP. He thought that the argument that the best sort of primary care for this client group was integration into general practice rested on too many assumptions: that patients wanted to be integrated; that services were available; and that the will was there on the part of local GPs to take on homeless patients. He also thought that the twin objectives of the schemes - to provide good quality primary care to homeless people and, wherever possible, to encourage them to register with local GPs - created a problem of 'mixed messages'. On the one hand, as a doctor he wanted to establish trust with a patient, but this conflicted with having to tell them to go and get treatment elsewhere. This could be construed as yet another rejection and homeless people were already sensitive to rejection by people in positions of authority.

Apart from clinical work in the centres, he also provided informal advice and support to centre staff, although he was less engaged in formal training sessions for new centre staff than other team members. He also sought the opinion of centre staff about how to develop the project's services. Like his predecessor, he also became involved in education and training activities for health services staff outside the project. He did a weekly surgery in ordinary general practice which he found important to enable him to maintain contact with a broader spectrum of patients and medical problems than he would encounter in the centres.

(iii)   Project co-ordinator

The project co-ordinator was contracted to the FPC to work 36 hours a week, but about a quarter of this time was spent on general FPC work and not on project-related activities. During the monitoring period the amount of his time spent on FPC work gradually increased to a point where he was spending in theory about 15 hours a week working on the project, but in practice considerably less. It is difficult to assess the full impact this may have had on the way the team worked and the way the project developed, but at the very least it must have restricted the amount of administrative and clerical support available to team members. In January 1988 he left the project and transferred to the FPC's Complaints Section full-time.

He saw himself as providing administrative support rather than acting as a co-ordinator. He preferred to be responsive to the directions of the project doctor and other team members rather than to take the initiative himself. He was mostly involved with record-keeping and correspondence-related duties. One of his most time-consuming tasks was maintaining the manual record system. He was also responsible for keeping a manual age/sex register of all patients using the project team's services. Along with the co-ordinator of the sister project in Camden he serviced the joint Steering Group set up to advise both projects.

(iv)   Alcohol counsellor

The alcohol counsellor was employed on the project part-time. She worked four days a week and split her time fairly evenly between the East London scheme and working for Inform(AL). She tended to spend little time at the project's administrative base. In February 1987 she estimated she was there for about three hours a week doing paperwork. By December this had increased to about six hours a week, but then included regular project meetings and seeing more clients there as well as doing paperwork.

Not all of the activities she undertook at the centres related specifically or exclusively to alcohol; she did general group work and counselling and tapped into her management skills to provide training and support for centre staff. Early on some of her workload could be described more appropriately as social work and she was relieved of these tasks when a social worker joined the project. In contrast, the departure of the CPN placed more demands on her time and she found herself doing more counselling.

During the monitoring period the balance of her workload changed; the training aspect of her role expanded and she saw fewer clients. She provided training for staff and volunteers in the centres in communication and counselling skills, group work skills and team building. She was pleased to be asked to give this support and felt that it was a good measure of the confidence and trust of the centre staff in the professionalism of the project team. She aimed to equip the staff to deal with more of their clients' problems themselves, instead of creating a dependency on her services. She considered this a better long-term approach, given the uncertain life of project and the fact that alone she could not possibly meet the demand for help with alcohol-related problems in the centres.

She also became involved in a variety of project-related activities outside the project's administrative base, for example with the Women's Forum organised by No Fixed Abode; the Day Centres' Forum (before it was dissolved); and St. Botolph's Advisory Group.

(v) Social worker

He hoped that his inclusion in the project would help people develop an awareness that providing health care services without looking at people's lifestyles and the social reasons for ill health was an inadequate approach. He intended to offer practical help to homeless people about housing, finance, benefits and so on. By doing this, he aimed to help steer the project towards providing a more holistic service. He wanted to offer continuity of work and thought he could best do this by establishing a regular presence at a number of centres. He visited a core group of three day centres and one large long-stay hostel. Much of what he did in the centres he described as 'problem-solving', by which he meant helping people to find solutions to the problems that beset their everyday lives. This work included: providing advice and support; making referrals, usually to housing agencies; and some, but not much, ongoing case-work with individual clients. He was rarely at the project's administrative base for more than about six to eight hours in any week and this time was spent on paperwork, attending team meetings and seeing clients.

His interest and involvement in resettlement work increased during the monitoring period. At the long-stay hostel he sifted people to see whether they were vulnerable under the Homeless Persons' Act and if they were, he would refer them to the Homeless Persons' Unit. He also worked closely with the hostel's resettlement team. They would refer people to him who they felt needed more support once they had moved out of the hostel. In two of the day centres he set up self-help groups aimed at people with accommodation. He had become aware that many of those he was seeing already had some form of accommodation, but nevertheless had severe problems in that they were in danger of losing it through isolation and lack of support. This was particularly common among people with alcohol problems.

The social worker provided training and support for centre staff and for workers in local agencies. He also retained and strengthened his involvement in a network of local organisations and agencies with an interest in homelessness.

(vi) Community Psychiatric Nurse

In general terms the CPN thought that his role in the team was 'to provide a comprehensive psychiatric nursing service to the homeless, undertaking assessment, identifying problems and subsequently deciding on the intervention to help tackle problems and achieve goals'. In practice he found these principles difficult to apply in the context of developing outreach work in the centres and it would appear that he found it difficult to adapt his hospital training and background to a community setting. We encountered a number of views as to why the role of the CPN in the project did not develop successfully, some of which hinged on personality factors and others of which related more specifically to the use of a CPN as a resource in this type of initiative.

The CPN himself considered that the social stigma relating to psychiatric work contributed to the reluctance of day centre staff to draw upon his services, even though they recognised the scope and need for them. They thought that he had a preference for being office-based and expected them to make referrals to him, instead of his coming to see clients in the familiar environment of the centres. There were differences of opinion between the CPN and other team members about how he should develop his role in the project. It was suggested that he should try and establish relationships with clients by assuming a more informal role, mixing with clients at the centres and taking part in day centre activities. He saw this type of intervention as inappropriate and unsatisfactory and it proved impossible to find a compromise which he was comfortable with and which also fitted in with the needs of the day centre workers and their clients.

Team dynamics

With perhaps one exception, each of the team members in East London thought that they had a special role in the project that could not be fulfilled satisfactorily by anyone else in the team, and this related to their professional expertise rather than their individual qualities. The second project doctor played down his special contribution to the team; although he acknowledged that he had specialist medical skills, he considered that, in the context of caring for homeless people, team members' roles were not as well-defined as their professional expertise might suggest.

At the beginning of the monitoring period there was a general consensus among team members and the FPC that leadership of the team, along with advice and support, was provided by the project doctor. This was largely because he had been the first member to be appointed and had been involved in discussions with the DHSS and the FPC about the composition of the team. He himself thought that it was also partly because he carried the title of 'doctor'. He was seen to have a strong personality and to be a good organiser and negotiator and it was recognised that these skills were important to get the project off the ground.

His successor continued the ethos of a doctor-led team, but in a much lower-key way. He saw his position in the project team as perhaps different from that of a GP in an ordinary primary health care team. Unlike a local GP he was not an independent contractor; he was a salaried employee like all the other team members. With the arrival of the new doctor, leadership, in the sense of professional direction, became less clear cut. He was generally seen by other team members as responsible for the administration and organisation of the project, but not for directing their work. They felt that professional direction was unrealistic for a number of reasons.

Generally speaking, the leadership role was poorly defined. This ambiguity did not seem to be an obstacle when the project was working well. However, team members speculated about what would have happened if they had disagreed violently. Suggesting that it might have been useful to have had the arrangements for decision-making and accountability more clearly spelt out, one team member observed, 'Are we a collective or are we a hierarchy?'

One way of establishing a team identity and a sense of belonging is to set up regular team meetings. A disadvantage arising from the incremental appointment of team members in East London over a long period was that initially the team had been too small to make meetings worthwhile. After the alcohol counsellor and the social worker had been appointed an effort was made to hold regular meetings on a weekly basis. As team members were involved in outreach work they were rarely in the office at the same time and this weekly slot was important to ensure that there was a fixed point when they did meet together and function as a team. Team meetings also provided a forum where people working in related fields could come along, both to learn about the project and to talk about their particular activities.

Camden pilot scheme

Structure and management

The team
The team in Camden comprised a salaried doctor, a nurse and a project co-ordinator. A proposal that it should also include health visitors did not work out in practice, mainly because of nursing management and funding difficulties. Funding was made available by the DHSS for dental and chiropody sessions if and when required.

The managers
The scheme was managed by the Camden and Islington FPC. They were the employing authority for the salaried doctor and the project co-ordinator, but not for the nurse. She was employed by Bloomsbury Health Authority and was accountable to the Director of Community Nursing and responsible to the Senior Nurse, District Nursing. Her accountability was further divided because she was also 'accountable' to the project doctor for her day-to-day work.

Premises and facilities
The project co-ordinator was initially based in the offices of the FPC. When the salaried doctor joined the scheme in June 1986, the project moved to premises in Chalton Street, NW1, where Bloomsbury Health Authority had made available three rooms in their child dental health

clinic for the team's use. The cost of these premises during the life of the pilot scheme was covered by the Health Authority. The team were given a microcomputer and software facilities for data management, spreadsheets and word processing. This gave them the facility to set up and maintain a computerised medical record system.

Outreach approach in practice

Locations for regular surgeries

The Camden team experienced major difficulties in finding locations for their services within the boundaries of their managing FPC, largely because there were few day centres in Camden for homeless people. If they had cast their net more widely they could have aproached a number of other day centres and hostels, but these were in the vicinity of Great Chapel Street Medical Centre, which was already offering services for homeless people. They felt this blocked off certain opportunities for developing their scheme because they did not want to tread on toes, nor did they want to duplicate services. To get the project off the ground, they set up regular surgeries in a centre located in a neighbouring FPC.

The project doctor and nurse established regular clinics in three centres during the monitoring period:

(i) *Arlington Drop-In Centre*, a day centre in Camden Town. Around half the users were sleeping rough, a further third were likely to be hostel dwellers and the rest were housed in some form of their own accommodation. The vast majority of users were men. The team approached this centre to discuss the health needs of their clients and two months later, in November 1986, the project doctor started to hold regular surgeries there twice a week. The project nurse attended during these surgeries and also held two further clinics a week on her own.

(ii) *West London Day Centre*, a day centre located within the geographical boundaries of Kensington, Chelsea and Westminster FPC. This centre had a history of providing health care for its attenders, of whom the majority were men but about 10 per cent were women. When the project doctor learned that the local GP providing a weekly surgery here wanted to give it up he took it on, even though the centre was outside the boundaries of his managing

FPC. He established twice-weekly surgeries in September 1986. Since at least 1979 this centre had employed a nurse who was part-funded by Bloomsbury Health Authority and she worked alongside the project doctor during these surgeries. The *project* nurse only visited this centre if their own nurse was away on surgery days. Again, for the purposes of our evaluation we considered the day centre nurse as a team member, with the proviso that she was an extra resource which could not be counted on elsewhere.

(iii) *The Simon Community Night Shelter*, a 22-bedded shelter near King's Cross station run by the Simon Community, which also had a number of residential group homes and did outreach work on the streets at night. Again, the vast majority of users were men. Most were overnight guests, some of whom used the shelter one night a week on a regular basis. The project doctor set up regular surgeries at this shelter two mornings a week, starting in November 1987. The project nurse worked with him at one of these surgeries and in addition visited the shelter twice a week on her own.

The project team had also hoped to start regular surgeries at a large long-stay hostel run by Camden council, but much to their frustration this plan never materialised. Before they could begin clinics the council had to arrange for a new door and toilet to be installed and at the end of 1987 the team were still waiting for these alterations to be made. They felt that they could have undertaken other clinics in the meantime if they had known how long the building work would take.

Homeless families

The Camden team did not set up surgeries in any hostels or hotels for homeless families, but they did collaborate with two health visitors, a dietician and a geriatric visitor to pilot a health information facility at a local hotel where homeless families were being placed. The aim of the facility was to link homeless families into whatever mainstream services they needed. The service started in July 1987 and the intention was to run it initially for six months, irrespective of the numbers who used it. In the event the service was discontinued. Take-up had been low, partly because the service had received little publicity and also because it had been badly sited in the basement of the hotel. More fundamentally, by the time the service had started, local councils had changed their policies regarding the placement of homeless families and were moving them out of the hotel.

Teamwork

Individual roles and work patterns

(i)   Project doctor
At the beginning of the pilot scheme the project doctor in Camden spent almost half of his working week on administrative tasks, mainly negotiating with statutory and voluntary agencies about potential sites for holding clinics. He was also heavily involved with the East London project team and with the evaluators in setting up a medical record system.

The serious difficulties encountered by the team in finding locations for outreach work limited the amount of time the doctor spent doing clinical work. In January 1987 he spent about 10 hours a week running surgeries in two centres; in November this had increased to about 14 hours a week because he had started visiting the Simon Community Night Shelter. Like his counterparts in East London, he confirmed that he tended to spend more time with patients listening to their stories than he would in general practice. Ordinary GPs work to a tighter time schedule, which also has to include home visits. To keep in touch with general practice, the project doctor also did one ordinary GP surgery per week.

He did not automatically recommend patients to register with a local GP if they were unregistered. Like the project doctors in East London, he often found it hard to tell someone that because they had an address they could not see him and would have to go and find a GP. This was a particular dilemma at West London Day Centre where attenders had got used to seeing a doctor at the centre long before the pilot scheme started and often regarded this doctor as their own 'GP'.

Working for the pilot schemes entailed a big adjustment for the project doctors from the pattern of general practice, where it is accepted the GP has a considerable amount of free time. In contrast, the salaried doctors working for the schemes had a fixed 40-hour week, and the doctor in Camden found it difficult to adjust to a routine which meant coming back to the office after doing clinics and finding tasks to do. He became involved in several local groups and committees, such as the Bloomsbury GP Forum and the Bloomsbury Homeless Persons' Steering Group (convened by the Health Authority). He also developed a number of teaching and research activities, some of which linked in with his honorary lectureship in the Department of Primary Care, University College and Middlesex Hospitals. For example, he became involved in teaching medical students who were doing their block of training about general practice.

He also thought that the project team should take on a more campaigning role and publicise what they were doing. In his view most of the information available about health care and homeless people was very general and anecdotal and he felt that the project team were uniquely placed to go beyond this and collect information about why homeless people were not using mainstream services.

(ii)   Project nurse

Initially the project nurse was out in the field for much of the time, contacting other agencies and people and trying to get the project off the ground. At the beginning of the project she also spent a considerable amount of time trying to organise the ordering of both basic supplies, such as saline solution and handwash, and pharmacy supplies because there was a general lack of clarity surrounding what procedures she should use and who should pay for them.

In addition to providing general nursing services to homeless people at the two centres where she established regular clinics, she also wanted to use her interest in health promotion and education for this client group and to develop some form of positive health programme. She envisaged running health sessions at the day centres in addition to the normal clinics, and also exploring whether there were any hostels in the area who felt they could benefit from an extra input from a health professional. With this in mind, during the monitoring period she visited two hostels on a weekly basis, one run by a voluntary organisation and the other by the local council. Her visits to these hostels started in January and July 1987 respectively.

She found it easier to get the message of health promotion across to people she saw in these hostels, where no doctor attended regularly, than she did at Arlington Drop-in Centre. People at the Drop-in Centre may have found it difficult to understand why they should take responsibility for their health and go elsewhere to register with a doctor when one already came to the centre. Also, because there was no doctor on the premises at the hostels, it may have been easier for residents to get away from the traditional doctor-patient relationship, which encouraged them to think about their health only when something was wrong. Nevertheless, to a large extent her expectations of the benefits she could bring to clients at these hostels were not met, but she concluded that her visits were probably justifiable in terms of the support they provided for the staff.

She also did some one-off sessions at the centres on various aspects of health education and promotion, and she judged the response to these to have been very mixed. She thought that videos were useful in addressing specific topics like AIDS, but were less effective when it came to more general topics such as disease prevention, nutrition, and rights of access to medical services. She did not provide any formal nursing care on the streets, but she did try to do some 'street work' with those people who she knew would never use the centres, offering them advice and information about local services and rights of access. Other commitments, and doubts about how effective this approach was, made it difficult for her to find the time and energy needed to do regular circuits round the streets of Camden.

(iii) Project co-ordinator

Initially the project co-ordinator spent much of her time making contacts and looking to see where the areas of need were. A priority had been to look for places where the project could establish clinics. Once the clinical outreach work had started one of her central tasks was entering patient records onto the computer and updating these records each time a patient saw the project doctor or nurse. She undertook the basic administrative work that was necessary to keep the project running and took charge of the petty cash. She also became involved in a number of project-related activities outside the administrative base. For example, she provided administrative services to both the Bloomsbury

Homeless Persons' Steering Group and a sub-group of the local Joint Care Planning Team (JCPT), which had been set up to look at homelessness.

Overall, she found her work interesting and fulfilling but for much of the time she felt under-occupied. She thought that when the pilot scheme had been designed too little thought had been given to what the co-ordinator would be doing once the project had got off the ground.

Team dynamics

The team in Camden was smaller than the East London team. Team members took responsibility for certain aspects of work and had their own areas of interest, but they did not emphasise the differences in their expertise. On the contrary, they thought that there were a lot of activities they undertook as a team where their roles were interchangeable, in theory if not in practice. The doctor obviously possessed skills which the others did not, but at the beginning of the project he had an open mind about whether a doctor with a prescription pad was the most appropriate resource for providing primary health care for homeless people, or whether it might not have been more useful to employ several district nurses.

Comparing their team with that operating in East London, the Camden team members speculated that, with a nurse who was also a health worker, they were able to offer a more overall health service to clients, as opposed to a social service. They did not think that the lack of a social worker had detracted from the service they offered because most of the centres were already able to provide this facility. Without having an alcohol counsellor or CPN working for their team, they had worked hard at building up good links with local alcohol agencies and with the health authority CPNs. They liked this approach because it linked their clients into the local agencies, instead of isolating them further by providing them with a separate service.

The Camden team tried to try and work in a non-hierarchical way and in practice team members considered there was no team leader. It was generally felt that the team was too small and individual members were off-site too often for any one person to assume leadership for the overall project. Instead, they all took leadership roles at different times and under different circumstances because they recognised that each was more able and qualified to take the initiative in some areas, but not in others. However, they were all conscious that outside agencies usually perceived and treated the doctor as the team leader.

Regular weekly project team meetings were established and provided a forum for team members to meet and discuss what they had been doing and their future plans. Although these meetings were never suspended, after a few months they dropped off to about once a month. It was apparent that the dynamics of a 'trio' were sometimes problematic. There was always the risk of one of the three feeling excluded and with team members spending much of their time away from the project's base, there was also the danger of working in isolation without consulting or informing colleagues. The risk of friction in relationships which is inevitable when people are brought together artificially in a team was exacerbated because the team felt isolated, both professionally and geographically, and individual team members had different employers and different lines of accountability. While no team members in Camden wanted a team leader, one person suggested that a group facilitator at team meetings would have been helpful, both to create a safe environment and to rein in individuals if the meeting seemed to be getting out of hand.

In assessing the schemes it has to be recognised that both teams had to contend with the stresses and problems of starting a new scheme, with a new team and an innovative way of working, while under close scrutiny and constrained by a limited time scale. All these factors were likely to compound the problems commonly experienced by people involved in multidisciplinary teamwork.

3   Profile of Users

This chapter gives a profile of *all* the people who used the services of the team members during the calendar year 1987. The extent to which they used the schemes and their reasons for consulting team members are examined in Chapter 4. The discussion in both chapters is based on information drawn from the medical record system set up in both project sites. We analysed the data on two different levels: (i) the total number of different *individuals* seen by each project team; and (ii) the total number of *consultations* made by these people during the year. Some people consulted once only, while others made numerous visits. It is important to bear in mind that the data describe only one aspect of team members' activities: direct care provision for individual clients.

The medical record system
The medical record system in both projects had two related components from which we collected information:

(i)   Medical record cards
A medical record card was created for each new user. The card was raised by whichever team member the person first contacted. The front of this card recorded the registration number and brief personal details. The rest of the card was used for notes relating to each consultation with the project doctor or with any other team member. In both schemes the cards were usually kept at the individual centres where clinics were established and not at the project's administrative base. The medical record cards were our main source of data about the *individuals* who used the pilot schemes: for example, their age; sex; place of birth;

accommodation status; and whether or not they thought they were registered with a GP. We identified cases by patient registration number; no name was recorded for use by the research team.

(ii) Contact sheet

Team members also recorded information on a 'contact sheet' about each consultation they had with a user. The contact sheet was marked out with columns in which team members entered codes summarising details about the user and the nature and outcome of the consultation. Individual team members kept their own contact sheets for each centre they visited. The contact sheets were our main source of data about *consultations* with team members and are discussed in Chapter 4.

Using the patient registration numbers on the medical record cards and the contact sheets we were able to combine the two sources of data, thus linking together the personal details of each patient with information about their first and subsequent consultations.

Problems in the medical record system

Although the numbering system for the medical record cards and contact sheets was discrete to each project, the system for recording information was the same. A major difference in the storage and retrieval of this information was that the Camden scheme was able to develop a computerised record system. Although the medical record cards were kept at the individual centres, this project also stored the information centrally on its computer. This gave team members quick and easy access to information about users. The East London project was restricted to paper record systems: in addition to using the medical record cards and contact sheets described above, a manual age/sex register of users was kept at the administrative base.

Devising a medical record system which satisfied our needs for the evaluation and was also acceptable to service providers in both project sites was not easy. We negotiated with team members for three months before arriving at agreed formats for the medical record card and the contact sheets. There were differences of opinion about the amount and kind of information it was feasible and acceptable to ask the doctors and other team members to record. Information that would have been useful to the evaluation was not necessarily seen by team members as relevant to providing care.

Every effort was made to ensure that the procedure for completing the contact sheets and record cards was systematic, both within and between teams. However, differences of interpretation concerning a few of the categories of information collected were unavoidable. We also had to accept the constraint that the service providers would use their professional judgment on how much information they felt able to ask individual clients. As they got to know users, they felt more able to ask about their social as well as their medical history, but they were particularly reluctant to ask too many questions on a person's first visit. In some cases, this meant that very little information was recorded. When users consulted more than once, some of the missing details were filled in at later visits.

Profile of users

Who used the pilot schemes and what do we know about their circumstances? From the medical record cards we were able to count the number of individuals who had consulted team members during the monitoring period and compile an aggregate picture of their personal characteristics and their type of accommodation, if any. We were also able to identify the proportion who thought they were registered with GPs. This picture is incomplete since information was not always entered on the record cards and this is indicated in the tables. There were three main reasons for missing data, the first being the most common: (i) team members exercised their professional discretion and did not ask users questions about their personal history; (ii) users were asked questions, but could not recall the required information; (iii) users refused to give their personal details.

Generally speaking, missing information was more of a problem in Camden than in East London, largely because one of the team members working for this project felt uncomfortable about asking users questions about their social, as opposed to their medical, history. However, the alcohol counsellor in East London was also apprehensive about recording information. She felt that, given the nature of the service she offered and the way she worked, it was not always appropriate for her to ask too many personal questions. In any case, she found it difficult to record information during counselling sessions because, in order to help clients feel relaxed and 'safe', she deliberately avoided carrying a note pad.

The population of users in each project site is discussed separately. Some of the similarities and differences between the two groups of users are commented upon, but direct comparison between the statistics for the two projects is difficult for several reasons: the size and composition of the two teams was markedly different; and the centres in the two areas through which the outreach work was channelled were dissimilar both in number and type. The outlets in City and East London included a detoxification unit and a short-stay hostel as well as several day centres and a crypt holding evening sessions for homeless people. In contrast, in Camden the clinics were held at two day centres and a night shelter.

City and East London Pilot Scheme

Numbers using the scheme
A total of 885 individuals used the City and East London Pilot Scheme one or more times during the 12-month monitoring period. Table 3.1 (p.46) shows the breakdown of this total by the day centre, night shelter or hostel where the person was *first seen* and a record card was raised. On subsequent visits these individuals might have used the project team's services at another centre covered by the scheme, but they would have retained their original patient registration number.

The most popular places for making contact with the scheme were St. Botolph's Crypt and Cable Street Day Centre, which were both busy centres where the project doctors held twice-weekly clinics; the clinics were held in the evening at St. Botolph's Crypt and during the day at Cable Street. Few people had first encountered the scheme at Tower Hamlet's Mission and the project doctor's service was eventually discontinued at this centre. Very few were registered as having first been seen at the project's administrative base, but this was consistent with the project's commitment to an outreach approach. A small number had first been seen by the alcohol counsellor at the local alcohol agency to which she was attached and where she worked part-time.

Table 3.1 (p.46) shows that the majority of users were men. Only 14 per cent (132) were women. Almost half these women had first used

37

the project at Providence Row, a short-stay hostel. The others had taken advantage of the scheme at one of the day centres. No women had used the service at Booth House because this was the detoxification unit for men only.

Age
The age range of users in East London was broad and is set out in Table 3.2 (p.46).

The East London team felt that, generally speaking, the homeless population in their area was more stable than in Camden and reflected more the stereotypical image of the homeless person as a middle-aged single male. Almost half the total number of users were aged between 35 and 54. Five per cent of users were past retirement age and the majority of these had used the evening clinic held in the local crypt, or had seen the team at whichever day centre they regularly attended.

However, 28 per cent of all the users in East London were younger than 35, and this gives some indication that homelessness is not confined to middle-aged single males. Indeed, 8 per cent of all the male users and just over a quarter of the women were aged under 25. Almost a third of those under 25 had first used the scheme at the short-stay hostel reflecting the high usage of the scheme by women at this centre. The others had made contact through one of the day centres (although most of these centres were not keen to encourage attendance by young people) or, for a tiny minority, the detoxification unit.

Place of birth, marital status, employment status
Table 3.3 (p.47) shows the place of birth of users. This information was known for 82 per cent of users. Just under half had been born in England; a further 17 per cent had originally come from Scotland or Wales, and 15 per cent from the Irish Republic. Otherwise few users were known to have come from outside the United Kingdom. The numbers from ethnic minority groups were notably low; for example, only 1.2 per cent of all users were recorded by team members as being of Afro-Caribbean (West Indies) or African origin. This reflects the fact that people from ethnic minority groups make little use of traditional day centres or hostels.

Team members were reluctant to ask about marital status and in any case this information appeared to be unreliable. Some people using the scheme were believed to be living with a partner but had not disclosed this. Others were technically married but lived alone. Eighty-four per cent of users said they were single, widowed, divorced or separated and only 3 per cent were recorded as being married. It can be assumed that the majority of users were living as single persons.

The majority, just over 70 per cent, were unemployed. Only 4 per cent were said to be in full-time employment and a further 6 per cent were in part-time jobs or had done casual work during the past three months. Again team members were reluctant to ask users about their job status and this information was not recorded in 16 per cent of cases.

Accommodation

With the exception of those at the detoxification unit, users were asked where they had stayed the night immediately before using the scheme, and the type of accommodation, if any, that they had at the time of their first consultation is recorded in Table 3.4 (p.47). Residents at the detoxification unit were asked what type of accommodation they had the night before admission to the unit. (It would have been inappropriate to record the unit as a category of accommodation because residents stayed there for one week only and were admitted specifically for the detoxification programme.) In contrast, those staying at the short stay hostel were living there for up to six weeks and in some cases longer. When they used the scheme their accommodation was recorded as 'short-stay hostel'. However, team members would record 'no fixed abode' when they knew that someone who saw them at the hostel was there for, say, only one night in two weeks, in order to have a bath.

Just under one third of those using the East London scheme were living rough, skippering or squatting. The vast majority of these were men (only 21 were women) and almost two-thirds were in the 35-54 age range. They had been seen mainly at the evening clinics in the crypt, or at the day centre which had twice-weekly clinics. A sizeable number in this category had been encountered by the project doctor in the detoxification unit. A further 2 per cent had slept at a local night shelter and 16 per cent were temporarily housed in short-stay hostels. Around 17 per cent were more settled and living in long-stay hostels.

A surprisingly high proportion of those using the East London scheme, 22 per cent, had some form of accommodation of their own, which included rented accommodation provided by the local council or a housing association. A major difference between the populations in East London and Camden generally was that in East London there had been much more resettlement among the local population, although those resettled often come back to use the day centres.

GP registration

There were two main reasons for wanting to know whether users were already registered with a GP. Team members needed to know because an objective of each project was, wherever possible, to encourage homeless people to use mainstream services. The evaluators wanted to explore the common belief that registration is difficult for homeless people and therefore we needed to know what proportion of those using the pilot schemes thought they were registered.

Almost half of the 885 people who used the East London project during the monitoring period thought that they were registered with a GP. However, this figure needs to be treated with caution. For the purpose of recording an entry on the medical record cards registration was interpreted as what the *patient* understood by registration. It was unrealistic to expect users to be able to distinguish clearly between different types of registration, so it is possible that this proportion includes some temporary as well as permanent registrations. It also refers to registration with a GP in London or elsewhere. In cases where the GP was outside London, the concept of the 'local GP' would be irrelevant to the user: for example, the GP would not be able to respond to emergencies or requests for home visits.

Forty-eight per cent of the men using the scheme said they were registered with a GP compared with 57 per cent of the women, who, of course, represented only 14 per cent of the users of the scheme. It has been suggested that people in the younger age groups for whom homelessness is a fairly recent experience are more likely to be registered with a GP than those who have become detached from mainstream provision through being homeless for some considerable time. Table 3.5 (p.48) shows that a higher proportion of all users under 25 were registered than of those in the 25-54 age range. However, those aged 55 and over were as likely to say they were registered as those under 25. The most likely explanation for the higher rate of reported GP registration among older users seemed to be that a greater proportion of those in their late 50s or older were 'settled' in East London, in that they had their own accommodation or were living in a long-stay hostel.

Generally speaking, compared with those who had no fixed abode, a higher proportion of those with hostel places or living in their own accommodation said they were registered with a GP. They accounted for almost two-thirds of the total who were registered. However, it must not be overlooked that just over a third of those who were sleeping rough or skippering also said that they were registered with a GP in London or elsewhere.

But how reliable was this information? We asked the FPC managing the project to confirm how many of the people using the scheme during the monitoring period were permanently registered with a GP on their General Medical List. We were not able to check whether any of the users of the scheme were registered with GPs in other areas. It was found that as many as 19 per cent of those who had used the scheme between 1 January 1987 and 31 December 1987 appeared on the FPC's records as being *permanently* registered with a GP in their area. Others may have been treated by local GPs on a temporary resident basis, but this information was not available from the FPC. Users who said they were registered with a GP but did not appear on this FPC's records may well have been permanently registered with a GP in another area.

Referral into the scheme

How did those who consulted team members in East London come to use the scheme in the first place? The record cards indicate that in most cases patients presented themselves at the clinics asking for help or approached individual team members. This includes cases where individuals were told about the service by a friend who had already come to trust the team and the services they offered. The situation at the detoxification unit was different because those who were admitted for the one-week detoxification programme had to have a routine medical examination and this was frequently done by the project doctor. Less than 3 per cent of all referrals to the team were known to be other than self-referrals: for example, referrals from centre staff or from statutory or voluntary agencies. In about 15 per cent of cases team members felt unable to ask about referral source.

Did users first seek help from the project doctor or from one of the other specialist team members? Approximately 42 per cent first had contact with one of the two salaried doctors who were employed sequentially by the project or with the American doctor who was seconded to the scheme. A further 16 per cent had first seen the Health Authority nurse who worked alongside the project team at one of the centres. Although she was not formally a member of the project team, for the purposes of collecting information about clients' use of the service we considered her as a team member. Of the remaining users, around 5 per cent had seen the alcohol counsellor first and just over 8 per cent had approached the social worker for help. Less than 1 per cent had first had contact with the community psychiatric nurse during the five months of the monitoring period in which he was in post.

Camden pilot scheme
Some of the information which we have about users in East London is not available for the Camden Project, largely because team members in Camden were particularly reluctant to ask users for information which they thought was irrelevant to the medical care they were providing. The main areas of missing data concern: marital status, which was not recorded in 79 per cent of cases; employment status, which was not completed in 60 per cent of cases; and source of referral into the project, which was recorded for 1 per cent of cases only.

Numbers using the scheme
The record cards show that a total of 576 individuals used the Camden pilot scheme one or more times during the 12-month monitoring period. A small number of patients consulted team members at two different centres, but the majority who used the scheme more than once did so at the same centre.

A breakdown of the use of the scheme by centre (Table 3.6, p.48) shows that 322 individuals were first seen at Arlington Drop-in Centre, 193 at West London Day Centre and 61 at the Simon Community night shelter. The figure for the night shelter is low because the team did not start regular clinics there until November 1987. No users were seen at the project's administrative base. Again, the majority of users were men: only 15 per cent were women, almost exactly the same proportion as that found in East London.

Age
The impression among both project teams was that the homeless population in Camden was generally younger than that encountered in the East End. This was not reflected in the use of the schemes, however. In fact, Table 3.7 (p.49) shows that the proportion of users under 25 was 4 per cent in Camden, as compared with 10 per cent in East London. This may be because younger people are likely to be fitter and in less need of medical and nursing care than older homeless people. In Camden, as in East London, around half the users were in the age-range of 35-54 years and about 5 per cent were over retirement age.

Place of birth, marital status and employment status
Table 3.8 (p.49) gives a breakdown of the place of birth of those using the Camden project. As in East London this information was available for 82 per cent of users. Just over a quarter of the total users were recorded as having been born in England, a proportion markedly lower than that found in East London. In contrast, the Camden project was used by a higher proportion of people born either in Scotland (23 per cent), or in the Irish Republic (22 per cent).

Accommodation
Table 3.9 (p.50) shows the type of accommodation that users had stayed in the night before their first contact with the scheme. The picture seems to support the impression of both project teams that the homeless population in Camden was more transient than in the East End. Around 39 per cent of users were living rough or skippering - a marginally higher proportion than that found in East London. Although many in this category were middle-aged men, almost a quarter of those using the scheme and aged under 30 were also living on the streets. Whereas in East London few women users were sleeping rough, in Camden almost a third of the women users were in this situation. Camden users were also more frequently housed temporarily in bed and breakfast

accommodation, and they were less likely to have their own accommodation. Few had hostel places, but no direct comparison can be drawn with the East London project; the Camden team did not include any hostels among their locations for clinics, whereas the East London team visited a short-stay hostel.

GP Registration

Fewer users in Camden than in East London said they were registered with a GP. Again this may reflect the greater geographical mobility among the homeless in the Camden area which makes registration with a 'local'GP difficult. Table 3.10 (p.50) shows that just over one third of those using the Camden project claimed they were registered with a GP. This compared with almost a half in the East End. The proportion of women users who said they were registered was almost 45 per cent compared with 33 per cent of the men. Reported registration with a GP was no more extensive among the younger users than among those in the older age groups.

As we found in East London, registration was more common among those who were more settled in hostels or who had their own accommodation than among those who were sleeping rough or skippering. Nevertheless, almost 30 per cent of those who were living on the streets claimed to be registered with a GP.

As in East London, we were not able to check the registration status of everyone using the pilot scheme, but we did ask the managing FPC to confirm how many users were known to be permanently registered with a GP in their area. We also asked Kensington, Chelsea and Westminster FPC to do a similar check because one of the centres visited by the project team was on their patch. We found that approximately 16 per cent of those people who had used the scheme during the monitoring period were *permanently* registered with a GP on the General Medical List of one or other of these FPCs. Again the FPCs were not able to provide us with information about temporary registrations.

Referral into scheme

Lack of information entered on the record cards prevents much comment about how people in Camden came to use the scheme in the first place. However, our general impression from talking to team members was that the majority of users were self-referrals, although some may have been guided towards the scheme by workers in the day centres or the local night shelter. The records do show that the project doctor was the first point of contact with the scheme for two-thirds of users but as we have explained, the records underestimate the amount of contact users had with the project nurse.

Table 3.1   All users of the East London pilot scheme (1.1.1987-31.12.1987) by place of *first* consultation and sex

column percentages

| | Total | Place of first consultation | | | | | | | |
		Cable Street	St Botolphs	Prov. Row	T.H. Mission	Booth House	Underwood Road	Inform-AL	Other
Sex									
Male	86	92	89	50	52	100	100	91	99
Female	14	8	11	50	49	-	-	10	1
Base: all users	*(885)*	*(246)*	*(255)*	*(111)*	*(31)*	*(131)*	*(10)*	*(21)*	*(80)*

Table 3.2   Age of all users of the East London pilot scheme: 1.1.1987-31.12.1987

column percentages

| | Total | Place of first consultation | | | | | | | |
		Cable Street	St Botolphs	Prov. Row	T.H. Mission	Booth House	Underwood Road	Inform-AL	Other
Age									
713	21	20	24	16					
25-34	18	15	15	27	13	21	20	24	16
35-44	27	25	29	20	13	46	10	-	20
45-54	22	23	26	15	29	20	20	14	21
55-64	12	18	14	5	13	9	-	10	10
65 and over	5	6	6	1	7	2	10	5	11
Dk	5	2	2	3	10	-	40	43	16
Base: all users	*(885)*	*(246)*	*(255)*	*(111)*	*(31)*	*(131)*	*(10)*	*(21)*	*(80)*

**Table 3.3   Place of birth of all users of the East London pilot scheme:
1.1.1987-31.12.1987**

column percentages

	Total	Cable Street	St Botolphs	Prov. Row	T.H. Mission	Booth House	Underwood Road	Inform-AL	Other
Place of first consultation									
Place of birth									
England	43	35	48	54	45	45	20	33	34
Scotland	14	12	14	13	26	24	20	10	8
Wales	3	2	4	3	-	2	10	-	1
N. Ireland	3	2	4	4	-	2	-	-	3
Irish Republic	15	13	16	14	13	19	-	-	20
Outside UK	5	3	6	6	-	6	-	-	11
DK	18	33	9	7	16	3	50	57	24
Base: all users	*(885)*	*(246)*	*(255)*	*(111)*	*(31)*	*(131)*	*(10)*	*(21)*	*(80)*

**Table 3.4   Accommodation of all users of the East London pilot scheme
1.1.1987-31.12.1987 at the time of *first* consultation**

column percentages

	Total	Male	Female
		Sex	
Type of accommodation			
Rough/skipper	30	33	13
Squat	3	3	4
Night shelter	2	2	2
Short-stay hostel	17	12	48
Long-stay hostel	17	20	4
Hotel, B&B	3	4	1
Own accommodation	21	21	23
Specialist (alcohol, drugs)	3	4	1
Other	3	3	4
DK	1	1	1
Base: all users	*(885)*	*(763)*	*(122)*

**Table 3.5   Proportion of all users of the East London pilot scheme
(1.1.1987-31.12.1987) who said they were registered with a GP
by age**

column percentages

		Age						
	Total	Under 25	25-34	35-44	45-54	55-64	65 & above	DK
Registered with GP?								
Yes	49	57	46	45	47	61	55	43
No	42	39	46	49	46	34	30	26
DK	1	1	2	1	-	3	2	-
No entry on record cards	7	3	6	5	8	3	13	31
Base: all users	*(885)*	*(92)*	*(158)*	*(239)*	*(197)*	*(110)*	*(47)*	*(42)*

**Table 3.6   All users of the Camden pilot scheme (1.1.1987-31.12.1987),
by place of *first* consultation and sex**

column percentages

		Place of first consultation		
	Total	Arlington Drop-in	WLDC	Simon Community
Sex				
Male	85	83	86	89
Female	15	17	14	12
Base: all users	*(576)*	*(193)*	*(322)*	*(61)*

Table 3.7   Age of all users of the Camden pilot scheme: 1.1.1987-31.12.1987

column percentages

| | | Place of first consultation | | |
	Total	Arlington Drop-in	WLDC	Simon Community
Age				
Under 25	4	6	3	2
25-34	19	22	17	20
35-44	26	23	26	34
45-54	24	20	27	23
55-64	11	7	15	7
65 and above	5	3	6	3
DK	11	19	6	12
Base: all users	*(576)*	*(193)*	*(322)*	*(61)*

Table 3.8   Place of birth of all users of the Camden pilot scheme: 1.1.1987-31.12.1987

column percentages

| | | Place of first consultation | | |
	Total	Arlington Drop-in	WLDC	Simon Community
Place of birth				
England	29	17	36	28
Scotland	23	25	21	23
Wales	2	1	3	2
N. Ireland	3	4	3	7
Irish Republic	22	25	20	21
Outside UK	4	3	5	2
DK	18	25	13	18
Base: all users	*(576)*	*(193)*	*(322)*	*(61)*

Table 3.9 **Accommodation of all users of the Camden pilot scheme (1.1.1987-31.12.1987) at the time of *first* consultation**

column percentages

Type of accommodation	Total	Sex	
		Male	Female
Rough/skipper	39	40	32
Squat	3	3	1
Night shelter	12	13	9
Short-stay hostel	5	4	6
Long-stay hostel	6	6	8
Hotel, B&B	11	11	13
Own accommodation	14	14	19
Specialist (alcohol, drugs)	-	-	-
Other	8	7	12
DK	3	4	1
Base: all users	*(576)*	*(491)*	*(85)*

Table 3.10 **Proportion of all users of the Camden pilot scheme (1.1.1987-31.12.1987) who said they were registered with a GP, by age**

column percentages

Registered with GP?	Total	Age						
		Under 25	25-34	35-44	45-54	55-64	65 & above	DK
Yes	35	33	33	33	36	47	33	27
No	52	63	58	61	51	47	56	24
DK	1	-	2	-	-	-	-	2
No entry on record card	12	4	6	6	12	8	11	47
Base: all users	*(576)*	*(24)*	*(110)*	*(149)*	*(140)*	*(64)*	*(27)*	*(62)*

4   Take-up of Services

To what extent were the team's services used in each area and what were the most common presenting problems? The discussion in this chapter is based on the *total number of consultations* made by users during the monitoring period.

We built up an aggregate picture of consultations with team members using the contact sheet information described in Chapter 3. The contact sheets provided details about users at the time of each consultation, such as their registration status, and also indicated the action taken by team members during each consultation. Team members were asked to record the outcome of each visit, which was defined as the 'terminating action' to that consultation: for example, referral to another team member; hospital referral; referral to GP; prescription; or dressing. Given that one of the objectives of the pilot schemes was, wherever possible, to get homeless people back into mainstream services, they were also asked to record whether or not they advised the user to register with a local GP. The problems of missing data which we encountered with the medical record cards also arose with the contact sheets.

Four major qualifications need to be taken into account when interpreting the extent of use of the project team's services as recorded on the contact sheets:

(i) In Camden this information tended to underestimate the amount of contact the project nurse had with patients and to overestimate the GP's involvement. This problem arose because of the way the contact sheets were completed when the doctor and nurse shared clinics. The project nurse did two clinics a week on her own at

Arlington Drop-In Centre and for these sessions she filled in her own contact sheets. However, during the two clinics a week at this centre that she shared with the project doctor he filled in one contact sheet in his name on behalf of them both. A similar situation occurred at West London Day Centre, where the nurse employed by the centre also shared two clinics a week with the project doctor. All of the consultations at these shared clinics were recorded in the name of the project doctor, with the result that his apparent input into these clinics was inflated, while the role played by the nurse was not recorded. In many cases it is likely that the doctor saw the patient in the first instance and made the diagnosis, but the nurse provided the treatment, for example dressing a wound.

(ii) In City and East London we had to allow for the fact that the alcohol counsellor did group work as well as individual counselling. Group activities could not be recorded on the contact sheets because these were intended for individual consultations. We therefore designed a separate record sheet for the alcohol counsellor to keep a systematic record of the group work she did in the centres.

(iii) It is important to take into account factors which reduced the potential number of consultations during the monitoring period. For example, locum cover was not always available during team members' holidays. In particular, the salaried doctors were entitled to take 30 days holiday, but no locum cover was available during this period. In City and East London there was also a four-week period when no doctor was in post and therefore no consultations were recorded. In addition, sessions had to be cancelled when for any reason one of the day centres was closed on a clinic day.

(iv) The contact sheets recorded consultations made during clinic times or when team members held regular sessions at the centres. However, some of the contact team members had with people at the centres was much more informal than this. They often stopped to talk to people as they walked around the centres and this casual contact was not recorded, even though they may have given help and advice.

City and East London pilot scheme

Number of consultations

The 885 individuals who used the East London scheme made a total of 3,198 consultations during 1987. As the majority of users were men, it is not surprising that almost 80 per cent of the total number of consultations with the team during the year were made by men. There was little difference between the age groups looked at as a proportion of all consultations made by male users.

In Table 4.1 (p.75) we show the total number of consultations broken down by the team member seen on each occasion and the centre where the consultation took place.

Approximately half of these consultations were made during the regular clinics held by one of the project doctors. A high proportion of the consultations, just over a quarter of the total, took place with the Health Authority nurse who was not officially a team member. She worked four afternoons at Cable Street Day Centre and during the monitoring period over half (57 per cent) of all the consultations made at this day centre were with her. The fact that she worked part-time at this centre and was therefore more available to attenders than the other team members helps to explain why she was involved in a relatively high number of consultations. Our interviews with clients also suggested that they tended to see her as a 'friend' as well as a nurse and frequently visited her for a general chat rather than for nursing care. Evidence from our interviews at this centre suggested that some men enjoyed having a 'pretty nurse' to talk to.

It would be pointless to try and compare the extent of team members' activity or the rate of consultations at different locations on the basis of the figures in Table 4.1 (p.75) because we would not be comparing like with like. As explained in Chapter 2, whereas the project doctor held regular clinics at particular centres, the other team members did some sessional work but also operated on a more ad hoc basis. Some team members were therefore more 'visible' or more often available than others. More specifically, the alcohol counsellor, who worked part-time for the project, also did group work which is not shown in this table because it records consultations with individual users only. A further complication was that team members did not necessarily visit the same centres, and this explains why there are some gaps in Table 4.1 (p.75); (no consultations are indicated when the team member did not provide a service at that centre).

Frequency of consultation

Just over half of all the people who used the scheme in the monitoring period did so once only during the calendar year (Table 4.2, p.76). Almost three-quarters of these users had consulted the project doctor.

The date of their *first* consultation in 1987 inevitably influenced the number of times these individuals sought help from the team during the twelve-month period. Generally speaking, the later in the year that users first consulted the team the less likely they were to have made further visits.

There are numerous other reasons which might explain why people used the scheme once only: for example, they may have got what they wanted at this visit and not have needed further help during the monitoring period; they may have moved on to another area; or they may have preferred to seek help from other sources, such as hospital accident and emergency departments. Some may well have been successfully referred back into mainstream provision or have decided to use the services of a GP in any case. That so few people at the detoxification unit used the scheme more than once is explained by the fact that most were resident there for just one week and, unlike other users, they had not chosen to seek help from the team in the first place; seeing the project doctor was a routine part of the detoxification programme.

Around 17 per cent of all users consulted twice during the year and 28 per cent consulted three times or more. Users did not necessarily see the same team member on different occasions. For example, they may have had a variety of medical and social problems over the twelve-month period and at different times required the help of the doctor, the nurse and the social worker.

There was not always a clear connection between the nature of the presenting problem and the team member consulted; for example, not all of the problems presented to the doctor could be described as medical. In some cases users may have consulted a team member simply because they were available at the centre at the time when help was needed. Others may have chosen to see a particular team member because they liked and trusted them or, in the case of the doctor, because of his 'title'. In a small number of cases, approximately 3 per cent of all consultations, team members had referred the user to a team colleague who they thought could be of more help. The majority of these referrals were made by the project doctor, most frequently to the alcohol counsellor, although some were directed to the social worker or the nurse.

Some users made extensive use of the scheme, as can be seen by the 5 per cent who consulted more than 12 times during the calendar year. The majority of these users had first made contact with the scheme early on in the monitoring period and during the 12 months these 47 individuals made between them 830 consultations - a quarter of all the consultations recorded by the team. Almost half these consultations were with the nurse employed at Cable Street Day Centre and just under a third were with the project doctor. It does not necessarily follow that those making heavy use of the scheme were more unhealthy than those consulting less. Some might have had multiple or chronic health problems, but others might have presented regularly simply because they wanted a general chat with someone sympathetic about their circumstances.

Nature of consultations: presenting problems and outcomes
What were the main types of problems that led users to seek help from the project team and how did team members respond to these problems? In particular, what action did they take on consultations? As the team was deliberately multidisciplinary and team members therefore offered different types of services, it was necessary to explore these questions separately for each professional discipline. The number of consultations recorded with the community psychiatric nurse were too few to warrant analysis, however.

(i) Consultations with the project doctors

(a) Presenting problems
A breakdown of consultations with the project doctor by presenting problem and clinic location is shown in Table 4.3 (p.77), which includes consultations with all three doctors employed on the project.

The following points should be considered in interpreting this table. Entries on the contact sheets were generally made by presenting complaint at the time of consultation, rather than by diagnosis. For example, a person who presented with dyspepsia would be recorded by the doctor under 'Gastrointestinal' even though the dyspepsia might have been brought on by an underlying drink problem.

Often the project doctors did not have access to a user's past medical history which might have indicated that what was actually wrong with them was different from the apparent presenting problem. In this respect their record keeping was different from that found in general practice; GP audits are usually based on diagnosis and outcome. The types of problems presented by users of the scheme are, therefore, not strictly comparable with the morbidity of the general population as recorded in general practice. It is also hard to make comparisons with statistics collected by other projects serving the homeless because, even though most tend to record by presenting problem, they use different bases for classifying this information.

The categories we use in Table 4.3 (p.77) are those agreed by the project doctors initially employed in the two areas as the basis upon which they would classify presenting complaints. Sometimes users presented with two or more complaints at the same consultation and in these cases two (or more) entries would have been made on the contact sheet for that consultation. For example, if the user with dyspepsia had also wanted attention for a skin rash, his consultation would have been recorded under 'Dermatology' as well as 'Gastrointestinal'. Wherever possible the doctors also attempted to record whether the complaint was a chronic condition or an acute episode. We have not used this breakdown in our table; in practice the distinction between 'chronic' and 'acute' was frequently hard to make and depended on each doctor's assessment at the time.

Sometimes people used the scheme several times because they needed 'repeat treatment' for a particular problem. This category needed to be handled carefully in order not to overestimate the incidence of presenting problems. For example, if a person consulted with a skin problem which required several repeat visits it would have overestimated the incidence of dermatological problems if each of these consultations had been recorded as a *new* case of dermatology. To avoid over-counting, the project doctors were asked to indicate whenever a consultation was for repeat treatment and also to describe which category of complaint the treatment referred to. This enabled us to distinguish between new cases of a particular category of complaint and repeat treatment for that complaint.

This distinction between new incidences and repeat treatment is included in Table 4.3 (p.77) where we show three figures against each category of presenting problem: (i) the percentage of consultations which involved new incidences of the problem; (ii) the percentage of consultations which involved repeat treatment; and (iii) the combined figure for new incidences and repeat treatment. As the difficulty with recording repeat treatment was not fully appreciated until several months after the monitoring period had begun, a number of cases involving this category were recorded early on without the nature of the problem being specified. As a result, in East London we know that 9 per cent of all consultations with the project doctor involved repeat treatment, but in approximately 22 per cent of these consultations (33 consultations) we do not know what the treatment was for. These 33 consultations are excluded from Table 4.3 (p.77).

What were the most common presenting problems seen by the project doctors in East London? Table 4.3 (p.77) shows that just over 17 per cent of all consultations with the doctor involved new cases of respiratory complaints and with the inclusion of consultations for repeat treatment, this figure increased to 19 per cent. Users presented with chronic conditions such as emphysema, old pulmonary TB, lung cancer and chronic bronchitis, as well as with acute bronchitis and minor illnesses such as colds, sinusitis and coughs. Given the life-style of many using the clinics, it was not surprising that a greater proportion of these consultations occurred during the winter months than in the summer; almost two-thirds of respiratory problems were recorded during these months. There was little difference between the proportions of male and female users who presented with new cases of respiratory problems (18 per cent and 16 per cent respectively), but respiratory complaints were more common among older users.

Other fairly common presenting problems were those categorised as 'Dermatology', 'Psychiatric' or 'Trauma'. Approximately 14 per cent of consultations involved a dermatological condition and the vast majority of these were new cases. These skin problems included acute rashes, infections and infestations, as well as chronic cases of psoriasis, seborrhoea, varicose eczema and leg ulcers.

A similar proportion of consultations, 14 per cent, involved a psychiatric problem. For some users this might have been an acute psychological disturbance (for example, following bereavement) but for the majority it involved some form of chronic psychiatric illness such as schizophrenia. A higher proportion of women users (18 per cent) were recorded as having presented with a psychiatric problem as compared to the proportion of male users (12 per cent). Psychiatric problems were also frequently encountered among younger users: 20 per cent of consultations involving people under 25 involved a new incidence of a psychiatric problem, again probably reflecting the higher proportion of women in this age group; and a similar figure was recorded for users in the 25-29 age group .

'Trauma' was also recorded in 13 per cent of clinic consultations. The vast majority of these incidences involved acute conditions which had recently happened: for example, broken or fractured bones following an accident or wounds following a stabbing.

A quarter of all clinic consultations were recorded as being 'Alcohol or drug related'. The vast majority of these involved alcohol abuse, but quite frequently those abusing alcohol also abused drugs like heminevrin (prescribed to aid withdrawal in alcoholics). Alcohol abuse was recorded across all age groups, but was less commonly recorded as a presenting problem for those users aged under 30 than for older users.

Entries under 'Alcohol-related' tended to be recorded pragmatically and differences of interpretation occurred between doctors. As a result, the figures for this category are not comparable between projects. The figures in East London suggest more alcohol problems than in Camden because for a time one of the doctors in East London was recording the 'hidden agenda' of drink problems as well as obvious cases where alcohol abuse was involved. A drawback to this approach was that as the doctor was asking about alcohol intake when putting together a patient's medical history, it was difficult for him to avoid prompting the user to talk about alcohol. His opposite number in Camden was using this category only if patients came in with an alcohol problem or alcohol formed a major part of their problem.

In almost 20 per cent of consultations the presenting problem could not be recorded under one of the pre-selected headings and the category 'Other' was used. This category includes a wide range of complaints, the most common being: insomnia, gynaecological problems, eye problems, hearing problems, epilepsy and generally feeling unwell. It also included those 5 per cent of consultations where insufficient information was recorded to allow a more appropriate entry.

(b)   Outcomes
What action did the project doctors take on consultations? Table 4.4 (p.78) gives a breakdown of all GP clinic consultations by outcome, defined as the 'terminating action' to each consultation.

Two general points should be considered in interpreting this table. Firstly, just as users may have presented with more than one problem, there may have been more than one outcome to each consultation. Secondly, the table underestimates the extent of advice that was given to users. The category of 'Advice only' was used when advice or counselling was the only outcome and no other action was taken.

The fact that there could be multiple entries both for the presenting problem and for action taken on consultation made it difficult for us to link the two sets of information. Where a single presenting problem was involved we could identify the outcome(s), but where users presented with two (or more) complaints and there were two (or more) outcomes, the system of recording information that we had negotiated with team members did not allow us to distinguish which outcomes related to which presenting problems. Where we make the connection between categories of presenting problem and outcomes, this is based on the 68 per cent of consultations with the project doctor where a single presenting problem was involved; this was a total of 1,110 consultations.

Just over half of all consultations with the project doctor resulted in a prescription or repeat prescription for medication. This was particularly common when the consultation involved a dermatological problem, a respiratory complaint or one of the conditions entered under 'Gastrointestinal'. Almost 13 per cent required some type of dressing, most frequently for a wound, but also for leg ulcers or some other form of skin problem. A similar proportion of consultations resulted in providing the patient with a medical certificate. In just over 17 per cent of consultations the user was asked to come back again, for example, for a change of dressing, a repeat prescription for medication, or for the results of a hospital investigation.

A sizeable proportion of all consultations with the doctor, 16 per cent, resulted in advice only. Advice was given on a wide range of social and medical issues including, for example: diet; drink problems; psychiatric problems; current use of tablets or other medicines; welfare benefits; how to register with a GP; and more general aspects of health education.

Consultations with the project doctor often resulted in referrals, either to other team members or, more frequently, to local GPs or to other agencies. Twelve per cent of consultations led to users being referred to a local GP, and this was often when people were already registered with one. Four per cent of consultations led to referrals to statutory or voluntary housing agencies including statutory housing agencies, direct access hostels, and specialist hostels (for example, those catering for people with mental health problems). Six per cent of consultations resulted in users being referred to other agencies including the DHSS; social services departments; workers at the centre where the clinic was held; agencies offering drugs, alcohol or mental health advice; AIDS counselling; opticians; dentists; and centres for delousing. The doctors reported difficulties in finding places for patients who needed detoxification. There were few facilities in London and these were overstretched. The problem was particularly acute for women with alcohol problems.

Fourteen per cent of all project doctor consultations (234 consultations) resulted in users being referred to hospital. Almost half these hospital referrals were for further investigation of the presenting problem. Some patients would have needed X-rays, not just for chest complaints, but also to check on injuries sustained in accidents or fights. Others would have been referred for blood tests. The project doctors, like all GPs, had direct access to these facilities and although they referred patients for investigation, it was on the basis that they came back to them for treatment. This category comprised problems they could investigate as GPs and did not need to refer to specialists. They retained responsibility for the patient.

The second doctor to be employed on the pilot scheme explained that his policy was to refer as little as possible to hospital consultants and direct access diagnostic facilities because he doubted whether many of the homeless people would go. He referred only those who he thought would keep the appointment and they tended to be the ones who were more settled. His impression was that for non-alcohol-related problems patients would keep appointments, but for alcohol-related problems they were less likely to do so. He was fairly confident that most of the people he referred were seen by the support service concerned; either he got feedback from the patient or he received a letter from the hospital or service agency.

Just under a quarter of hospital referrals were to outpatients' departments. In these cases patients would have been given a letter for an appointment with a doctor in the appropriate specialty. The purpose of a further 9 per cent of hospital referrals was to get the patient admitted for treatment.

Ten per cent of hospital referrals were to an accident and emergency department, although an entry recorded under this category could be confusing because it might actually have been a referral for admission, but the hospital might have declined to accept the patient over the telephone. This category of hospital referral also included users who had taken overdoses of drugs, when casualty is the usual admission route.

(ii)   Consultations with the nurse

(a)   Presenting problems

Table 4.5 (p.79) gives a breakdown of all consultations with the health authority nurse employed at Cable Street Day Centre by presenting problem.

The nurse spent a lot of her time *talking* to patients as well as providing nursing services. Just over half of all the consultations with her involved the user seeking general advice about a social or medical problem. Advice was sought by all age groups but it was a particularly common feature of consultations made by younger users; for example, three-quarters of the consultations made by those under 25 involved the user asking for advice. Moreover, of the 40 per cent of consultations where the 'Other' category was used, over half consisted of the user visiting the nurse for a 'general chat'.

Other common complaints for which the nurse's help was sought were those which were categorised as 'Dermatological', and our impression was that skin problems also accounted for a sizeable proportion of the visits for repeat treatment.

Just over a quarter of all consultations with the nurse were recorded as alcohol or drug related and again most of these consultations involved alcohol rather than drug abuse. While few of the consultations made by users under 30 involved alcohol, over half the consultations made by users in the 35-39 age group were recorded as alcohol or drug-related (55 per cent).

(b)   Outcomes

The most striking feature revealed by Table 4.6 (p.80) is that in 41 per cent of the consultations the nurse provided advice only and took no further action. This is consistent with the finding that with this client group she spent much of her time talking and not providing traditional nursing service. Nursing care, predominantly in the form of dressings for wounds or for chronic skin complaints, was evident in just under a third of nurse consultations.

The professional limitations of the nurse's role are also reflected in the table: for example, only 2 per cent of consultations resulted in referrals to hospital and less than 1 per cent resulted in a medical certificate being issued. Nurses cannot prescribe drugs and in the 18 per cent of consultations where 'prescription' of medication was recorded, this meant 'handing out' medication such as paracetemol. Referral to a GP occurred during 11 per cent of consultations; occasionally this was to the project doctor, but more often the user was recommended to register with a local GP.

(iii)   Alcohol counsellor

(a)   Presenting problems

The information recorded by the alcohol counsellor was less comprehensive than that compiled by other team members and needs to be interpreted with caution. In particular, in almost half of all consultations with the alcohol counsellor the age of the users was not known. A breakdown of consultations by presenting problem is given in Table 4.7 (p.81).

The categories of presenting problem used by the alcohol counsellor were different from those designed for the doctors and the nurse and were selected to reflect her type of work. It needs to be repeated that these figures record *individual* consultations only and do not indicate the extent of group work that was undertaken. A further proviso in interpreting the figures is that around 60 per cent of all the consultations with the alcohol counsellor were not alcohol-specific; she also provided more general advice (in about 22 per cent of consultations) and counselling for a variety of social problems, particularly before the social worker was appointed to the project.

Just over 40 per cent of consultations involved an element of continuation counselling; in about a third of these the main problem was alcohol related. Just under a quarter of consultation were acute episodes and required some form of crisis intervention; almost two-thirds of these concerned alcohol abuse. Overall, approximately 40 per cent of all consultations with the alcohol counsellor were alcohol, or very occasionally drug, related.

(b) Outcomes

As Table 4.8 (p.82) shows, almost two-thirds of all consultations with the alcohol counsellor resulted in a repeat appointment. In the majority of these cases the presenting problem was recorded as 'continuation counselling'. In the 32 per cent of cases where she had recorded 'To come again' the outcome of the session had been more vague. The option to make further visits had been left open, but no repeat appointment had been made.

The alcohol counsellor commented that referring clients on to support services had become easier once she had got to know the centre staff and had built up a network of contacts in the various statutory and voluntary agencies. The support services to which she made most frequent referrals tended to be those catering for alcohol-related, social or housing problems. Unfortunately, the staff in these agencies were usually overstretched and she often found it difficult to get hold of a client's social worker or the relevant housing worker. She also found it difficult to get a client accepted by any of the local hospitals for detoxification unless they had clear medical reasons for needing this facility. She confirmed the view of the project doctor that the lack of detoxification facilities for women was particularly acute.

(c) Group work

The alcohol counsellor undertook group work in the centres she visited, as well as doing one-to-one counselling. In total she held around 60 group sessions during the twelve-month monitoring period. A few of these were one-off sessions, but more often groups were established which met regularly on a fortnightly or monthly basis.

Some of the groups were categorised as 'support' groups; for example, at one hostel she established a 'support' group for residents which met on a fortnightly basis, and enabled residents to raise grievances and previously unspoken issues around living in a residential project. Other groups were categorised as 'therapeutic'; an example of these was the group established at one of the day centres which allowed members to share and discuss their alcohol problems. The purpose of some of the groups was simply to get users or residents to come together and discuss issues of common concern: for example, housing, alcohol abuse, and budgeting.

Little information was collected about group members. This was because the alcohol counsellor thought it inappropriate to ask attenders for any personal details. The size of the groups ranged from only two people up to a maximum of 14 members. The 'therapeutic' and 'support' groups tended to be small, with between two and five people in the group. Once the group was established, at any one session there would be several core members who attended on a regular basis and one or two new clients. The general discussion groups were usually larger and these too would often have a core membership of regular clients.

The majority of clients attending the group sessions were male, but the alcohol counsellor worked hard at getting women users or residents involved. Women's groups, which provided them with a safe environment in which to discuss 'women's issues', were established at two of the centres towards the end of the monitoring period.

(iv)   Social worker

(a)   Presenting problems

Consultations with the social worker are broken down in Table 4.9 (p.82) according to presenting problem.   Once again different categories of presenting problem were agreed in advance with the social worker in order to reflect the types of problems he was likely to encounter.

Not surprisingly the most common category concerned 'Accommodation'; almost two-thirds of people consulting the social worker had sought help with their housing problems. These included people in all age groups but it is not possible to be more specific because age was not recorded in approximately 41 per cent of these consultations.

The social worker also received a sizeable number of requests for help with welfare benefits, accounting for at least 15 per cent of consultations with him. The 'Other' category was used for a broad range of largely social rather than medical problems, including practical help required in dealing with other agencies; requests for help with clothing or furniture; bereavement; children in care; and users who simply wanted someone to talk to.

Approximately 16 per cent of consultations with the social worker were alcohol, or more rarely drug, related.   As with other team members, this category was recorded pragmatically.   A consultation was likely to be recorded by the social worker as 'Alcohol-related' if it was relevant to the user's reason for seeking help; for example, if it affected their ability to find accommodation or cope with resettlement.

(b)   Outcomes

Almost half the consultations with the social worker resulted in advice only, as can be seen from Table 4.10 (p.83). Advice was provided on a wide range of topics, the most common being: gambling; cash benefits; furniture; clothing; alcohol; and accommodation.

During the course of the monitoring period the social worker found himself becoming increasingly involved in housing work, particularly resettlement, and this is reflected in the number of referrals to housing agencies which accounted for just over a quarter of the consultations with him. Most of these referrals were to the Local Authority Housing

Department or to direct access hostels, but a few involved voluntary housing agencies or specialist hostels. The most significant change in his referral pattern during the monitoring period was that he made an increasing number of referrals to Tower Hamlet's Homeless Persons' Unit. However, he would only send people to this Unit if he was confident that they were entitled to help. He knews that single homeless people would be subjected to a long period of scrutiny to find out whether they were entitled to the service and they found this a harrowing experience.

Not all his referrals, however, concerned housing. Eleven per cent of consultations resulted in referrals to other agencies: namely local offices of the DHSS; social services departments; and agencies offering alcohol advice.

Camden and Islington pilot scheme

Certain factors must be taken into account when interpreting the data from the Camden scheme. As already explained,the consultation statistics in Camden tended to underestimate the extent of contact the nurses had with users and overestimate the action on consultations taken by the doctor. Also, as described in Chapter 2, not all the work undertaken by the project nurse was clinic-oriented. She visited several centres on a more informal basis with the purpose of talking to users and residents about health education. This activity was not captured on the contact sheets.

Number of consultations

In Camden a total of 576 individuals used the team's services in the monitoring period and during these twelve months they made a total of 2,022 consultations. Just over 80 per cent of all consultations were made by men.

In Table 4.11 (p.83) we give the total number of consultations broken down by the team member seen on each occasion and the location where the consultation was made. Separate data are shown for consultations with the project nurse and with the nurse who was not actually employed by the project, but worked alongside the project doctor at West London Day Centre. A small number of consultations took place with a locum GP and with an agency nurse and these have been amalgamated with the figures for the project doctor and project nurse respectively.

Just over half of these consultations took place at the regular clinics held by the project doctor with the project nurse in attendance twice a week at Arlington Drop-in Centre or with the nurse working alongside him twice a week at West London Day Centre.

The project nurse, when working alone and not sharing a clinic with the doctor, was involved in just under a quarter of all consultations. Her greatest input was at Arlington Drop-in Centre, which she visited throughout the entire monitoring period. Almost half of the consultations recorded at this centre were with her and our interviews with clients showed that she was well liked and regarded as a 'friend' as well as a nurse. She did not start going to the Simon Community night shelter until November 1987 and she did not visit West London Day Centre.

A quarter of all the consultations recorded by the Camden team during the monitoring period were made with the nurse at West London Day Centre at times when she was working there alone and not assisting at the twice-weekly clinic with the doctor. She was a member of staff at this centre and was readily available to users. Forty-five per cent of all the consultations made at this centre were with her, excluding her involvement in the shared clinics.

Frequency of consultation

How frequently did users in Camden see one or other of the team members during the monitoring period?

Table 4.12 (p.84) shows a similar pattern of use in Camden to that found in East London. Around 58 per cent of people who used the scheme during the monitoring period did so once only. Again, generally speaking the later in the year people first used the scheme, the less likely they were to have made further visits. Of those who had made a single visit, 57 per cent had consulted the project doctor; the rest had either seen the project nurse or the nurse attached to West London Day Centre.

Just under 14 per cent of users had used the scheme twice and the remaining 28 per cent had used it three or more times - very similar proportions to those found in the East London scheme. Approximately

5 per cent of all users had been seen by the project doctor or nurse more than twelve times during the calendar year. All of these had initially made contact with the scheme in the first half of the monitoring period, and during the year had made between them a total of 483 consultations - almost a quarter of all the consultations recorded by the project team.

Nature of consultations: presenting problems and outcomes
What were the main types of problems that led users in Camden to seek help from the project team and what action did team members take on consultations? We look first at the experience of the project doctor and then at the nurses.

(i)   Consultations with the project doctor

(a)   Presenting problems
A breakdown of consultations with the project doctor by presenting problem and clinic location is shown in Table 4.13 (p.85). The points that need to be considered in interpreting this table have been given for the equivalent table for the East London project (Table 4.3, p.77). We make the distinction between new cases of each category of presenting problem and repeat treatment, as well as giving the combined figure.

A general difference between the two pilot schemes is that in each category of presenting problem the Camden doctor recorded a higher incidence of repeat treatment than his counterparts in the East London project. This difference is marked when consultations involving repeat treatment are looked at as a proportion of all doctor consultations. In Camden 34 per cent of all consultations with the doctor during the monitoring period involved repeat treatment, whereas in East London only 9 per cent of doctor consultations were entered as repeat treatment.

Many factors could have contributed to this difference. The most likely explanation is that the doctors varied in their policies towards repeat treatment. We know that one of the doctors in East London rarely coded for repeat treatment because, when this was necessary, he encouraged users to get treatment from a local GP rather than use the scheme.

If we look at new cases of presenting problems, the most common medical problems encountered by the doctor were those recorded as 'Respiratory' or 'Dermatology'. Almost 10 per cen of consultations involved a respiratory complaint and this figure increased to just over 12 per cent when repeat treatment was included. A marginally higher proportion of female users than male users sought help because of a respiratory illness.

Dermatological conditions accounted for just over 16 per cent of consultations, but a good number of these were for repeat treatment; for example, dressings for leg ulcers. In ordinary general practice a GP would usually see leg ulcers once and then refer the patient on to a district nurse for subsequent dressings. Therefore although it might have appeared that the doctor was seeing many leg ulcers in the day centres, this might have been because the same people were always seen by the doctor for repeat treatment.

Just over 10 per cent of consultations involved a psychiatric problem. Thirteen per cent were recorded as being alcohol or drug-related and the vast majority of these involved alcohol abuse. We have explained the differences between the doctors in recording this category; in Camden it was used only when the patient presented with an alcohol problem or alcohol formed a major part of the problem.

In just under 10 per cent of GP clinic consultations the user had sought some form of general advice from the doctor rather than wanting help with a physical problem. In some cases this could have been advice about a drinking problem or a psychiatric problem. In others, the user might have wanted help with obtaining a bus pass or asked for a medical card to use as a means of identification.

The category 'Other' was used in just over 17 per cent of consultations. It covered a wide variety of medical and social problems, as in East London.

(b)   Outcomes

A breakdown of all project doctor consultations by outcome, defined as the 'terminating action' to each consultation, is given in Table 4.14 (p.86). The same general comments apply to this table in East London (Table 4.4, p.78). There is the additional point that Table 4.14 (p.86) may overestimate the amount of work undertaken by the project doctor. We do not know the extent to which the nurses and not the doctor were involved in the 'terminating actions' to consultations during their shared clinics.

Approximately 20 per cent of the consultations with the project doctor in Camden were recorded as involving more than one presenting problem and in these cases, the consultation may have resulted in more than one outcome.

A prescription or repeat prescription for medication was the most common outcome to consultations with the doctor in Camden, accounting for 60 per cent of his consultations. This was particularly common when the presenting problem was a respiratory or dermatological condition and was higher than in East London. In practice the doctor prescribed drugs in the same way as a GP, but he tended to give drugs for less time than he would in general practice. Instead of prescribing a month's supply, he would be more likely to write out a prescription for a week or two weeks at a time. He thought that patients often preferred this because it meant that they would need to see him again and they actually wanted this contact. Also, it gave him more control over the supply of drugs and reduced the risk of their passing into the wrong hands, either because they were stolen from the unsuspecting owner, or because they were deliberately sold.

Fifteen per cent of consultations with the doctor ended with his giving the patient *advice only* and no other treatment. As in East London many consultations on other matters also involved an element of advice giving.

Dressings were supplied at 10 per cent of consultations, either for skin complaints such as leg ulcers or, more commonly, for some type of wound or injury. A similar proportion of consultations resulted in the patient being given a medical certificate.

Patients were referred to a local GP less frequently in Camden than in East London; in just under 3 per cent of consultations compared to around 12 per cent in East London. One reason for this difference might have been the fact that fewer users in Camden said they had their own GP. Team members in Camden might also have been less optimistic than their East London colleagues about the willingness of local GPs to take on homeless people. The project doctor explained that in general practice his level of referrals to other support services had been low and he continued this pattern while working for the project, largely because he thought this particular client group would have difficulty keeping appointments.

Very few referrals were made to housing agencies - only 2 per cent of consultations. However, around 9 per cent of consultations involved referrals to agencies other than those dealing exclusively with housing. The Camden team did not have an alcohol counsellor and just over a third of these referrals were to agencies which gave help and advice to those with a drink problem.

Seven per cent of all consultations (78 consultations) with the doctor in Camden resulted in the patient being referred to hospital compared to the equivalent figure of 14 per cent in East London. The project doctor said that there were practical difficulties in referring homeless patients to hospital. If they did not have an address it was difficult to know where to send notification of their appointment, and by the time of their appointment they might have moved on.

A third of all hospital referrals in Camden were for further investigation of the presenting problem, with the project doctor retaining responsibility for the patient, whereas just under a third involved the patient being admitted to hospital for treatment. Two patients were admitted to Wytham Hall. (This charitable establishment is run by a community of doctors, administrators and medical students in West London aiming to provide a sick bay for men who, because of homelessness, cannot be cared for during periods of acute illness.)

(ii) Consultations with the nurses

(a) Presenting problems
Table 4.15 (p.87) gives a breakdown of all consultations with the project nurse and the nurse employed by West London Day Centre by presenting problem.

A sizeable proportion of all consultations with the nurses, almost 22 per cent, resulted in the user coming back for repeat treatment. In Table 4.15 (p.87) this total for repeat treatment has been broken down by category of presenting problem.

The pattern of problems seen by the nurses in Camden was in many ways similar to that experienced by the nurse who worked alongside the East London project team. They spent a lot of their time talking to users seeking advice about a social or medical problem or simply wanting a chat, as well as providing nursing care. Users were recorded as wanting general advice in almost 20 per cent of all nurse consultations. Advice was sought by users in all age groups but, as in East London, it was particularly common among younger users; almost half the nurse consultations made by those under 30 involved asking for advice.

Other common complaints for which the nurses' help was sought in Camden were categorised either as 'Dermatology' or as 'Trauma'. About 19 per cent of consultations involved skin problems, but over half of these were for repeat treatment; for example, dressings for leg ulcers. Just over 17 per cent were classified as 'Trauma'; and the majority of these were injuries which had been recently sustained.

Between them the nurses categorised just over 8 per cent of consultations as alcohol or, more rarely, drug-related. In 16 per cent of consultations they came across problems which were entered under the 'Other' category described above.

(b)   Outcomes

Table 4.16 (p.88) gives a breakdown of action taken by the nurses on consultations. It does not record their involvement in clinics shared with the project doctor.

Generally speaking, the picture was similar to that encountered in East London. A third of all the consultations with one or other of the nurses resulted in advice only and no further treatment. There was a marked difference between the consultations at Arlington Drop-in Centre and those elsewhere; the proportion of consultations at this centre ending in advice only was almost double that recorded for the other two centres. Many factors may have contributed to this, including the nature of presenting problems encountered at the centres and the approach taken by the two nurses. Table 4.15 (p.87) shows that the proportion of users at this centre whose *presenting problem* was recorded by the nurse as 'general advice' was also markedly higher.

Almost a third of consultations required basic nursing care, often in the form of dressings for leg ulcers and wounds. Just under a quarter resulted in a prescription or repeat prescription, but as in East London this did not mean that the nurses were able to prescribe drugs.

Their referral activity was not extensive. In 6 per cent of cases the patient was referred to the project doctor and a similar number of referrals were made to local GPs. The project nurse explained that she did not recommend all the people whom she saw to register with a GP if they were not already registered. It would depend on their reason for coming to see her. As she put it, if they came in for 'a two-minute plaster job' then broaching the subject of GP registration might be inappropriate. There was also a more general issue to consider, that when people came to see the nurse for first aid they welcomed a general chat, but did not expect or want a lot of questions. Half of the small number of referrals to agencies other than those dealing with housing problems were to agencies which provided alcohol advice.

Acceptability

It is commonly believed that homeless people do not fit into ordinary general practice because their appearance or behaviour is 'unacceptable'. We asked team members in both project sites to record at each consultation how acceptable *they* thought users of the pilot schemes would be in an ordinary GP's surgery.

Team members used a simple three-point scale; whether they thought the 'acceptability' of the patient in a GP's surgery would be 'good', 'fair' or 'poor'. Their assessment was based on a number of subjective factors, including opinions on appearance and behaviour, and took into account the likely 'acceptability' of the patient to the GP, the GP's receptionist and to other patients in the waiting room.

We expected that 'acceptability' would be a difficult concept to explore and so it proved. However, the exercise of recording this information was valuable in that it highlighted the fact that different professionals have different views about what is or is not acceptable. It also underlined the fact that individuals may be 'acceptable' on one occasion and quite 'unacceptable' on another. 'Acceptability' is not a constant factor in either sense. This raises important issues which must be taken into account when discussing the potential or actual integration of homeless people into mainstream services.

Team members differed among themselves in their assessment of individuals. For example, a patient whose acceptability was rated as 'good' by the alcohol counsellor may on the same day have been rated as 'fair' or 'poor' by another team member less used to individuals with alcohol problems.

Team members who saw the same user more than once may have rated them differently on separate occasions. The rating may have depended on the user's state of drunkenness or sobriety at the time. It may also have been influenced by how well the team member knew the person; as team members got to know patients they tended to give them higher scores because they overlooked some of the aspects of appearance or behaviour which might have been off-putting initially.

It was thought that the vast majority of users of the schemes would be acceptable in general practice. In City and East London the acceptability of 70 per cent of users was rated as 'good' at the time of their *first* contact with the pilot scheme. In Camden the equivalent figure was 65 per cent. In both project areas less than 6 per cent of users were rated as 'poor' in terms of their likely acceptability to ordinary GPs.

In making any comment on team members' ratings of patients' acceptability, we must take into account the fact that they had a commitment to working with this client group, and their assessment of who would be acceptable in general practice might well have been more generous than that of an ordinary inner-city GP. Nevertheless, their assessment that over two thirds of users in both project areas would be 'acceptable' in general practice is an important finding which must be taken into account when discussing whether or not homeless people can be integrated into mainstream health care services.

Table 4.1   Proportion of total consultations by users made with each member of the East London team: 1.1.1987-31.12.1987

column percentages

	Total	Cable Street	St Botolphs	Prov. Row	T.H. Mission	Booth House	Underwood Road	Inform-AL	Other
Team member seen									
First project doctor	16	9	30	25	61	36	6	-	2
Second project doctor	32	25	67	28	26	63	13	-	1
'Temporary' doctor	3	<1	2	33	-	-	-	-	1
CPN	<1	-	-	5	-	1	-	-	1
Alcohol counsellor	9	5	2	10	8	-	26	100	14
Social worker	11	4	-	<1	5	1	56	-	82
Health authority nurse	28	57	-	-	-	-	-	-	-
Base: all consultations	*(3198)*	*(1577)*	*(653)*	*(255)*	*(85)*	*(151)*	*(47)*	*(105)*	*(325)*

Table 4.2 here

Table 4.2 Frequency of use of the East London pilot scheme during 1.1.1987–31.12.1987, by month of first consultation

column percentages

| | Total | Month of first consultation in 1987 | | | | | | | | | | | |
		Jan	Feb	March	April	May	June	July	Aug	Sept	Oct	Nov	Dec
Number of consultations per patient in calendar year													
one	55	34	50	50	47	60	55	75	75	57	71	70	83
two	17	11	18	19	30	13	18	22	11	27	10	19	15
3-12 times	23	36	29	29	23	22	24	3	14	16	19	11	3
more than 12 times	5	20	4	2	-	4	3	-	-	-	-	-	-
Base: all users	(885)	(179)	(101)	(86)	(43)	(68)	(76)	(36)	(28)	(82)	(62)	(67)	(41)

Table 4.3 **Breakdown of all consultations with the East London project doctors, by presenting problem: 1.1.1987-31.12.1987**

*column percentages**

				Place of consultation			
	Total	Cable Street	St Botolphs	Prov. Row	T.H. Mission	Booth House	Other
Presenting problem							
Respiratory	19	14	23	19	34	10	-
New	*17*	*14*	*20*	*18*	*32*	*10*	-
Repeat	*2*	*<1*	*3*	*1*	*1*	-	-
Cardiovascular	2	1	2	1	1	3	-
New	*1*	*1*	*1*	-	*1*	*3*	-
Repeat	*1*	-	*1*	*1*	-	-	-
Gastrointestinal	9	9	7	10	8	12	-
New	*7*	*8*	*6*	*8*	*8*	*11*	-
Repeat	*1*	*1*	*1*	*2*	-	*1*	-
Musculoskeletal	9	9	8	8	11	7	25
New	*8*	*7*	*7*	*8*	*11*	*6*	*25*
Repeat	*1*	*2*	*1*	-	-	*1*	-
Dermatology	14	13	17	7	14	7	19
New	*13*	*12*	*16*	*7*	*14*	*6*	*19*
Repeat	*1*	*1*	*1*	-	-	*1*	-
Psychiatry	14	13	11	27	16	7	50
New	*13*	*12*	*10*	*23*	*16*	*7*	*50*
Repeat	*1*	*1*	*<1*	*4*	-	-	-
Trauma	13	14	15	7	23	7	6
New	*13*	*14*	*15*	*7*	*23*	*7*	*6*
Repeat	*<1*	*<1*	*<1*	-	-	-	-
Alcohol/drug related	26	23	17	7	31	97	31
New	*26*	*23*	*17*	*7*	*31*	*97*	*31*
Repeat	-	-	-	-	-	-	-
Medical certificate	3	2	3	5	3	-	-
New	*3*	*2*	*3*	*5*	*3*	-	-
Repeat	-	-	-	-	-	-	-
Chiropody/dental	7	7	9	4	4	-	-
New	*7*	*7*	*9*	*4*	*4*	-	-
Repeat	-	-	-	-	-	-	-
Other medical	20	26	16	25	12	10	44
New	*19*	*23*	*15*	*24*	*12*	*10*	*44*
Repeat	*1*	*3*	*1*	*1*	-	-	-
General advice	8	7	8	12	27	1	6
New	*8*	*7*	*8*	*12*	*27*	*1*	*6*
Repeat	-	-	-	-	-	-	-
Base: all consultations with							
project doctor	*(1631)*	*(535)*	*(641)*	*(217)*	*(74)*	*(148)*	*(16)*

* The columns add to more than 100 per cent because more than one presenting problem was possible at each consultation.

Table 4.4 **Breakdown of action taken by East London project doctors on all project doctor consultations: 1.1.1987-31.12.1987**

*column percentages**

| | Total | Place of consultation | | | | | |
		Cable Street	St Botolphs	Prov. Row	T.H. Mission	Booth House	Other
Outcome							
Referral to hospital	14	16	14	11	16	16	31
Referral to GP	13	14	15	4	32	1	6
Referral to team member	5	6	4	6	11	1	13
Advice only	16	22	14	21	10	1	13
Prescription	52	41	52	55	42	95	63
Nursing/dressing	13	13	18	1	22	1	25
Medical certificate	12	3	4	8	5	93	6
Referral - housing	4	3	4	8	3	1	19
Referral - agency (excl. housing)	7	8	6	8	8	1	6
To come again	17	21	20	8	20	-	38
DK	1	1	1	1	1	2	
Base: all consultations with project doctor	*(1631)*	*(535)*	*(641)*	*(217)*	*(74)*	*(148)*	*(16)*

*   The columns add to more than 100 per cent because more than one outcome was possible at each consultation.

Table 4.5   Breakdown of all consultations with the East London nurse, by presenting problem: 1.1.1987-31.12.1987 (Cable Street day centre only)

column percentages*

	Cable Street day centre
Presenting problem	
Respiratory	9
Cardiovascular	5
Gastrointestinal	9
Musculoskeletal	10
Dermatology	27
Psychiatry	4
Trauma	6
Alcohol/drug related	27
Medical certificate	<1
Chiropody/dental	8
Other medical (eg general chat)	40
General advice	54
Repeat treatment for any category of presenting problem	14
Base: all consultations with (health authority) nurse	*(901)*

*   The column adds to more than 100 per cent because more than one presenting problem was possible at each consultation.

Table 4.6 **Breakdown of action taken by the East London nurse on all nurse consultations (Cable Street day centre only): 1.1.1987-31.12.1987**

column percentages*

	Cable Street day centre
Outcome	
Referral to hospital	3
Referral to GP	11
Referral - team member	1
Advice only	41
Prescription	19
Nursing/dressing	30
Medical certificate	<1
Referral - housing	2
Referral - agency (excl. housing)	3
To come again	11
DK	<1
Base: all consultations with (health authority) nurse	*(901)*

* The column adds to more than 100 per cent because more than one outcome was possible at each consultation.

Table 4.7   Breakdown of all consultations with the East London alcohol counsellor, by presenting problem: 1.1.1987-31.12.1987

column percentages*

	Place of consultation: all centres visited by alcohol counsellor
Presenting problem	
General advice/information	28
Crisis intervention	22
Continuation counselling	41
Relapse	6
Trauma	1
Alcohol/drug specific	40
Medical certificate	4
Repeat treatment	32
Chiropody/dental	1
Other	17
Base: all consultations with alcohol counsellor	*(288)*

*   The column adds to more than 100 per cent because more than one presenting problem was possible at each consultation.

Table 4.8   Breakdown of action taken by the East London alcohol counsellor on all alcohol counsellor consultations: 1.1.1987-31.12.1987

column percentages*

	Place of consultation: all centres visited by alcohol counsellor
Outcome	
Referral to hospital	1
Referral to GP	1
Referral - team member	1
Advice only	8
Repeat appointment	62
Referral - housing	4
Referral - agency (excl. housing)	8
To come again	33
Base: all consultations with alcohol counsellor	*(288)*

*   The column adds to more than 100 per cent because more than one outcome was possible at each consultation.

Table 4.9   Breakdown of all consultations with the East London social worker, by presenting problem: 1.1.1987-31.12.1987

column percentages*

	Place of consultation: all centres visited by social worker
Presenting problem	
Accommodation	60
Welfare benefits	15
Employment	2
Psychiatry	2
Gambling	1
Alcohol/drug related	16
Other	16
Base: all consultations with social worker	*(359)*

*   The column adds to more than 100 per cent because more than one presenting problem was possible at each consultation.

Table 4.10   Breakdown of action taken by the East London social worker on all social worker consultations: 1.1.1987-31.12.1987

column percentages*

Outcome	Place of consultation: all centres visited by social worker
Referral to hospital	2
Referral - team member	2
Advice only	48
Referral - housing	28
Referral - agency (excl. housing)	12
To come again	13
DK	1
Base: all consultations with social worker	*(359)*

*   The column adds to more than 100 per cent because more than one outcome was possible at each consultation.

Table 4.11   Proportion of total consultations by users made with each member of the Camden team: 1.1.1987-31.12.1987

column percentages

		Place of consultation		
Team member seen	Total	Arlington Drop-in	WLDC	Simon Community
Project doctor	53	48	55	70
Project nurse	22	52	-	30
'Centre' nurse	25	-	45	-
Base: all consultations	*(2022)*	*(794)*	*(1130)*	*(98)*

Table 4.12 here

Table 4.12 Frequency of use of the Camden pilot scheme during 1.1.1987-31.12.1987, by month of first consultation

column percentages

	Total	Month of first consultation in 1987											
		Jan	Feb	March	April	May	June	July	Aug	Sept	Oct	Nov	Dec
Number of consultations per patient in calendar year													
one	58	34	54	36	61	42	50	77	58	76	74	73	92
two	14	17	8	21	19	21	14	12	18	12	11	13	5
3-12 times	23	32	29	37	14	33	31	12	25	12	14	15	3
more than 12 times	5	17	9	6	6	4	5	-	-	-	-	-	-
Base: all users	(576)	(102)	(65)	(52)	(36)	(24)	(42)	(26)	(40)	(41)	(35)	(48)	(62)

**Table 4.13   Breakdown of all consultations with the Camden project
doctor, by presenting problems: 1.1.1987-31.12.1987**

column percentages

	Total	Place of consultation		
		Arlington Drop-in	WLDC	Simon Community
Presenting problem				
Respiratory	13	16	11	15
New	*10*	*10*	*9*	*15*
Repeat	*3*	*6*	*2*	-
Cardiovascular	7	3	10	7
New	*2*	*2*	*2*	*6*
Repeat	*5*	*1*	*8*	*1*
Gastrointestinal	10	8	12	6
New	*6*	*6*	*7*	*4*
Repeat	*4*	*2*	*5*	*2*
Musculoskeletal	11	7	13	15
New	*6*	*5*	*6*	*13*
Repeat	*5*	*2*	*7*	*2*
Dermatology	16	21	13	19
New	*10*	*9*	*9*	*12*
Repeat	*6*	*12*	*4*	*7*
Psychiatry	11	7	13	15
New	*7*	*5*	*3*	*9*
Repeat	*4*	*2*	*10*	*6*
Trauma	7	8	6	12
New	*7*	*8*	*5*	*12*
Repeat	*<1*	-	*<1*	-
Alcohol/drug related	13	14	13	16
New	*13*	*14*	*12*	*16*
Repeat	-	-	*1*	-
Medical certificate	9	7	11	6
New	*9*	*7*	*11*	*6*
Repeat	-	-	-	-
Chiropody/dental	3	2	2	3
New	*3*	*2*	*2*	*3*
Repeat	-	-	-	-
Other medical	17	17	18	9
New	*11*	*11*	*10*	*9*
Repeat	*6*	*6*	*8*	-
General advice	10	11	10	1
New	*10*	*11*	*10*	*1*
Repeat	-	-	-	-
Base: all consultations with project doctor	*(1073)* **	*(379)*	*(625)*	*(69)*

*   The columns add to more than 100 per cent because more than one presenting
problem was possible at each consultation.

**   Excludes 49 repeat consultations for which no presenting problem was specified.

Table 4.14 Breakdown of action taken by Camden project doctor on all project doctor consultations: 1.1.1987-31.12.1987

column percentages

		Place of consultation		
Outcome	Total	Arlington Drop-in	WLDC	Simon Community
Referral to hospital	7	5	9	1
Referral to GP	3	4	2	6
Referral to team member	<1	-	<1	-
Advice only	16	21	14	9
Prescription	60	51	65	67
Nursing/dressing	10	17	5	17
Medical certificate	11	8	13	6
Referral - housing	2	1	3	1
Referral - agency (excl. housing)	9	10	9	7
To come again	12	10	14	15
DK	1	-	1	-
Base: all consultations with project doctors	*(1073)*	*(379)*	*(625)*	*(69)*

*   The columns add to more than 100 per cent because more than one outcome was possible at each consultation.

Table 4.15 Breakdown of all consultations with Camden nurses, by presenting problems: 1.1.1987-31.12.1987

column percentages

Presenting problem	Total	Place of consultation Arlington Drop-in	WLDC	Simon Community
Respiratory	5	5	4	7
New	*4*	*4*	*3*	*7*
Repeat	*1*	*1*	*1*	*-*
Cardiovascular	2	1	2	-
New	*1*	*1*	*1*	*-*
Repeat	*1*	*-*	*1*	*-*
Gastrointestinal	8	8	8	10
New	*6*	*7*	*5*	*7*
Repeat	*2*	*1*	*3*	*3*
Musculoskeletal	6	7	4	17
New	*4*	*5*	*3*	*7*
Repeat	*2*	*2*	*1*	*10*
Dermatology	19	24	13	41
New	*8*	*7*	*9*	*14*
Repeat	*11*	*17*	*4*	*27*
Psychiatry	10	8	12	3
New	*6*	*5*	*6*	*3*
Repeat	*4*	*3*	*6*	*-*
Trauma	17	10	23	14
New	*15*	*9*	*21*	*4*
Repeat	*2*	*1*	*2*	*-*
Alcohol/drug related	9	5	12	7
New	*6*	*5*	*7*	*7*
Repeat	*3*	*-*	*5*	*-*
Medical certificate	2	2	1	-
New	*1*	*2*	*1*	*-*
Repeat	*1*	*-*	*-*	*-*
Chiropody/dental	2	2	5	-
New	*2*	*2*	*5*	*-*
Repeat	*-*	*-*	*-*	*-*
Other medical	16	13	19	21
New	*14*	*9*	*17*	*21*
Repeat	*2*	*4*	*2*	*-*
General advice	19	35	7	7
New	*18*	*34*	*7*	*7*
Repeat	*1*	*1*	*-*	*-*
Base: all consultations with nurses	*(949)*	*(505)*	*(415)*	*(29)*

*   The columns add to more than 100 per cent because more than one presenting problem was possible at each consultation.

Table 4.16   Breakdown of action taken by Camden nurses on all nurse consultations: 1.1.1987-31.12.1987

column percentages

		Place of consultation		
	Total	Arlington Drop-in	WLDC	Simon Community
Outcome				
Referral to hospital	5	2	7	-
Referral to GP	6	9	3	4
Referral to team member	6	11	2	17
Advice only	34	47	24	24
Prescription	22	8	33	21
Nursing/dressing	32	30	33	48
Medical certificate	<1	-	1	-
Referral - housing	1	1	1	-
Referral - agency (excl. housing)	4	2	6	-
To come again	15	10	18	24
DK	1	1	1	-
Base: all consultations with project doctors	*(949)*	*(415)*	*(505)*	*(29)*

*   The columns add to more than 100 per cent because more than one outcome was possible at each consultation.

5 Voice of the Consumer

The previous chapter showed the nature and extent of use of the pilot schemes during the monitoring period and provided a profile of all users of the project teams' services during the year. This chapter looks in more detail at the views of homeless people about primary health care services and how they use them. There are many problems involved in the measurement and use of consumer opinion (see Locker and Dunt, 1978) and one study of particular interest for our population has addressed the difficulties of collecting data from residents of a common lodging house (Shanks, 1981). Although we took into account these problems when collecting and interpreting the data, we were convinced that the story needed to be told from the consumers' point of view and that their perceptions of the pilot schemes were an essential component of the evaluation.

Profile of homeless people interviewed

Sampling and interview procedure

We interviewed 190 users or potential users of the pilot schemes during the monitoring period. This survey was done on a quota sampling basis. Given the type of people with whom we were concerned, it was impossible to find a suitable sampling frame which would have enabled us to select a random sample. (Information about our sampling and interview procedure is contained in Appendix 1.)

100 interviews were carried out in June 1987 and a further 90 were completed in November 1987. This was intended to give us the opportunity of looking at any seasonal variations and to see whether knowledge of the schemes had increased over the period. In June the

89

overall number of interviews was split evenly between the two schemes: fifty from each. In November we interviewed fifty people in Camden, but in City and East London the number was reduced by ten because one of the clinics previously run under the pilot scheme had been closed down.

All interviews took place on the premises of the day centres, night shelters and hostels where the project doctors had established regular clinics. In Camden our 100 interviews were divided equally between the two day centres where clinics were held. In City and East London we interviewed 20 people in each of four centres where clinics were held and 10 in the other centre where the regular clinic was discontinued in June 1987.

We interviewed an equal number of users and non-users of the project teams' services in all the centres because we wanted to see whether there were any noticeable differences in the perceptions, expectations and general patterns of use of primary health care services between those who had used the pilot scheme's services and those who had not. A *user* was taken to mean someone attending the day centre, night shelter or hostel who had used services provided by one or more of the project team members at that centre, or at one of the other centres visited by the project teams. A *non-user* was defined as someone attending the centre but who had not so far used any of the services provided by the pilot scheme.

Although the sites for the interviews and the quota controls were determined in advance, the final selection of people for interview was left to the interviewers, who were carefully briefed about contact and interview procedure. This briefing, however, could not completely prepare them for the culture shock they experienced on their first visit to a centre. A typical initial reaction is vividly captured by one of the interviewers in her notes:

> From the moment of leaving the Tube there seemed to be nothing but shuffling old men in grey overcoats moving slowly towards the crypt. Just total culture shock - so many, it seemed, in such a small area accentuated by the low ceilings. It seemed like stepping back into something medieval.

Surprisingly few people refused to talk to us about their health care but it was often difficult to get them to focus on the questions. Instead of giving specific answers, individuals often related snippets of their life-story to illustrate their views or their experiences of health care. Some of these stories were compelling to listen to but they were time-consuming. This has a bearing on their use of health care services because, if they had difficulty in concentrating on direct questions posed by the interviewer, it is probable that they may have problems in an ordinary GP's surgery where the GP may not have the time or inclination to listen.

The sample

A brief description of those included in the sample provides the context for the ensuing discussion of their views about health care services and how they use them. The overall sample included 171 (90 per cent) men and 19 (10 per cent) women, reflecting the fact that very few women used the centres where the clinics were held.

Age

The age profile of the sample is shown in Table 5.1 (p.124). The ages of those interviewed were widely spread, ranging from 9 per cent of the sample aged under 25 through to 5 per cent who were 65 or over. The 'door policy' of each centre formally determines the lower end of the age range of users and residents. Three of the centres specifically stated they could not accept people under 16 years of age, one centre had a minimum age limit of 18, and another said it preferred not to admit people under 25 (although we interviewed several people at this centre who were below this age limit).

Place of birth

As shown in Table 5.2 (p.124), the majority were born in the United Kingdom or were from the Irish Republic. Of the total sample, 46 per cent were born in England or Wales, 24 per cent were born in Scotland and a further 19 per cent were from the Irish Republic. A breakdown of these figures on a project basis shows a similar pattern for both schemes. The 7 per cent whose place of birth was outside the United Kingdom represented a wide range of countries, including United States of America, Canada, Hong Kong, Germany, Poland, Holland, Nigeria, Brazil and South Africa.

Accommodation

To give some insight into their housing difficulties, respondents were also asked to describe the sort of accommodation, if any, they had stayed in the night before the interview (Table 5.3, p.125).

Of the total sample, 27 per cent said that they had been sleeping rough or skippering and a further 9 per cent were living in a squat. The numbers sleeping rough or skippering were higher in Camden (36 per cent) than in East London (18 per cent). They included people of all ages, including several who were over 65. Some respondents sounded resigned about their condition, like this man in his fifties in East London who said he usually spent the night:

> Under the car park. It's really snug under the railings and there is no one there but me. I pull my rug over me and I'm quite warm.

Others, typified by this man in his forties in East London, were less phlegmatic:

> I was sleeping rough under a flyover... a Catholic sister found me a place with an Irish fellow, otherwise I'd have frozen. I can't believe the weight I've lost. I'd have died in another couple of days.

For one young man in Camden, like many of those sleeping in the locality, home consisted of 'two cardboard boxes and a sleeping bag in Lincoln's Inn Fields'.

Hostels, either short-stay or long-stay, provided a base for 23 per cent of those interviewed and a further 4 per cent were in hotel or bed and breakfast accommodation. The standard of hotel accommodation was generally regarded as low, as summed up in this comment by a male in his sixties in East London:

> It's called a hotel but it's a doss house. There's no cooking facilities. It's so bloody freezing cold in winter. That's why I come to these places [day centres]. As soon as I'm up, I'm out walking.

A further 12 per cent of the sample, again fairly evenly spread across the age range, were staying with friends or relatives.

We were surprised to find that about a quarter of those interviewed said they had their own accommodation, and this figure was similar for both projects. Few of these people were under 35 and most were in the 35-64 age range. Twelve per cent of the sample said they were in a council flat, a further 8 per cent also had a flat but not necessarily a council flat, 4 per cent were staying in a bedsit or lodgings and of the remainder, two people were living in their own houses and one in a caravan. Typically they continued to use day centre facilities because they lacked the emotional, practical or financial support necessary to cope on their own in independent accommodation. They felt lonely and isolated and wanted to spend their time in a warm environment in the company of their friends.

Employment

We asked users or residents whether or not they had a job and, as expected, we found that the majority (88 per cent) were unemployed (Table 5.4, p.125).

Respondents frequently volunteered additional information about their employment history and it was apparent that many had not had a job for years and were not confident about their ability to find employment. This problem was illustrated by one unemployed man in East London who explained, 'I wouldn't know where to begin. I see these people going all over the world - I wouldn't even be able to start packing.'

Contact with relatives

As an indicator of whether they had any kind of support network, we also asked them whether they had any relatives with whom they were in contact (Table 5.5, p.126).

Many were hesitant about answering this question and it evoked particularly strong feelings on the part of those who had no such contact. Just over half of the sample (54 per cent) came into this category and a typical response was that of the man who said emphatically, 'Oh God, no!'. Some explained that they had no relatives, but most had simply become estranged from relatives for a variety of reasons and either did not want to see them again, or felt unable to do so. A particularly sad case was the young man in Camden whose parents refused to have anything to do with him. Reflecting on his own persistence in trying to resume contact with them, he said, 'You can't give up, you must keep trying'. He had been trying for nine years since he was 17 years old. Of the 45 per cent of people interviewed who were in contact with relatives, almost half had seen or spoken to a relative in the previous week, and just over one in ten of them had had some contact during the past month. The relatives most often mentioned were mother and/or father, sister or brother.

Homeless people and primary health care services: how they use them and how they view them

Registration with general medical practitioners

There has been little first-hand evidence from single homeless people themselves on the difficulties they may encounter in registering with a GP, and indeed little evidence on the factors involved. In our interviews we explored these specific issues, as well as more general questions about their experiences of primary health care services.

We asked the people in our sample whether they were registered with a GP in London or elsewhere (Table 5.6, p.126). We did not ask them to distinguish between permanent and temporary registration because our pilot study confirmed the findings of an earlier survey carried out in Manchester (Health Care for Homeless People Team, 1984) that to do so created confusion for respondents. We were also unable to check the validity of this information because of the constraints of confidentiality. Although the figures may not therefore accurately reflect the proportion who were permanently registered with GPs, they do show people's perceptions about whether or not they were registered, and consideration of these perceptions is important to understanding their use of health care services.

We found that 60 per cent of the overall sample thought that they were registered with a doctor, but the proportion registered was markedly lower in Camden (51 per cent) than in East London (70 per cent), reflecting the proportions found to be registered among the client population as a whole (see Chapter 3). We observed considerable variation between the individual centres but, while this was a rich source of case study material, the numbers of people involved were too few to enable further analysis at this level.

Across the different age groups the proportions registered with a GP were very similar, but there were some marked differences when the sample was broken down by place of birth. The proportion of those born in Scotland who said they were registered with a doctor was 67 per cent whereas the equivalent figures were smaller for those born in England and Wales (59 per cent) or the Irish Republic (47 per cent). Perhaps, however, they were registered with a doctor in Scotland, which is not a lot of use when you live in London.

Not surprisingly the level of GP registration was much lower among those sleeping rough, skippering or living in a squat than it was for those who were living in hostels or hotels, or who had their own accommodation (Table 5.7, p.127). Of the 52 people sleeping rough or skippering just over a quarter (14) said they were registered with a doctor but nearly three-quarters (38) were not registered with a GP in London or elsewhere. However, 85 per cent of those in their own accommodation said they were registered with a doctor.

We asked the 114 people who said they were registered who the GP was and where the surgery was located. Sixty-five per cent (74) were able to name the GP with whom they thought they were registered and the most interesting feature of the resulting list was that it contained the names of 61 different doctors. Only one doctor was mentioned more than once. In this case, 14 people claimed to be registered at his practice in East London, and three of them were interviewed at Arlington Drop-in Centre in Camden and not at a centre in East London. Over 80 per cent of those who said they were registered named a doctor in London. We asked the small number who were registered with GPs outside London whether they had tried to get on the list of a doctor near where they were currently staying. None of the 19 people concerned had done so.

We were interested to know whether the 76 (40 per cent) of the people in our sample who said they were not registered had tried to register with a GP within the past year and if so, whether a GP had refused to take them on his list. We found that over 80 per cent of them said they had made no attempt to get themselves registered. Only 13 people had tried to register and of these, 8 said that a GP had refused to take them. Although in three of these cases the GP had apparently claimed that his list was full, the homeless people involved, like this man attending the Arlington Drop-in Centre in Camden, thought they had been refused either because they were of no fixed abode, or because they did not have a medical card:

> Yes well, they reckoned it was full up, like. If you're homeless they don't want to know. If you're homeless they just say go to the emergency ward at the hospital.

But did they want to be registered? Was it important to them? We asked the 76 people who were not registered whether they in fact wanted to be registered with a GP. Thirty-two people said they would like to be registered but were often unsure about what would make it easier for them to do so, or they thought they could not register because they had no fixed address. As one man at West London Day Centre explained, 'Well I'm no fixed abode you see, so I probably couldn't register'. One person had a drug problem and insisted this had prevented him from finding a GP - 'There's not many that aren't scared off tackling a drug problem. I don't know any doctors who would entertain me in this area.'

Few people had firm ideas about how registration could be made easier for them but several respondents thought that a permanent address or a medical record card or some other proof of identity was essential for registration. One person suggested that a more durable medical card would be helpful - 'A plastic card with an identification number would be handy. I don't know my NHS number. I'm always losing pieces of card. A plastic card would be different, it would last longer.' The numbers involved were small, but those unregistered and aged under 35 were keener to be registered with a GP than their older counterparts.

Just over 50 per cent of the people in our sample who were unregistered insisted that they did not want to register with a GP, and most provided a number of reasons why they held this view. Around half of them said they were fit and healthy and could not see the point in registering with a doctor unless and until they were sick. Typical comments were - 'I haven't really got any health problems, touch wood. Otherwise it's irrelevant...' and, 'There's nothing wrong with me. Why do I need to register?' For others their mobility and the uncertainty about where they would be in a week or a month's time was the main reason for not registering - 'You are in one place one time, a month later somewhere else. If you tried to register with a GP each time you would always be changing GPs.'

Several people admitted that they had had bad experiences with GPs, and having been rebuffed, had now given up trying to register. A case in point was the man at Cable Street Day Centre who said apologetically:

> I can't be bothered. I couldn't care less. Next time I want a
> GP they'll put me in a wooden box. Sorry if that's not the
> answer you want.

Some, like this man in Camden, preferred to use hospital casualty departments - 'I'm all right. If I have any problems I go to hospital. There are enough hospitals in London to keep me happy.' But a number of people shared the view of the man at Arlington Drop-in Centre who told us - 'There's no need. I can always see the doctor here if I'm ill.' They saw no point in registering with a local GP when they could more conveniently use the services of the project doctor when he visited the centre. This is an important factor in assessing the impact of the pilot schemes.

A commonly held perception of the health care experiences of the single homeless is that they *do* want to register with GPs, but that they are frequently turned away by doctors when they seek medical care. This reluctance of GPs to take them on has been explained in terms of fears of abuse, disruption and unreliability (Leighton, 1976), hostility from other patients (City and Hackney CHC), excessive workload (DHSS, 1981) and transience (Bone, 1984). The picture that emerged from our survey, however, was not one of homeless people demanding to be registered and being turned away by GPs. Around 17 per cent of those who were unregistered *did* want to be registered, and it is important to consider why a number of those who had tried had been refused. But the clear message that emerged from our interviews was that for many homeless people, as indeed for many housed people, registering with a GP was not seen as a priority. As other recent studies have found (NFA Day Centres, 1987), many single homeless people feel they have no need of medical care and may have low expectations about their health or may be wary of GPs as a result of a previous unhappy experience with primary care (Liverpool CHC). If they are in temporary accommodation, registering with a new GP may also increase their sense of rootlessness by severing their links with another area which they have identified as home (SHIL Sub Group, 1987).

Use of primary health care services

Registration with a GP is one indicator of whether or not the single homeless have access to a GP through the usual channels, but it says little about the quality of care that individuals receive or indeed whether they actually *get* care at the times when they need it. For single homeless people who are not registered with a GP close to where they are staying, the difficulties of obtaining adequate primary health care are likely to be greater. We wanted to get some insight into the way single homeless people use primary health care services so we asked all those in our sample whether they had wanted to see a doctor in the past year: if they had, we talked to them about the last occasion on which they had sought medical care. (Table 5.8, p.127).

Just over two-thirds of all the people interviewed said that at some point during the previous twelve months they had wanted to see a doctor. The proportion was marginally higher among those who had said they were registered with a GP (75 per cent) than among those who were not (62 per cent). Fewer of those aged between 45 and 54 had wanted to see a doctor during this period, but otherwise there was little difference between the age groups in their demand for medical care. Of those who had wanted to see a doctor, 33 per cent had done so during the week before the interview; 48 per cent had done so more than a week but less than six months before the interview; and 18 per cent were referring to events which had occurred more than six months before.

What sorts of health problems had caused them to seek medical attention? In a few cases they gave more than one reason and it proved unrealistic to try to disentangle which was perceived as the main complaint.

Respiratory disorders were clearly the commonest reasons for people seeking medical care and were mentioned by 18 per cent of those who had wanted to see a doctor. These conditions included bronchitis,

TB, colds, flu, sinusitis, coughs and a variety of nose and ear problems. As Table 5.9 (p.128) indicates, other commonly mentioned problems could be grouped under the general diagnostic categories of gastrointestinal, dermatology, trauma, musculoskeletal and psychiatry. Additionally, 11 per cent of those who had sought medical care admitted that their problem had been alcohol related.

Gastrointestinal problems for which people wanted medical attention included a variety of stomach complaints, stomach ulcers, constipation, piles, diarrhoea or vomiting. Dermatological conditions comprised all manner of skin problems, rashes, infestations, septic wounds, leg ulcers, cuts, grazes and eczema. Those people whose reasons for consulting a doctor were classified under trauma had been involved in accidents, falls or fights and had broken bones, fractures or sprains, or had sustained injuries such as a cut lip or bruising. Musculoskeletal problems usually referred to conditions such as arthritis. Those who said that they were suffering from depression or some type of nervous disorder are included in the table under the general heading of psychiatry.

Other people had wanted to see a doctor because they had problems with their feet, eyes or teeth and several said they had just felt 'generally unwell'. We also talked to a number who had wanted drugs, pills or routine injections, or simply a general medical check-up.

The majority of those who had wanted to see a doctor during the past year had managed to get medical care, although this was not necessarily from a GP. Several people had failed to see a doctor, even though they had wanted to, and their attitudes varied considerably. Some were resigned about their situation and, like this man at Cable Street Day Centre, had not even tried to see a doctor when they felt ill - 'I had no medical card, no identification. So I didn't try. They always turn you away.' Others had had similar experiences to this young man in Camden who had sought care from a variety of different sources and was angry and frustrated about being turned away:

> I was in and out of emergency places and they didn't want to know, so I said 'fuck it' and didn't bother. I think the emergency places are the biggest load of crap. If you're drunk they don't want to know you. You can't get a letter. That's why you get all the dossers in the emergency wards.

99

> They've nowhere else to go. You get so fucking frustrated, and they don't understand.

Sources of primary health care

Where do single homeless people go when they want to see a doctor? The 124 people in our sample who had succeeded in finding a doctor had used a number of different sources of care (Table 5.10, p.129). On the *last* occasion that they had wanted to see a doctor 39 per cent had consulted a local GP and in most cases this had been a GP in London. The majority of these people had already said that they were registered with a GP in London or elsewhere. A further 13 per cent had been seen by a hospital doctor, either in out-patients or in an accident and emergency department and a few had attended Great Chapel Street Medical Centre.

Just over a third had chosen to use the doctor who provided a service at the day centre, night shelter or hostel which they attended. This tendency was more marked among those people we interviewed in centres in East London than it was in the two centres in Camden. In most cases the doctor concerned was one of the salaried doctors working for the pilot scheme, but several people in Camden had used the doctor at The Passage, which is another centre for homeless people in Victoria. We also found that just over half of those who had used the project doctor were already registered with a GP. What we do not know is how relevant this registration was to their current circumstances.

The overwhelming majority (over 90 per cent) of those who had succeeded in finding a doctor assured us they had not encountered any difficulties in being seen. Having to queue and to cope with a long wait were the main problems described by the few who said they had encountered difficulties.

We asked people how satisfied they had been with the treatment they had received on their last visit to a doctor. In particular, we wanted to know whether they had felt able to tell the doctor all they wanted to about their health and whether he or she had given them sufficient time to talk about their problems. The level of satisfaction was strikingly high - 83 per cent (103) of those who had seen a doctor in the past year were satisfied or very satisfied with the treatment they had received, but this may have been because their expectations of care were generally low. It also has to be remembered that 35 per cent of these people were talking about their level of satisfaction with the doctor's services provided under the pilot scheme and were not referring to treatment provided by a local GP or an accident and emergency department.

Only a few of those who had seen a doctor in the last year were dissatisfied and in most cases this was because they were unhappy about the type of treatment given (several had been refused pills or drugs) or thought that the treatment had not worked. Some, like this 40-year-old man in West London who had had difficulties with a local GP, also complained about the doctor's attitude towards them and their presenting problem:

> I only asked for a couple of days supply of pills. I lost my temper. He talked to me as if I wasn't there. He was talking down to me, not at me, as if all alcoholics were morons.

Another complaint among those who were dissatisfied with their treatment was that the doctor concerned had been reluctant to examine them. Talking about his experience in the accident and emergency of a London hospital, this man at Cable Street Day Centre explained:

> I couldn't walk or sit down. I waited fifty minutes in bad pain. I tried to explain to the nurse, but the doctor only gave me a few seconds and refused to see me. There was no examination, nothing.

Several had mixed feelings about the treatment they had received or thought they had been given unrealistic advice. One of the older residents we interviewed at Booth House Detoxification Centre gave a bleak picture of the problems confronting the homeless alcoholic who was trying to give up drink. Illustrating the force of peer group pressure he said:

> He told me to keep away from drink - this is difficult. I'm coerced - physically even, you wouldn't believe it - my mates at the Mission, they don't like it if I don't drink. The night before I came here they insisted I had to go out and drink with them. They didn't want me to come in here.

This picture was reinforced by another resident at Booth House who, at the age of 31, seemed to have little to look forward to:

I don't really need medical help, only with this problem. It's worse than AIDS or cancer. It's a terrible thing to have. I was going to be married three years ago and it all went wrong and I started to drink. I've tried to stop. I'd stopped for about a month before this time and here I am at the Salvation Army. We used to joke about them and here I am. If there is a God then that is my only hope. I'll kill myself next time - I tried last week.

While it was clear that many people had felt able to tell the doctor all they wanted to about their health, although in practice this may have been very little, almost 20 per cent insisted that they had experienced difficulties in talking to the doctor about what was troubling them. The doctor was often perceived as being too busy, not interested in them as a temporary patient or only interested in their specific presenting problem. Some, like this man we spoke to at the Detoxification Centre, were anxious that if they did open up about *all* their problems the doctor would be deterred from taking them on - 'I was too shy to talk about it. I thought he wouldn't take me on so I didn't tell him about my problems.' Doctors seemed to have been particularly unsympathetic towards those with alcohol problems, according to our respondents. Another resident at the Detoxification Centre told us - 'He gives me pills and all that, but he's not interested in alcoholism. He thinks it's self-inflicted.'

Our conversations with residents at Booth House revealed the difficulties these men had experienced in getting admitted to a detoxification centre and highlighted the general lack of facilities available for alcoholics who want help in coming off drink. As one resident explained:

I stole something and ended up in court and put on probation. If that hadn't happened I can't see how I would have been admitted. The facilities for alcoholics who want therapy are appalling. If you are a weak personality you will give up.

He continued:

I feel there should be more facilities available to alcoholics who want to stop drinking. And more publicity on the problems caused by drink. A lot is ultimately up to yourself, but if you get into a critical situation you need help.

Residents were appreciative of the help provided by the Salvation Army but some, like this 35-year-old man, found the disciplined routine and environment of the unit difficult to cope with:

It's very hard to get into these places. There aren't enough of them. Too hard to get in. You wait too long. I do believe too that these places are too full of forced religion. That's my personal view. Definitely they take you off the sleeping tablets too quickly, and you're just coming off the drink. At the same time, I do think they're marvellous places. When you're in trouble they're definitely a haven. Alcoholism is an illness. I don't think you should have to say your prayers. It should be treated as an illness. I've seen geezers climbing up the wall here because they've had no tablets.

We wanted to obtain a more comprehensive picture about where single homeless people go when they have a health problem, so in addition to asking them about their *last* visit to a doctor we also asked all those in our sample whether or not they had sought medical care on any other occasion in the past year. Just over a third of the sample had done so and, as Table 5.11 (p.130) shows, they had used a wide range of sources as well as consulting a local GP. We also found that those who had seen a doctor in the past year tended to have used other sources of medical help as well.

Some had been unsuccessful in getting treatment and, like this man at St. Botolph's Crypt, felt they had been turned away because of their appearance and their lack of an address - 'I walked into a surgery in Hammersmith and the GP told me I was a tramp and he didn't want me at his surgery. I was very upset.' Not all had necessarily wanted to see a doctor. A particularly articulate young man with psychiatric problems had strong views about the type of help he needed and felt that this could be provided more effectively by the community psychiatric nursing service:

I find the community psychiatric nursing service is what I need, not a doctor. You don't need to see a doctor but rather a person you can confide in. I see the CPN system as the

103

most supportive you can get. The only problem is that you have to approach them in office hours and you don't get emergency numbers.

We also asked whether or not they had received or asked for help from any other statutory or voluntary agencies during the previous year (Table 5.12, p.131). The majority said they had sought help from other agencies. Some of these, most obviously local DHSS offices and Local Authority Housing Departments, provided specific financial benefits or housing services. But other agencies or projects were mentioned which dealt with alcohol, drugs or mental health problems, for example, the Alcohol Recovery Project and the Compass project. These were seen as alternative sources of help and advice on *health*-related matters. Perhaps this is not surprising since the single homeless in our sample had reported particular difficulties in finding GPs who were sympathetic to these problems.

While many had contacted a number of different agencies during the past year, we should not overlook the fact that 21 per cent of the total sample said that they had used no other agencies. Typically those in this group were either keen to assert their independence or, like this man in his fifties in East London, were resigned to coping alone - 'They're for the youngsters really aren't they? When you get to our age you've learnt you've got to help yourself. It's no good turning to anyone else.'

Use of hospital services
A thorough investigation of the use of secondary (i.e. hospital) care by homeless people was outside our remit. However, we wanted to throw light on the types of difficulties non-registration with a GP creates for homeless people in need of hospital care, and so we asked everyone whether or not they had stayed overnight in hospital during the past five years. We stressed *admission* to hospital because we wanted to exclude one-off visits to hospital accident and emergency departments to obtain primary care.

Admission to hospital

As Table 5.13 (p.131) shows, 55 per cent of the total sample (104) had been admitted to hospital during this period. Around two-thirds of them said they had been treated in London hospitals.

A considerably higher proportion of those who said they were registered with a GP had spent time in hospital compared with those who were not registered: 65 and 41 per cent respectively. When we looked at the age profile, hospital admission had been more common among the younger people in our sample than for those aged over 35.

We asked all those who had been hospitalised to talk to us about the circumstances surrounding the last time they had been admitted. The range of problems which had caused hospitalisation are shown in Table 5.14 (p.132), where it can be seen that the pattern of presenting problems is quite different from that relating to primary care shown in Table 5.9 (p.128).

Some form of trauma was by far the predominant reason for being admitted. This included injuries sustained in accidents or falls and sometimes through fights or assaults. Supporting our observation that Arlington Drop-in Centre in Camden Town was in a notably tough environment, we found that broken bones and fractures, sprains and other accidental injuries were particularly common among people attending this centre, compared with the other centres included in our survey. Some of the circumstances in which trauma had occurred were unusual, like this man in East London who said - 'I fell out of a tree and broke my wrist and damaged my pelvis'. Typically, as with this young man, their injuries were alcohol-related - 'I was drunk at the time and blacked out on the escalator. I woke up in hospital.'

Not surprisingly, a strikingly high proportion of the residents we interviewed at Booth House Detoxification Centre had been hospitalised in the past five years because of alcohol-related problems. As illustrated by this 42-year-old man who was admitted to hospital suffering from alcohol abuse and hypothermia, there is a risk that intolerance towards drunkenness can lead to more serious health problems being overlooked - 'The police didn't know whether to prosecute me for drunkenness or take me to hospital. Luckily they did the latter or I'd have died.'

Among those who had been admitted to hospital because of psychiatric problems there were some particularly disturbing cases where people had found it difficult to get help when they wanted it, like this young man at West London Day Centre - 'I tried to kill myself. I needed a rest. I had lots of problems. It's the only way I can get help. I have to do something drastic to get help.'

We wanted to know how people had been admitted to hospital and, in particular, whether or not their admission had followed a visit to a GP. In 74 per cent of cases a GP had not been involved. This was largely because some of form of trauma was often the reason for being hospitalised and many people, like this 35-year-old man at Cable Street Day Centre, had been picked up off the streets and taken to hospital by ambulance - 'I was knocked down when I'd been much the worse for drink I'm afraid. I was taken to hospital by ambulance.'

In addition to these emergency cases, some people had been taken to hospital by a friend or relative, by a member of staff at the centre or by the police. A very few had just turned up on their own at a hospital and had been admitted on the spot. In about a quarter of cases a GP had been involved before admission and in almost all these cases the person was registered with a GP.

The overwhelming majority (94 per cent) said they had not experienced any difficulties in being admitted to hospital. For many who had been admitted as emergency cases this was not an issue. They often could not remember much about the incident other than waking up in a hospital bed. For a tiny minority, like this young man in East London, getting admitted to hospital had not been easy:

> The London Chest Hospital were annoyed because I hadn't gone through the usual channels. I was spoken to like a moron. They're quite surprised when they find you can communicate. When they see your address they tend to react in a certain way. They don't like people who don't conform to their system.

Discharge arrangements

Half of those who had been admitted to hospital had been discharged in under a week. Bearing in mind that discharge arrangements and after-care can be a problem if the patient has no home to go to and no

106

GP to notify, we asked people where they had gone when they were discharged. We also asked whether anyone had discussed this with them.

As Table 5.15 (p.133) shows, at the time of their *last* admission to hospital, which could have been at any time in the previous five years, 40 per cent (42) of all those concerned had had a home of their own to be discharged to. This was marginally more true for those aged under 35 than for the older people we interviewed. However, the circumstances of many appeared to have deteriorated since then. At the time of our interview with them, over half of these people no longer had a home and were sleeping rough, skippering, squatting or living in hostel or bed and breakfast accommodation.

Twenty-four per cent had had a hostel place or hotel to go to and several had been able to stay with friends or relatives. But as many as 16 per cent had had nowhere to go on discharge from hospital and had gone straight from being an in-patient to living on the streets or skippering. For many in this category the future had looked dismal. There was also an element of black humour among the homeless alcoholics who had been discharged back onto the streets, captured by this 50-year-old man in East London - 'As soon as I came to I discharged myself. All I had on was pyjamas. A taxi-driver took me back. Anywhere, the first off-licence.'

Around two-thirds of those who had been in hospital said that they had not talked to anyone at the hospital about where they would go on discharge. This was not necessarily the fault of hospital staff. Like this man in his late forties who had been an in-patient at the London Hospital, some chose not to discuss their discharge plans - 'I could have gone to speak to someone but I didn't. It was my decision'. If they had discussed the issue of their accommodation on discharge, the majority had talked to a hospital social worker or to a doctor. Not all were happy about the counselling or advice they had received. Some complained about lack of support and understanding, like this man in West London - 'If you're dirty or trampish they don't want to know. Same with the nurses. If you're a dosser they don't even want to talk to you.'

Use and perceptions of the pilot schemes

Knowledge and use of the pilot schemes

To what extent did homeless people know about or use the services provided by the pilot schemes, and how satisfied were they with these services?

As explained earlier, our quota sample was designed to include an equal number of users and non-users of the pilot schemes. Table 5.16 (p.134) looks at the 95 *users* only and shows which services they said they had used. In both places a small number of people had been to see more than one team member.

Take-up of services by users

In East London we found that 76 per cent of users had been to see the doctor currently in post and that 33 per cent had seen his predecessor before he left the project in March 1987. There is some overlap here because a small proportion of them had seen both doctors. Few people interviewed had used the services provided by the other team members and, of those who had, 10 had seen the health authority nurse who worked alongside the project team in Cable Street Day Centre, 3 had sought help from the social worker and one had talked to the alcohol counsellor. In Camden, 74 per cent of users said they had been to see the project doctor, just over a third had seen the project nurse who visited Arlington Drop-in Centre and a slightly higher proportion had used the nurse at West London Day Centre who worked alongside the project doctor. Except for the four people we spoke to at Tower Hamlets Mission who had been to see the nurse at Cable Street, all those who had used the services provided by the pilot schemes had done so at the centres where they were being interviewed.

Awareness of services by non-users

Our general finding was that even among non-users of project services there was a relatively high level of awareness about the facilities available and the people providing them. Just over half the 50 people in our sample in East London who said they had *not* been to see the project doctor were nevertheless aware that his services were available if they wanted to use them. Similarly, roughly half the 77 people in the sample who had not used the health authority nurse, the social worker or the alcohol counsellor said that they knew that these services were available. In Camden just over two-thirds of the 62 people in our sample who had not used the project doctor (but may have seen a project nurse) confirmed that they knew about the doctor's services. A similar proportion of the 61 people in the sample who had not seen a nurse attached to the project (but may have seen the doctor) were aware that the nursing service was available through the centres.

We had thought that the level of awareness about the services might be higher when we interviewed in November because the schemes had been established longer. However, this was not the case. Although the numbers involved are far too small to draw firm conclusions, we found that both in East London and in Camden the proportion of non-users interviewed who did *not* know about the project doctor's services was marginally higher in November than in June. This was also found when they were asked about the services provided by the other team members. This may be more a reflection of the shifting population of potential clients attending the centres than an indication that awareness of project services had somehow declined. If this is the case, it may point to the need for a *continuous* advertising effort on the part of service providers and staff in the centres and other places where potential users congregate.

Services provided by the pilot schemes: the consumers' view

To find out what they thought about the medical service offered and why they used it we asked all those who had been to see one or more of the project doctors to talk to us about the *last* time they had used this service. The ensuing discussion concerns only those 77 people (40 in East London and 37 in Camden) who had been to see the project doctor.

In both areas nearly all those who had used the medical services provided by the pilot scheme had seen the project doctor in the six-month period before the interview, and roughly a third of these had done so in the week before the interview. For 80 per cent of users in centres in East London this was the first time they had seen the project doctor, but in Camden a notably higher proportion had used the service on earlier occasions.

Reasons for using the pilot schemes
We asked people how they had come to know about the project doctor's services. A few had been referred to the doctor by one of the nurses working with or alongside the project team, but the majority had heard about the service simply by being at one of the centres visited by the doctor and mixing with people who had already used it. Often they said they had seen a notice advertising the medical service on a board or door in the centre, or that centre staff had suggested they see the doctor. For one user in East London the presence of a doctor in the centre was unmistakeable - 'You could smell him as soon as you walked through the door'.

The situation for residents at Booth House Detoxification Centre was exceptional. As one resident explained - 'The staff told me about the doctor, but it's automatic if you come in here'. When they arrive at this centre, all residents have to have a routine medical check by a doctor. This will be done either by the project doctor or by another doctor visiting the unit, depending on which day of the week they are admitted.

We also wanted to know why people had gone to see the project doctor at the day centre, night shelter or hostel rather than use any other source of medical care. Was it primarily because they were not with registered with a GP? Generally speaking, we found this not to be the case. Just over two-thirds of the total number of users said that they were registered with a GP and in most cases, their GP was in London. There was, however, a noticeable difference between the two project sites. Perhaps reflecting the more transient population in West London, a much smaller proportion of people who had used the project doctor in Camden said they were registered with a GP compared with those who had been to see the project doctor in East London; the figures were 43 per cent and 78 per cent respectively.

Why had people who were already registered gone to see the project doctor instead of consulting their own GP? For one or two the fact of their registration was irrelevant to their current circumstances. They had moved on and their GP was simply too far away. However, irrespective of registration status, the overwhelming reason given for using the medical service at the centres was its convenience. Typically people who had used the service said that it was 'handy at the time', or that, as they were often in the centre, it was easier to see the doctor there than to look for one elsewhere. They did not have to make an appointment and so long as they were prepared to wait, they would eventually get to see the doctor. This guarantee of being seen was an important incentive to try the pilot scheme for those who had experienced rejection by a local GP or a casualty department. As this man in Camden told us:

> I use the doctor here because I'm on the fucking streets. If you come in here and you see the doctor's coming, you stay. Without collapsing on the street, you're wasting your time going to a casualty department.

In weighing up the impact of the pilot scheme on local GPs, it is noteworthy that one young man in East London said that he had started using the project doctor because he thought his own GP was unhappy about treating him since the pilot project had been set up - ' Dr........ was not open when I wanted him and I heard he was getting funny about seeing us when we had the project doctor'.

Among those in our sample who had been to see the project doctor, respiratory disorders and dermatological conditions were the commonest reasons for seeking help, along with feeling generally unwell or wanting a routine check-up. It was common for those who were already registered with a GP in London only to use the medical service provided at the centres when they had a minor problem. As this young man at Cable Street Day Centre explained - 'I only go to see any other doctor than my own GP if it is trivial. Because the last time I used one I was given penicillin which I'm allergic to.' For more serious complaints they would go to their own doctor.

The reported treatment provided by the project doctors reflected the nature of the presenting problems and differed little between the two projects. In about a third of cases pills or tablets had been prescribed and these included vitamins as well as aspirin and antibiotics. For those with dermatological conditions it was common for the doctor to prescribe skin cream or ointment or a special shampoo. Others had been given liquid medicine, eye drops and, in a couple of cases, asthmatic inhalers. Ten per cent of users said that they had been given a good medical examination and 17 per cent told us that the doctor had given them advice or simply talked to them about their drinking habits, their diet or more generally about caring for their health. In a few cases the patient had been referred to their own GP for further treatment or had been sent to hospital for an X-ray or possibly a blood test.

Satisfaction

In both project sites the overwhelming majority said they were satisfied with the care provided by the project doctor as Table 5.17 (p.135) shows. This high level of satisfaction may well have been a genuine reflection of the quality of the service provided, but we should not overlook the possibility that it also reflected the generally low expectations of those using the service. People we interviewed may also have been reluctant to criticise the facilities or those providing the services for fear that they would lose access to them or that the service might be shut down.

Many, like this man in West London, said that it was the convenience of the service that was attractive - 'You don't need to make an appointment with him. You might have to wait two days to see another doctor. It's no good waiting two days and being half-dead, is it?'

Access to the project doctor was also seen to be relatively simple compared with registering with a local GP. Several people we spoke to, like this man at Arlington Drop-in Centre, would have liked to have been able to register with the project doctor - 'It's a pity I couldn't register with him. It's too much buggering about with other doctors, filling in forms and so on.'

A complaint about local GPs and casualty departments had been that they were rarely willing to give homeless people a thorough check-up. In contrast, about a quarter of the people who had used the project doctor either in Camden or in East London said that what they liked about the service was that the doctor had bothered to give them a thorough medical examination.

The personality and style of the doctors working for the pilot schemes was also an important factor influencing people's use of the schemes. It was often unrealistic to try to disentangle what people felt about the service from their feelings about the project doctor. In contrast to some of the negative comments they had made about local

GPs or doctors in casualty departments, people frequently explained that they liked using the project doctor because they trusted him and felt that he understood their circumstances. This did not mean that the project doctors were necessarily 'soft' on their patients. On the contrary, as this comment by a user in Camden illustrates, caring could involve firmness and straight talking - 'He's a nice bloke. He seems a very caring person. He says "John, you're going to be dead if you don't stop drinking soon".'

Dissatisfaction

Only a very few said that they were dissatisfied with the service they had received or had mixed feelings about it and, on the whole, they had more to say for themselves than those who were satisfied. Their complaints tended to be linked closely to their personal problems and it was those with addiction problems who were most likely to be critical. One young man who described himself as a drug addict and an alcoholic complained vigorously that he had found the project doctor unresponsive to his demands:

> I went in there because I'm a drug addict and alcoholic and he won't refer me to a fucking addiction centre or alcohol clinic. He'll put a bandage on me but he does fuck all else. I don't know how he could improve. That's the sort of doctor he is you know.

Another dissatisfied user thought that because he had admitted that he was an alcoholic, he had not been given the treatment he wanted:

> He could improve by first of all examining people, a physical examination, instead of just listening. Seems to me the first thing he asks is, 'Are you an alcoholic?', and if you say yes, the block is on.

Overt criticism of the structure and operation of the service was rare among users, but several people, like this man at West London Day Centre, suggested a number of changes which they thought would improve the service:

> If you were able to register with him it would be better. If he prescribed drugs more it would be better. People could be

113

informed more. I had been coming here for some time before
I knew about the doctor being here.

Similarly, a user at Arlington Drop-in Centre criticised the lack of
publicity about the scheme and also identified a possible problem
concerning confidentiality of the service:

> There's no advertisement of the service they give, either in
> the Centre or in any of the Camden council journals. Camden
> council does not notify the people who sleep outside enough
> about the service. It should be put in the Arlington House
> Newsletter. The seats in front of the doctor's surgery should
> be brought forward a few feet so no-one can listen to you
> when you are in there. Some of them do, you know. If
> you've got a woman in there, some of them try to listen
> through the door.

For some, like this woman at West London Day Centre, it was the
non-availability of the doctor on certain days that was frustrating - 'The
only real problem is no service on a Friday. You go all the way up the
stairs and no-one is there.' To solve this problem, another user at this
centre suggested - 'It would be good if the doctor came in more often.
We class him as our doctor but we can only see him for a few hours.
Basically you never know when you're going to need him. The centre's
open five days a week. If the doctor could come in five days as well
that would be good.'

Communication with the doctor

We asked users whether or not they had felt able to tell the project doctor
all they wanted to about their health and also whether he had given them
sufficient time to do so. In both schemes we found that most people
had felt able to talk to the doctor about their health problems. Of the
few who had been unable or unwilling to do so, all but one were already
registered with a GP. Like this man at Cable Street, it was not so much
that they found the project doctor unapproachable that stopped them
talking to him, but rather that they preferred to confide in their own GP
- 'I would reserve all the details for my appointed doctor. It's more
efficient, satisfactory for my own doctor to have all the information on
his files.'

Another Cable Street user was worried about the confidentiality of the project service and this had made him reticent about describing his problems - 'I wouldn't tell the doctor here about my health problems because I have a relationship with my own GP. There is no relationship, no trust here. I don't know who he might talk it over with when I come out of the office.' The fact that the doctor was male prevented one young female user from feeling comfortable enough to talk about what was really worrying her - 'I wasn't able to tell him but I'm on penicillin as I had an itch down below. It was too embarrassing.'

While most people felt able to talk to the project doctor about their health, only about half the people who had used this service felt able to discuss problems or difficulties which were not strictly medical. A few, like this young man at Cable Street, said that the temporary nature of the service meant they had not had time to establish a relationship with the doctor - '...because I don't really know the man. He is a sort of circuit doctor. Here one minute, not the next'. This criticism was echoed by another user at Cable Street who told us - 'Travelling doctors haven't got the time to sit down and discuss problems. It's not their fault when they've got fifty outside, mostly alcoholics, and the others are the same problems over and over again.'

Just under a quarter were adamant that it was their decision not to discuss their personal business with the doctor. In contrast, one or two wanted the doctor to inquire more about their general welfare and to take a more active role in sorting out their housing problems, like this man at Providence Row Refuge who suffered from asthma:

People should be allowed to stay here longer than six weeks. Where will I go? I think the doctor should have more authority on when you leave. He should go more into your welfare I think. How can I leave here with nowhere to go with my chest?

And some, like this man at Cable Street, chose not to discuss personal problems with the doctor because they thought their dubious reputation in the day centre circuit was too well known for them to get any help - 'I know I'd get no help. He knows me too well from what he's heard from the others.'

Nursing services

We also sought users' views about the nursing services provided by the pilot schemes. As the East London Project did not formally employ a community nurse the majority of these users were interviewed in Camden. A total of 47 people had either used the project nurse who visited Arlington Drop-in Centre or had seen one of the two nurses who worked alongside the project teams. One of these extra nurses was based at West London Day Centre in Camden and the other worked part-time at Cable Street Day Centre in East London. Once again we asked users to talk about the *last* time they had been to see the nurse.

The majority of people who had used the nurse were self-referrals. As with the project doctor service they had learned about the nursing facilities simply by being at the centres where a nurse was available. At West London Day Centre the pilot scheme had been grafted onto an existing health care facility and people were used to seeing a nurse there, as this man explained: 'There is a notice on her door. I've been coming here for six years so I know about the service'. A couple of people had been referred by the project doctor and in a few cases day centre staff had steered attenders towards the nurse.

Well over two-thirds of the users we spoke to had seen the nurse on several occasions and some described themselves as 'regulars', who popped in to see her for a chat or a laugh and a joke. When we asked them to recall their last visit we found that the most common reasons for seeing the nurse were to get help with a dermatological complaint or respiratory problem or simply to talk to her and perhaps have something explained about their health. Several had gone to the nurse because they had felt generally unwell and one or two had wanted treatment for blisters on their feet or for conditions like athlete's foot.

Just over a quarter of users said the nurse had given them cream, ointment or shampoo. Around 15 per cent had been given plasters or dressings and a similar number said they had been supplied with tablets or some other medicine. We found that simply listening to people's problems and offering advice was an important aspect of the nurses' role. Almost a quarter of users said that the benefit they had received from seeing the nurse was that they had had a 'general chat' and that she had tried to sort out their problems.

Without exception, everybody said they were satisfied with the service they had received from the nurses attached to the pilot scheme. Furthermore, the overwhelming majority also said that if they had a minor complaint they would be happy to see the nurse instead of going to see the doctor. Although several people said they liked the service because of its convenience, the majority of users were keen to talk to us about the personal qualities of the nurses and tell us what wonderful people they were. Typical comments were - 'She treats you like a human being' - and - 'She's an angel in disguise, she's a saint'.

Users often acknowledged that the day centres were difficult places to work in, particularly for women, and this increased their regard for the nurse, as this man at West London Day Centre said - 'She's doing a great job because she works here. You must have something special in you to work here. Something special in the heart.' The nurses were also seen as good listeners and people felt relaxed enough to talk about their problems, as this man at Cable Street said - 'She's got a very nice attitude. You're not frightened to tell her anything. She draws it out of you, medical problems or anything else.' And at Arlington Drop-in Centre the nurse was often respected as a friend as well as a nurse - 'You can take the mickey out of her. She's got to put up with all of this in the centre. I've never seen anyone argue with her. She came with us on a day out. You can see her as a nurse and as one of the lads.' A similar comment was made about the nurse at West London Day Centre:

> The nurse here is good because she goes that bit further than just giving you medical help. She's friendly, she knows everyone by name. You trust people who know you and psychologically you're half way to being cured if you believe she can help you. We could all just queue up down at the medical mission but its just a conveyor belt down there. And another reason is she's got clout. You tend to see the nurse first. She'll tell you if there's something wrong and if you should see the doctor. She can also get on to the hospital and get you in there if you're bad enough, otherwise they just turn you away.

Other team members
We were not able to explore the consumers' view of the services provided in East London by the alcohol counsellor or the social worker because too few people in our sample had used these services. The one man interviewed who had used the alcohol worker was a resident at Providence Row Refuge and had been referred to the project by staff at the Refuge for counselling about an alcohol problem. We spoke to only three people who had referred themselves to the social worker and they had wanted advice about housing. One was put in contact with a housing association, another was referred to the local authority housing department and the third was given help with obtaining furniture. A particularly illuminating comment made by one of these users about the role of the social worker was that he provided the *motivation* needed to try and change things - 'I tend to plan what I need to do but often don't do it. It adds structure to life, making appointments. Without the social worker I might not have gone ahead with the move to Tower House.'

Special or integrated services?
A persistent theme in discussions about improving health care provision for homeless people is whether homeless people need special services or whether the aim should be to integrate them into mainstream GP services. The consumers' voice is rarely heard in this debate, so we asked all the people in our sample whether they would prefer to be registered with a local GP and visit the surgery or to use the special medical services provided at the day centre, night shelter or hostel.

Our general finding, as shown in Table 5.18 (p.135), was that there was no overwhelming preference stated either for special facilities or for integrated services. Almost half the people we spoke to said that they would prefer to be registered with a local GP and visit the surgery when they wanted health care, but a third said they preferred to use the special medical services provided at the centres. We also found that around 12 per cent had no clear idea about which type of service they wanted, and a small proportion wanted access to both types of provision. A few, like this man sleeping rough in West London, showed no interest in using any type of health service provision - 'I'm never ill. All you need is to keep your head warm, eat good food and wear a good pair of shoes. With that, you don't need doctors.'

We found that three-quarters of those who said they would prefer to be registered with a GP and use the surgery were *already* registered with a GP. This did not necessarily mean that they did not value the services provided by the pilot scheme. Just under half of them had also used the services provided by one or more team members. Young people under 35 at the centres tended to prefer to use mainstream GP services. Those who said they would rather use the special medical services provided at the centres were fairly evenly spread across the age groups. Two-thirds were not registered with a GP, and a similar proportion, but not necessarily the same people, had used one or more of the services provided by the pilot scheme.

There were some notable differences between the two schemes. A larger proportion of people interviewed in East London said they would prefer to be registered with a local GP. This may have reflected a number of interrelated factors: that the population was less transient, that GPs in East London were more willing to take on homeless people and that people felt more able to find a local GP. Indeed, as we have seen, 70 per cent of people we spoke to in East London centres were already registered with a GP compared to only 51 per cent of those we interviewed in Camden.

The proportion of people preferring to use the special medical services provided at the centres was higher in Camden than in East London, but this difference was largely accounted for by the preferences of those attending West London Day Centre, rather than by users of Arlington Drop-in Centre. A health care service had been available at West London Day Centre for a number of years and people had become used to the convenience and familiarity of seeing the doctor or nurse at the centre, rather than seeking care elsewhere.

We asked people to tell us their reasons for their preferences or why, in some cases, they wanted access to both types of service. Those who said they would prefer to register with a local GP talked a lot about the advantages of continuity of care, particularly the fact that their GP would know their past medical history. As this woman at Providence Row Refuge told us - 'They've got all my information about my tablets and things and I don't need to explain'. They also thought that it would be easier to form a relationship over time with a local GP than with the visiting project doctor who was not at the centre every day. One young

119

man in East London who was registered with a GP, but had also used the pilot scheme, explained:

> I would prefer registration with a local GP because here there is no back-up. The prescription is written before you get in there. He sees so many people. There is no time to relay with your own GP for your history. The diagnosis is there and then. There is no time to build up a relationship. Its like a conveyor belt.

Those who had been refused pills or tablets by the project doctor seemed to think that a GP would be more likely to give them the treatment they wanted, as this young man in West London explained, - 'It would be easier with a GP. I could get "downers" from a GP. The doctor here doesn't give you tablets. I've heard that he doesn't prescribe tablets.' A similar complaint was made by an 18-year-old male in East London who had used a local GP as well as the project doctor and decided that the GP was better because 'he gives me pills for my headache that work'. He admitted that he had in the past been admitted to hospital after taking an overdose of tablets. And it was because he thought that a GP would be more likely than the project doctor to give him drugs that another man in West London said he would like access to both special and GP services:

> Because you see the project doctor is a good doctor but he won't give me any valium to steady my nerves if I try to come off the drink. He won't give me any heavy drugs. He doesn't trust me. He thinks I'm going to drink on top of them. I've got to go to Dr....... to get the drugs what bring me off the drink.

Another perceived attraction of being registered with a local GP was that he would be available at times when the project doctor was not. One non-user at Providence Row Refuge commented - 'You can see a GP any time. The doctor isn't here very often.' Similarly, a user of the pilot scheme in West London who was sleeping rough observed - 'Well, if I was bad I'd register with a GP because the project doctor wouldn't be able to come out in the middle of the night. That's the only reason I'd register.' The 'round the clock' availability of a GP gave some people a feeling of security, as this man in West London Day

Centre said - 'I suppose I would have a sense of security knowing there is a doctor I can go to at any time of the day or who would come to me if necessary.'

Some people who were already registered with a GP felt it would be unfair of them to use the pilot scheme. Like this man at Cable Street, they saw the scheme as necessary only for those who did not have a doctor - 'I'm registered with a local GP. Its only fair to make arrangements to see him, rather than burden someone else.' In any case they were also unsure whether they would allowed to use the scheme, as this man at Arlington Drop-in Centre explained:

Well if I didn't have my own doctor I'd have to use this address. It's a nice thing that there is something like this for people coming down to London. I'm only a few hundred yards from my own GP and I know him. I don't know whether I'd be accepted here. I wouldn't tell the doctor here I had a GP of my own. He'd say I should go to my own GP. I'd have to use a false name if I saw the doctor here. I suppose if I had a little accident I would pop in to him or see the nurse if I had a cut or something, but if I thought I had anything serious like blood pressure I'd go to my own GP.

There was also a tendency to think that a local GP would have wider skills or better facilities at his surgery than was possible within the day centres, night shelters or hostels. Several people we spoke to were registered with GPs based in health centres and, like this man in West London, were appreciative of the other facilities that these centres could offer - 'I've only been with the new doctor six weeks. But there is also a counselling service at the health centre which I find helpful. I have confidence in the centre so far. You would need to ask me again in two years' time.'

Among the third of the sample who preferred to use the special medical services provided at the centres rather than register with a GP, two-thirds had actually used the project doctor's services. The main arguments in favour were that the special service was quick and convenient and that the service was better because the project doctor was more interested than an ordinary GP. Typical comments were -

'It's easier, you don't have to queue up. It's pretty quick' - and 'It's handy, no other reason. It's on the doorstep.'

For some, it was simply an extension of their day centre routine - 'You can just take your cup of tea and sit near the door'. This factor was particularly important for those, like this man at Arlington Drop-in Centre, who felt desperately uncomfortable about sitting in a GP's surgery - 'The doctor's surgery in ...... Street is very small and crowded with people. It's very claustrophobic and I dread the idea of sitting there waiting on my turn.' And as a user in East London commented - 'These services are specially for people like us, aren't they?'

Alternative sources of medical care

If the services provided by the pilot schemes were withdrawn where would those currently using the schemes obtain health care? To get some idea of the answer to this question, in November we asked homeless people who had used the project doctor where they would have obtained medical care if this service had not been available. About a third said they would have tried a casualty department or gone to their own GP. The rest were less confident about finding alternative sources of care or showed a disturbingly low level of concern about taking care of their health. As with this man in Camden, finding accommodation was frequently a greater priority than finding a GP - 'My only problem is finding accommodation. Anything else would have to come after that. I keep telling myself that if I became ill I would go to the police and hope they could tell me where to go. I tend to sleep near police stations.'

It was obvious that many of those using the pilot scheme would simply not bother to seek medical care if the service was shut down. This man at Arlington Drop-in Centre had had experiences with the NHS which had alienated him from the system - 'I'd probably not have bothered, just let the eye heal up by itself. To tell you the truth, I wouldn't have wanted to use other doctors after some of the experiences I've had.'

Some of the more capable and articulate people we spoke to, like this man at Arlington Drop-in Centre, thought they would be able to find a GP if they had to, but they were less optimistic about some of their colleagues - 'If I got really bad with drink then it'd be up to me to go and find a GP. But there are some here who can't read or write. They wouldn't know what to do.'

Perhaps, as our survey suggests, more homeless people could be encouraged to make better use of GP services and perhaps these services could be made more flexible to accommodate the needs of homeless people. But is there nonetheless a case for special provision of services for the minority who for one reason or another cannot or will not negotiate the system? We leave the last word to another regular at Arlington Drop-in Centre who made a plea for - '...more centres like this for people who won't go to hospital or to doctors at all. If they didn't have the doctor and nurse here they would just rot'.

Table 5.1   Age profile of homeless people Interviewed

column percentages

| | Total | Project | | City and East Centres | | | | | Camden Centres | |
		City & East	Camden	Cable Street	St Botolphs	Prov. Row	T.H. Mission	Booth House	Arlington Drop-In	WLDC
Age										
Under 25	9	10	9	10	10	25	-	-	10	8
25-34	21	20	21	10	20	25	10	30	22	20
35-44	31	33	28	30	30	20	40	50	30	26
45-54	21	14	27	20	10	10	20	15	32	22
55-64	14	16	12	20	20	15	20	5	8	16
65 & over	5	3	7	5	5	-	10	-	-	14
DK/refused	3	6	-	10	10	5	-	-	-	-
Base: all	*(190)*	*(190)*	*(100)*	*(20)*	*(20)*	*(20)*	*(10)*	*(20)*	*(50)*	*(50)*

Table 5.2   Place of birth of homeless people Interviewed

column percentages

| | Total | Project | | City and East Centres | | | | | Camden Centres | |
		City & East	Camden	Cable Street	St Botolphs	Prov. Row	T.H. Mission	Booth House	Arlington Drop-In	WLDC
Birthplace										
England & Wales	46	46	47	50	55	30	60	40	30	64
Scotland	24	22	26	25	20	15	20	30	36	16
N. Ireland	3	4	2	5	5	10	-	-	2	2
Irish Republic	19	19	19	10	10	25	20	30	24	14
Outside UK	7	8	6	10	10	15	-	-	8	4
DK/refused	1	1	-	-	-	5	-	-	-	-
Base: all	*(190)*	*(90)*	*(100)*	*(20)*	*(20)*	*(20)*	*(10)*	*(20)*	*(50)*	*(50)*

Table 5.3   Accommodation details of homeless people interviewed

column percentages

	Total	Project		City and East Centres					Camden Centres	
		City & East	Camden	Cable Street	St Botolphs	Prov. Row	T.H. Mission	Booth House	Arlington Drop-In	WLDC
Accommodation										
Sleeping rough/ skipper	27	18	36	20	25	5	10	25	26	46
Squat	5	2	7	5	5	-	-	-	10	4
Hostel/night shelter	2	-	4	-	-	-	-	-	8	-
Hostel, short-stay	14	29	1	15	15	95	-	5	-	2
Hostel, long-stay	9	13	6	15	15	-	20	20	4	8
Hotel/B&B	4	2	6	-	5	-	-	5	4	8
Own	25	24	25	25	20	-	60	35	30	20
Other	12	9	15	20	5	-	10	10	18	12
Base: all	*(190)*	*(90)*	*(100)*	*(20)*	*(20)*	*(20)*	*(10)*	*(20)*	*(50)*	*(50)*

Table 5.4   Employment details of homeless people interviewed

column percentages

	Total	Project		City and East Centres					Camden Centres	
		City & East	Camden	Cable Street	St Botolphs	Prov. Row	T.H. Mission	Booth House	Arlington Drop-In	WLDC
Employed	6	6	6	-	5	15	-	5	10	2
Unemployed	88	89	87	95	80	85	90	95	88	86
Retired	5	3	7	5	5	-	10	-	2	12
DK	1	2	-	-	10	-	-	-	-	-
Base: all	*(190)*	*(90)*	*(100)*	*(20)*	*(20)*	*(20)*	*(10)*	*(20)*	*(50)*	*(50)*

Table 5.5   Proportion of homeless people who were in contact with relatives

column percentages

		Project		City and East Centres				Camden Centres		
	Total	City & East	Camden	Cable Street	St Botolphs	Prov. Row	T.H. Mission	Booth House	Arlington Drop-In	WLDC
Contact with relatives?										
Yes	45	50	41	30	35	60	40	80	52	30
No	54	48	59	70	55	40	60	20	48	70
Refused	1	2	-	-	10	-	-	-	-	-
Base: all	*(190)*	*(90)*	*(100)*	*(20)*	*(20)*	*(20)*	*(10)*	*(20)*	*(50)*	*(50)*

Table 5.6   Proportion of homeless people registered with GPs

column percentages

		Project		City and East Centres				Camden Centres		
	Total	City & East	Camden	Cable Street	St Botolphs	Prov. Row	T.H. Mission	Booth House	Arlington Drop-In	WLDC
Registered with GP in London or elsewhere?										
Yes	60	70	51	60	55	75	70	90	62	40
No	40	30	49	40	45	25	30	10	38	60
Base: all	*(190)*	*(90)*	*(100)*	*(20)*	*(20)*	*(20)*	*(10)*	*(20)*	*(50)*	*(50)*

Table 5.7 Proportion of homeless people registered wth a GP broken down by accommodation details

column percentages

		Accommodation status							
	Total	Rough/ Skipper	Squat	Hostel/ Night Shelter	SS Hotel	LS Hostel	Hotel B&B	Own	Other
Registered with GP in London or elsewhere?									
Yes	60	27	33	75	70	72	50	85	70
No	40	73	67	25	30	28	50	15	30
Base: all	*(190)*	*(52)*	*(9)*	*(4)*	*(27)*	*(18)*	*(8)*	*(47)*	*(23)*

Table 5.8 Proportion of homeless people who had wanted to see a doctor in the past year

column percentages

		Project		City and East Centres				Camden Centres		
	Total	City & East	Camden	Cable Street	St Botolphs	Prov. Row	T.H. Mission	Booth House	Arlington Drop-In	WLDC
Had wanted to see a doctor	69	68	71	55	70	70	50	85	80	62
Had not wanted to see a doctor	31	32	29	45	30	30	50	15	20	38
Base: all	*(190)*	*(90)*	*(100)*	*(20)*	*(20)*	*(20)*	*(10)*	*(20)*	*(50)*	*(50)*

Table 5.9 Main problems causing homeless people to seek primary care

column percentages*

Problem	Total	Project		City and East Centres				Camden Centres		
		City & East	Camden	Cable Street	St Botolphs	Prov. Row	T.H. Mission	Booth House	Arlington Drop-In	WLDC
Respiratory	18	21	15	36	14	14	40	18	15	16
Cardiovascular	4	3	4	-	7	-	20	-	5	3
Gastrointestinal	9	11	7	18	7	14	-	12	5	10
Musculoskeletal	7	3	10	9	-	7	-	-	13	6
Dermatology	8	11	6	9	21	7	-	12	8	3
Psychiatry	8	11	4	9	-	21	-	18	5	3
Trauma	8	2	14	-	7	-	-	-	13	16
Alcohol related	11	11	10	9	-	-	20	29	10	10
Chiropody	3	7	-	-	21	-	20	-	-	-
Dental	2	2	1	-	7	-	-	-	-	3
Eyes	2	-	3	-	-	-	-	-	3	3
Generally unwell	5	5	4	18	-	7	-	-	5	3
Med. certificate	3	5	1	-	-	14	20	-	3	-
Drugs, pills	8	8	7	-	7	21	-	6	8	6
Check-up	5	10	1	9	7	7	-	18	-	3
Other	10	7	13	18	-	7	20	-	10	16
DK	3	-	4	-	-	-	-	-	3	6
Base: all needing a dr in past year	*(132)*	*(61)*	*(71)*	*(11)*	*(14)*	*(14)*	*(5)*	*(17)*	*(40)*	*(31)*

*   As respondents may have presented with more than one problem columns will not add up to 100 per cent.

Table 5.10 Sources of primary care used by people who had seen a doctor in the past year

column percentages

	Total	Project City & East	Camden
Source of care			
Doctor visiting project centre	35	42	28
Local GP - London or elsewhere	39	40	37
Doctor in A&E dept or hospital outpatients dept	13	9	16
Gt Chapel Street Medical Centre	2	2	3
Doctor in another centre for homeless	4	4	4
Prison doctor	1	-	1
Other	2	-	3
DK	5	4	6
Base: all who had seen a doctor	*(124)*	*(57)*	*(67)*

Table 5.11   Range of primary health care services used by homeless people in the past year

*column percentages**

	Total	Project City & East	Camden
Source of care			
Local GP London or elsewhere	10	14	6
Salaried dr working for pilot scheme	5	2	7
Gt Chapel St Medical Centre	1	-	1
Hospital A&E or outpatients	14	9	18
Psychiatric hospital	3	3	2
Alcohol agency	2	2	1
Dr at other centre for homeless	1	1	1
Mobile X-ray unit	1	-	1
Prison dr	1	1	-
Other	3	2	3
No other source of care used	65	61	56
Base: all	*(190)*	*(90)*	*(100)*

*   As respondents may have mentioned more than one service columns will not
add up to 100 per cent

130

Table 5.12   Other agencies contacted for help or advice

*column percentages**

		Project		City and East Centres					Camden Centres	
	Total	City & East	Camden	Cable Street	St Botolphs	Prov. Row	T.H. Mission	Booth House	Arlington Drop-In	WLDC
Social workers	26	30	23	50	15	35	30	20	24	22
Local DHSS offices	63	68	59	45	85	80	50	70	50	68
LA housing dept	20	22	18	15	30	20	20	25	16	20
Housing advice	14	11	16	20	10	10	10	5	16	16
Alcohol advice	11	13	8	5	-	5	-	50	8	8
Mental health advice	4	3	5	5	-	5	-	5	10	-
Drugs advice	4	2	5	-	-	5	-	5	8	2
Church	2	-	4	-	-	-	-	-	2	6
Other agency	3	2	4	5	-	-	-	5	2	6
Not sought help from any agency	21	18	24	30	10	15	30	10	34	14
Base: all	*(190)*	*(90)*	*(100)*	*(20)*	*(20)*	*(20)*	*(10)*	*(20)*	*(50)*	*(50)*

*   As respondents may have mentioned more than one agency columns will not add up to 100 per cent

Table 5.13   Proportion who had stayed overnight in hospital during the past five years

column percentages

		Project		City and East Centres					Camden Centres	
	Total	City & East	Camden	Cable Street	St Botolphs	Prov. Row	T.H. Mission	Booth House	Arlington Drop-In	WLDC
Yes	55	57	53	60	40	55	40	80	64	42
No	45	43	47	40	60	45	60	20	36	58
Base: all	*(190)*	*(90)*	*(100)*	*(20)*	*(20)*	*(20)*	*(10)*	*(20)*	*(50)*	*(50)*

Table 5.14   Main problem causing homeless people to be admitted to hospital

*column percentages**

		Project		City and East Centres				Camden Centres		
	Total	City & East	Camden	Cable Street	St Botolphs	Prov. Row	T.H. Mission	Booth House	Arlington Drop-In	WLDC
Problem										
Respiratory	5	-	9	-	-	-	-	-	6	14
Cardiovascular	1	2	-	-	13	-	-	-	-	-
Gastrointestinal	7	6	8	8	13	9	-	-	6	10
Musculoskeletal	-	-	-	-	-	-	-	-	-	-
Dermatology	3	2	4	-	13	-	-	-	-	10
Psychiatry	11	16	6	8	13	36	-	13	3	10
Trauma	43	39	47	58	25	27	50	38	63	24
Alcohol related	17	25	9	-	13	18	-	63	6	14
Drug related	7	8	6	-	-	36	-	-	9	-
Gynaecology	5	6	4	8	-	18	-	-	3	5
Generally unwell	3	4	2	8	-	-	25	-	-	5
Other	12	12	11	8	25	-	25	13	9	14
Base: all who had been admitted to hospital in past 5 years	(104)	(51)	(53)	(12)	(8)	(11)	(4)	(16)	(32)	(21)

*   As respondents may have mentioned more than one problem columns will
     not add up to 100 per cent

Table 5.15   Accommodation on discharge from hospital

column percentages

	Total	Project City & East	Project Camden
Accommodation on discharge			
Home	40	37	43
Hostel	20	29	11
NFA/Streets	13	6	21
Hotel/B&B	4	4	4
Friends/relatives	9	8	9
Skip	3	6	-
Squat	1	-	2
Other	9	8	9
DK	1	2	-
Base: all who had been admitted to hospital in past 5 years	*(104)*	*(51)*	*(53)*

Table 5.16   Use of services provided by the pilot scheme

column percentages*

	Project	
	City & East	Camden
Project services		
City & East:		
Project doctor (1)	33	
Project doctor (2)	76	
Nurse (not team member)	22	
Alcohol counsellor	2	
Social worker	7	
Camden:		
Project doctor		74
Nurse		36
Nurse (not team member)		38
Base: all who had used one or more of the services provided by pilot schemes	*(45)*	*(50)*

*   As users may have seen more than one team member columns will not total 100 per cent

Table 5.17 Satisfaction with the medical service provided by pilot scheme

column percentages

		Project	
	Total	City & East	Camden
Very satisfied	35	35	35
Satisfied	49	50	49
DK/mixed feelings	6	8	5
Dissatisfied	5	8	3
Very dissatisfied	4	-	8
Base: all who had seen a project doctor	*(77)*	*(40)*	*(37)*

Table 5.18 Preference for special or integrated services

column percentages

		Project		City and East Centres				Camden Centres		
	Total	City & East	Camden	Cable Street	St Botolphs	Prov. Row	T.H. Mission	Booth House	Arlington Drop-In	WLDC
Preferred service										
Integrated: Register with local GP and use surgery	49	53	46	55	60	55	40	50	50	42
Special: Pilot schemes	31	22	38	10	30	25	30	20	30	46
Both special and integrated services	4	6	3	15	-	-	20	-	6	-
Neither special nor integrated	4	6	3	5	10	10	-	-	6	-
DK	12	13	10	15	-	10	10	30	8	12
Base: all	*(190)*	*(90)*	*(100)*	*(20)*	*(20)*	*(20)*	*(10)*	*(20)*	*(50)*	*(50)*

6 Views of the Providers

What did the service providers involved in the pilot schemes think about the current provision of primary health care for homeless people in their locality and what was their assessment of the impact of the schemes? Did they think that some form of special and separate provision for homeless people should continue after the initial funding for the projects expired in March 1989? In this chapter we explore these and related issues from the viewpoints of the team members working on the two projects and the chairmen and administrators of the Family Practitioner Committees responsible for managing them.

Team members

Current provision of primary health care for homeless people

There was a consensus among team members in both areas that for a variety of reasons homeless people had difficulty obtaining primary health care. From their experience, it seemed that the problem lay both with service providers and with homeless people themselves. With few exceptions local GPs were thought to be reluctant to take on patients who were homeless. One team member argued that the right of GPs to refuse to register people was 'far too strong a privilege' and worked against the access of client groups, like the homeless, to medical care because they were thought to be difficult and time-consuming patients. Team members had also found that among the homeless population health expectations were generally low and registering with a GP was often not a priority.

It was thought that the system within the National Health Service was not flexible enough and that mainstream services were not geared to meeting the needs of the homeless. We were told that the problem was not simply one of access to these services, although this was a very real obstacle. There was also the key issue of 'narrow thinking' among policy makers and service planners. In particular, one team member was critical of 'the presumption that homeless people will fit into an appointment system like anyone else and be able to feed and clean themselves like anyone else'. Team members were keen to dismiss the stereotypical image of the vagrant, and insisted that by no means all the homeless were dirty and smelly. Nevertheless, they were aware that those sleeping on the streets did have difficulty in keeping themselves clean. As a consequence, this section of the homeless population found it very difficult to walk into a GP's surgery because of the stigma attached to their appearance and the likely reaction of other patients in the waiting room.

At the beginning of the monitoring period we asked team members whether they thought that homeless people in their locality needed special and separate provision of primary health care services. The majority view was that integration was the ideal goal and that special services carried the risk of segregating homeless people further from the rest of society. However, given their views on the inflexibility of current provision, they were unsure about how realistic this aim was in the short term. We were reminded that the homeless population was not an homogeneous group and that some sections would be more easily integrated than others. In particular, it was generally felt that people living in hostels for any length of time should be registered with local GPs, whereas the unsettled lifestyle of those on the streets made registration more problematic. Most agreed that there would always be some in this client group who for one reason or another could not or would not use mainstream services.

There was a consensus view that if more homeless people were to use ordinary GP services there was a great deal of educative and promotional work to be done, both with GPs and with the homeless. Homeless people had to be motivated to look after their health and convinced of the value of registering with a GP. However, there would be no point in raising their expectations unless GPs were willing to take them on. Consequently, work had to be done to educate GPs about the needs of homeless people and to rid them of their images about homelessness. If GPs were to take on a greater proportion of homeless people, they would also need adequate support and back-up from ancillary services.

Assessment of the pilot schemes

What did team members think were the objectives of the pilot scheme they were involved with and did these objectives deal with the problem as they saw it?

In both areas the aims of each pilot scheme were interpreted very broadly, and objectives for the project as a whole were overlaid with personal objectives. Two objectives were thought to be central: to provide a better and co-ordinated primary care service for homeless people in the short term; and in the longer term, to assist the integration of homeless people into mainstream services. Individual team members placed different levels of emphasis and expectation on these two objectives.

They also identified a number of other objectives according to their own perceptions of the scheme and their particular areas of interest. These included:

- highlighting the problem of homelessness and health care;
- finding out more about the needs of this client group in order to be able to match services more appropriately to these needs;
- establishing links with local health care providers and helping them to overcome their prejudices about homeless people;
- highlighting the need for training day centre and hostel staff about how to deal with the health care needs of their clients;
- letting homeless people know about and develop confidence in their rights of access to primary health care.

Not all team members shared all these views. Individuals' objectives also shifted over time as they became more familiar with their work and became more realistic, and in some cases more pessimistic, about what they could achieve in the lifetime of the project.

We thought it important to find out what the team members thought were the strengths and weaknesses of the schemes. We wanted to know their views on the management and structure of the schemes, as well as the approach to service delivery.

Strengths of the pilot scheme

In East London individual team members emphasised a number of positive factors about the team as a whole and the way it worked:

- team members were committed to the needs of this client group;
- they went out to meet homeless people in their own environment instead of expecting homeless people to come to them;
- the team was multidisciplinary and looked at people's social and emotional needs as well as their physical ailments;
- their approach was flexible, in that they responded to the needs of clients and day centre staff.

The project was considered important for many reasons, but three particular aspects were highlighted:

- it provided a service for a client group who were not well served by mainstream services;
- it had good links with and offered support and training to local voluntary agencies, particularly those centres participating in the scheme;
- the existence of the project drew the attention of statutory and voluntary agencies to the problem of homelessness and health care.

In Camden, team members thought that the major strengths of the project lay both in its service element and in the fact that it raised the profile of the health care needs of homeless people. They believed it was important that the project had been set up specifically to provide homeless people with a decent standard of service by people who treated them with respect, and had not been established as a 'hole in the corner service'. They were able to establish trust with people who used their clinics and could act as their advocate in relation to mainstream services.

Generally speaking, they thought that their client group was a very appreciative one and that staff in the centres were very glad to have their services available. They had helped some individuals who otherwise would not have received health care. Having a salaried GP with funding from the DHSS, instead of an independent contractor, was considered an advantage in one important respect: the project doctor had not been subject to the incentive to see as many patients as possible in order to increase his income.

Camden team members emphasised the importance of their project in two further respects:

- they were collecting data about the health care needs and experiences of homeless people which would be more reliable than the anecdotal information which was currently available;
- they gave homeless people another voice, which was linked into local statutory authorities and ultimately the DHSS.

Weaknesses of the pilot scheme

Many of the weaknesses described by members of both project teams were traced back to the structure, organisation and management of the projects. In particular, there was concern about what they thought to be a lack of support and direction both centrally from the DHSS, and from the joint Steering Group. They were aware that, as a result of several changes of staff at the Department, responsibility for the project had changed hands, but they said that poor communication had meant that they did not always know who had taken over. At times they had felt that there was no-one who had an interest in their problems or their future. They also felt that the Steering Group had had little management input.

The most common criticism about the management of each project was that there was in fact no real management structure. Most team members thought that the fact that they were employed by different authorities had proved to be a major weakness. In East London it was suggested that had there been a common employer this might well have alleviated to some degree the effects of having to function at various stages with fewer members than their assigned complement. It would also have made line management clearer and given staff a better understanding of their accountability, to each other and to the employing authority.

In some respects, changes in the membership of the team were also thought to have been detrimental. In particular, the delay in replacing the community psychiatric nurse in East London was identified as a major problem which had affected both the way the team worked and the services they could provide. The change of project doctor in April 1987 had also created a temporary hiatus and had upset some of the people using the service because they did not understand why the doctor they knew was leaving, and they had felt rejected.

Team members identified a number of crucial weaknesses in the infrastructure of the projects. It was generally considered that insufficient thought had been given to how the teams would operate and where they would get their supplies. These problems were thought to have been heightened by the fact that several authorities were involved and that they had been poor at communicating and collaborating with each other. The first project doctor in East London described how he had to 'box and cox' for supplies and explained that this had been unnecessarily time-consuming. He felt that the quality of service had been limited by bureaucratic problems and by the poor facilities available in some of the centres. Similar problems were also experienced in Camden although their overriding problem was finding sites in which to hold clinics. There was also criticism that the projects had not been publicised enough and that, as a result, they were not sufficiently well known among local health care providers.

Another cluster of weaknesses concerned team members' working environment. All the team members in both areas had experienced professional isolation and lack of professional support. In some respects, it seemed that there were parallels here between team members and the homeless people they served. Just as homeless people tended to be marginalised by society, team members were isolated from the community of their peers. One team member in East London observed that he was considered 'an anomaly' by his employing authority which showed a distinct reluctance about taking any managerial responsibility for him in terms of supervising his work. In Camden the team also complained about geographical isolation: they felt isolated from other FPC and DHA staff.

In addition to lack of peer support, the project doctors were also worried about the atrophy of their general clinical skills because they saw a skewed population compared to that seen in general practice; hence the fact that they each took on at least one session a week in ordinary general practice. The fact that they had no financial means to operate independently from their respective FPCs was a general source of frustration for some team members. Their finances were wholly managed through the FPC and one team member in East London commented that, while it might seem trivial to an outsider, the fact that his team did not even have their own petty cash float was a continual irritation.

A more fundamental weakness associated by team members with both projects was that they were not part of mainstream primary health care as it existed in Tower Hamlets or Camden. The teams were concerned that they were an imposed group and that their presence could undermine the uptake of local services by homeless people for two main reasons: first, as they had already pointed out, it was possible that clients who had established a relationship with them would then be reluctant to register with local GPs; second, there was the risk that in both localities the projects would become known as the 'service for the homeless' and other professionals would off-load on to them their general responsibility for homeless people.

Success of the pilot schemes
How successful did team members think the projects had been and what were their criteria for measuring success? In East London, team members tended to assess the impact of the project on two sets of consumers: (i) the homeless people using the day centres, night shelters and hostels; (ii) the centre staff.

So far as homeless people were concerned, they judged the project to have been successful in that it provided a good standard of care to people who normally had difficulty in obtaining health care. They were able to cite numerous cases where users had received prompt attention to their problems when otherwise they might have had to comb the streets for help. It was also thought that by providing a service which homeless people found acceptable and easily accessible they had contributed to raising individuals' expectations of health care and their rights in this respect.

However, they found it difficult to go beyond this and comment on the extent to which the project had improved the health status of individuals. As the doctor pointed out, outcomes were notoriously hard to measure in general practice. He had all the difficulties of ordinary GPs, and in addition had to contend with the fact that the client group was not a stable population. In particular it was very difficult to measure outcomes concerning morbidity because the clientts he saw at the centres often did not know their medical history and he rarely had access to their notes.

Team members in East London believed that they had been a useful resource which centre staff could call on when they needed training and support. They thought that indirectly this must have improved the services that the centres could offer clients. They also thought that the project had acted as a catalyst in bringing some of the centres closer together; for example, it was suggested that their involvement at the Salvation Army Detoxification Unit had resulted in its having better contact with other local agencies.

In Camden there were differences of opinion about how successful the project had been. One team member itemised a number of positive outcomes and these included:

- setting up clinics which were running well and were on the whole well attended; forging links with other agencies and organisations;

- getting involved in planning future services for the homeless (for example, through involvement with the Joint Care Planning Team);

- raising the profile of the health care problems experienced by homeless people.

Although it was impossible to measure, it was also hoped that the project had taken some of the pressure off the local casualty department and that, as a result, casualty staff would be less intolerant of the homeless people they encountered. They found it useful to refer homeless people to the project instead of trying to find a local GP willing to take them on.

However, while not denying the value of the project to those who used its services, other team members were less convinced about the extent of its achievements and were more vocal about the lack of success in certain areas. One view was that the *amount* of input rather than the *quality* had been inadequate. This comment related to the difficulties and delays the project team had experienced in trying to set up clinics. Another observation was that the project had been too 'clinic oriented' and that more time could have been spent on health education and health promotion.

While both project teams felt they had made progress in working towards the objective of providing a good quality service for homeless people that in the main had not existed before, they acknowledged that they had been generally less successful in working towards the other main objective in setting up the projects: namely, getting people to use mainstream services. There were a number of reasons why they felt this way. In particular, our attention was drawn to the potential conflict between these two objectives. Providing a more comprehensive and better service for homeless people in the short term involved building up relationships with people, who might then be reluctant to transfer their trust to a local GP.

More specifically, the doctors were conscious of a problem of 'mixed messages'; medical etiquette and practical commonsense required that they build up trust with their patients in the centres, but the long-term objective of the project meant that they should be telling these patients to seek medical care elsewhere. They were concerned that some patients would interpret this as yet another rejection and would fail to seek care anywhere. In East London, the social worker commented that there was an advantage in having a non-medical team member trying to get people to register because this avoided the mixed messages problem. When he referred people to a GP they were less likely to feel rejected because they knew that he was not 'refusing' to give them medical care.

Recommendations for future developments

We wanted to hear team members' views on what they thought should happen to the pilot projects after the initial period of funding expired in March 1989. In particular, we wanted to know whether they thought that the project in their locality should be continued, either in whole or in part, or whether their experiences had encouraged them to think there were better ways of improving the provision of primary care services for the homeless.

In East London there was general agreement that some sort of specialist care team needed to continue, but individuals had different ideas about its ideal format and the extent to which team members should be integrated into mainstream provision. Several people thought that instead of employing a salaried doctor, the medical service component should come from general practice locally. The argument for doing this was thought to be particularly strong with regard to residential centres, such as the Detoxification Unit, where individuals had an address and could be easily located. Only one team member dissented from this view. She could see the value of bringing in local GPs, but as a team member she liked working with one doctor.

Those team members who advocated using local GPs instead of a salaried doctor still thought it was necessary to provide medical care on an outreach basis in the centres because the projects had made little progress in linking homeless people into mainstream services. They could see a number of advantages in local GPs undertaking these surgeries. In particular, it would avoid the problem of 'mixed messages' as described by the project doctors. If local GPs could initially build up relationships with people by coming to see them at the centres, they could then try and draw them back into mainstream services by encouraging them to continue that relationship in the context of the ordinary surgery.

Several suggestions were made as to how local GPs could be remunerated for this work. One view was that they should become visiting medical officers to the various centres. Another suggestion was that they could be paid a set sum for each session held at a centre and, in addition, could claim a temporary resident fee from the FPC for each patient seen. Alternatively, if patients were seen regularly they could be permanently registered. It was appreciated that this could raise issues of medical etiquette because people seen at the centres might already be registered elsewhere.

There was a general consensus among the East London team that, while the project doctor's job could and should be absorbed into more flexible mainstream provision, the tasks performed by the other team members needed to be retained and performed by a specialist team. But to overcome the problem of professional isolation this team would need more support and backing than the current team members had experienced. It was thought that the problems of the single homeless were given a low priority by statutory agencies and that their interests were best served by workers separate from these agencies who could act as their advocate. Moreover, it was felt that there was in any case little hope of the social work element being taken over by the social services department precisely because the latter was already overstretched and the single homeless were likely to be low on its list of priorities for allocating resources.

In Camden there was concern that the service should not be stopped abruptly after three years, but there was also a consensus among team members that the project should not continue in its present form. They too felt that ideally local practices should take over the clinics that the project had established in the centres, but they were not optimistic that local GPs would be interested in taking them on. They also thought there was a risk attached to handing the clinics over to mainstream providers; even if several local GPs were persuaded to take them on, there was no guarantee that they would retain them and homeless people might find themselves back in the same position vis-a-vis health care as they were before the project started. Another alternative which was suggested was to retain a salaried doctor to undertake the clinics, but to attach the post to a local practice.

If the project were to be discontinued, there were conflicting views among team members about the best way of providing nursing services for homeless people in Camden. One person thought that ordinary district nurses working for the health authority should visit the centres and take over their share of homeless clients. Another recommendation was for a core nursing group within the health authority who specialised in this client group.

Although the Camden team were not in favour of continuing a special and separate service for homeless people, their experiences led them to recommend the appointment of health advisory workers or facilitators. They thought that these workers should be attached to existing day centres or health centres and not set up in isolation as the project team had been. It was envisaged that these workers would have a vital role to play both in drawing homeless people into mainstream services and in encouraging existing services to become more flexible. Their main task would be to go into the centres and provide health education in the very broadest sense: advising clients on how to register and how to use services.

Bearing in mind that the projects were essentially *pilot* schemes, we were interested to know team members' views on whether or not they thought that this approach to improving the provision of health care services for homeless people was a useful one to develop elsewhere. In both projects, team members had mixed feelings about initiating similar schemes in other areas. With the proviso that there would need to be sufficient numbers of both single homeless people and centres through which to channel the services, most team members thought that schemes like theirs *could* be set up elsewhere. However, given their views on the weakness of the schemes and their comments about the future of their own projects, they were not sure whether the same models *should* be transferred to other areas. One view was that the approach embodied by the scheme was useful as a short-term pump-priming exercise to focus attention on the problem and to initiate an improvement in services. Another view was that resources could be better spent on trying to support and encourage existing professionals to see the homeless population in their locality as part of their responsibility.

The East London team felt that the homeless population in their area was more stable than in Camden and reflected more the stereotypical image of the homeless person as a middle-aged single male. It was likely that around 70 per cent of the homeless people using the centres had been in the area for more than four years. They were mobile within the locality, in that they moved around between the day centres, but not outside it. As a result, the East London team thought that, compared to their Camden colleagues, they had been more able to offer continuity of care. They imagined that the Camden project was dealing with young people who had recently come to London and with families in bed and breakfast accommodation.

The Camden team were not in fact seeing families in bed and breakfast, but they too thought that the homeless people they saw were generally younger and more transient than those encountered in the East End. They speculated that many of these people were likely to be fitter than those seen by the other team and would need less medical and nursing care. Although a large number had drink problems, they were not likely to be in the area long enough to want to do anything about their addiction problem.

The managers
We asked the chairmen and administrators of the two Family Practitioner Committees managing the projects for their views on existing provision for homeless people in their locality. At the end of the monitoring period we also asked them what they thought about the progress and achievements of the pilot projects. In Camden there had been a change of FPC chairman during the life of the pilot scheme.

Current provision of primary health care for homeless people
In both areas provision for homeless people was regarded as inadequate, but respondents differed in their strength of feeling about this and about how they perceived the problem. They also had conflicting views about whether or not special and separate provision was necessary for this client group, or whether resources and effort should be directed at trying to integrate them into mainstream provision.

One view was that existing provision was patchy and unsystematic and depended far too much on the goodwill of certain GPs who carried more than their fair share of the workload. There was concern that the problem was a low priority for many health care providers and service planners who were happy for other people to deal with the problem informally because this avoided giving homelessness visibility or legitimacy.

In East London the more general point was made that although the NHS does not cater well for homeless people it also does not meet the needs of other sections of the population, such as Bengali families, who have difficulty using the system. The FPC had to think of ways of reaching all these disadvantaged groups, not just the homeless.

Another view was that the existing system within broad limits could deal with emergencies, but did not go much beyond this. Homeless people could get general medical care when something was wrong with them, but it was difficult to think of a way in which their contact with the system could go beyond that particular episode to ensure continuity of care.

Local GPs and registration

In both areas the FPCs were aware that there were problems in getting local GPs to take on homeless people. Although a good number of GPs indicated a willingness to treat individuals who were homeless, in practice only a very few took on substantial numbers of homeless patients. It was thought that the problem was largely one of attitudes and inaccurate images about the client group.

GPs were thought to be reluctant to register homeless people at their practices because they believed these individuals would disrupt the quality and type of service they were seeking to provide for the bulk of their patients. They were also thought to be anxious about getting inundated with a case-load of difficult patients with insatiable demands. Observing that some GPs were particularly concerned that treating homeless patients would entail having to cope with large numbers of drug addicts and other people with threatening behaviour, one FPC Administrator commented that this was a misconception; most in this client group were well behaved and only became demanding when they were constantly rejected.

There was, however, recognition that among the homeless population there were many who would be time-consuming and unrewarding patients and this presented a very real problem for over-loaded inner-city GPs. It was thought likely that in smaller practices resistance arose as much from a lack of time and facilities as from intolerant attitudes towards the client group. Moreover, the FPC chairmen and administrators were convinced that not all of the problem lay with the GP. They thought that for a variety of reasons homeless people were often unaccustomed or unwilling to use local GPs.

We asked whether the FPCs took the view that a person's lack of accommodation affected their ability to register with a GP, bearing in mind the NHS (General Medical and Pharmaceutical) Regulations. We were told that it was all a matter of *interpretation* and that lack of accommodation need not affect a person's ability to register. An address was asked for because this showed that the person was residing in the area and gave somewhere to send their medical card. However, these were simply bureaucratic requirements. A GP could send the medical card care of someone else, or the homeless patient could collect it from the surgery. Neither FPC Administrator took the view that lack of an address automatically precluded registration. However, being realistic about current practice, they suspected that a convenient way for GPs to avoid facing up to the problem was to insist on a home address.

The pilot scheme
What were the views of the FPC chairmen and administrators on the pilot schemes as a way of improving services for homeless people? We wanted to know what they thought about the management and structure of the schemes as well as their views on the approach to service delivery.

First of all, we asked them to clarify for us how they interpreted the objectives of the schemes. Some emphasised the practical contribution the schemes could make to health care for the homeless: for example, the projects were set up to channel people towards registering with GPs as well as meeting their immediate needs; and they were designed to provide care to those who would otherwise fall through the net. Other views highlighted the experimental nature of the projects and their value in finding out more about the extent and nature of the problem. Another common theme was that the projects were intended to increase general awareness and stimulate a broader response to the needs of the homeless. This was important because respondents thought that the pilot schemes could not be seen as a permanent solution. There was also some doubt about the extent to which a one-off project could seriously influence the number of people being drawn back into mainstream services.

Management structure and staffing
Our general impression was that the FPCs had found it difficult to incorporate managing the one-off schemes into their staffing and administrative structures. Line management was a key problem. The administrators had felt it inappropriate for them to be personally involved in managing and supervising project team members on a regular and frequent basis. However, the staffing structure of the FPCs meant that there was no-one else available at a middle-level grade to do this. This problem was exacerbated by the fact that the FPCs in any case were not the employing authorities for all team members; for

example, in Bloomsbury the Administrator felt unable to manage the nurse as she was responsible to Bloomsbury Health Authority.

Both FPCs believed this problem of line management had contributed to the feelings of isolation experienced by team members and the lack of support and direction that they had complained about. There was also some concern that not enough thought had been given to the co-ordinator's role. In both projects the co-ordinators had been under-occupied with project work once the projects had got off the ground. It was suggested that in retrospect this post had possibly been too highly graded and that perhaps there was a need for clerical/ secretarial help rather than for a project co-ordinator. In one area the co-ordinator was described as 'looking for a more positive role which did not exist', but it was not altogether clear why this role could not have been developed more creatively.

Another problem relating to the FPCs' staffing structure was that in one FPC the task of managing the pilot scheme had become particularly time-consuming. The Administrator, who had been enthusiastic about the project at the outset, said, 'I quickly learnt how much of my time and my staff's time would be taken up with the scheme'. In particular, we were told that because the project had to be separately budgeted and accounted for, the workload of the accounting officer had increased considerably.

In the other locality there was concern as to the extent to which the project had actually been managed at all by the FPC. The Administrator admitted that the FPC had perhaps underestimated the extent to which there would need to be 'entrepreneurial management' by the FPC. They had assumed that there was so much need to be met that once the project was set up team members would be inundated with work. They had not anticipated that they would have to take on a 'missionary' role to sell the project. We were told that there were already too many people 'fishing in the pond' with no co-ordination and the FPC should have done more homework about who was already involved.

A general problem identified in both areas was a certain amount of difficulty in getting things done because so many other authorities were inevitably involved. In the words of one Chairman, 'the management structure was Byzantine'. A number of authorities had been drawn into the schemes by the DHSS, but in practice they seemed to have little commitment to working together. This problem had manifested itself in a number of different ways: in particular, difficulty in acquiring premises, appointing staff, and organising general and pharmaceutical supplies. The FPCs could not take unilateral action on these issues because they were not the sole authority involved.

There was also some concern that the projects had been allowed to drift away from their original objectives, but that these objectives were in any case unclear. For example, in Camden the first clinic had been set up outside the FPC's locality. However, because the team had found it so difficult to get sites within the FPC area it had seemed inappropriate for the FPC to veto this opportunity. It had been thought rather more important to show support and interest to the team.

The Joint Steering Group was thought to have had little impact on the management structure in either area. Our respondents found it hard to find a purpose for this group and saw it largely as a Departmental tool, set up because it was felt that the schemes ought to have a steering group, without giving much thought to what useful role it could or should perform. There was no working relationship between the FPCs and the Steering Group, but it should be borne in mind that during this period FPC Administrators were in dispute with the Department about FPC gradings and salaries and were not attending meetings and other events organised by the Department. This included meetings of the Joint Steering Group.

A particular shared criticism was that it had been a mistake to set up one Steering Group responsible for both projects. One Administrator commented, 'I don't see how you can get consensus from people involved in two entirely separate projects dealing with totally different people. The discussion will inevitably be in the abstract rather than about specifics and it is only when you start to talk about specifics that you begin to move forward.' In East London a sub-group of the FPC had been set up to manage that project only. We were told that an important aspect of this sub-group was that, through the one co-opted member, it brought into play the influence of the Department of General Practice at St. Bartholomew's Hospital and this was largely a positive influence.

Salaried doctors

A distinctive feature of the staffing of the schemes was that they employed salaried doctors. We were interested to know what advantages the managers of schemes thought there had been in using salaried doctors instead of independent contractors and whether they had discovered any disadvantages. More generally, we wanted their views on whether they now supported the use of salaried doctors to improve the provision of health care for homeless people.

There was agreement that at the time the projects were set up there had been no other choice but to use salaried doctors because there had not been enough willing and committed GPs in either area to channel the initiative through the independent contractor service. It was thought that as GPs retired and younger doctors were coming onto their lists this situation was gradually changing. An advantage in appointing salaried doctors to the schemes was the knowledge that these people wanted to do the job for what it was: a particular job with a specific client group and at a set salary. If independent contractors had been used, the FPCs would have had the problem of trying to work out an arrangement for payment.

However, it was also apparent that there had been a number of disadvantages in using salaried doctors. As explained in Appendix 2, there was controversy over the fact that the grading for the post was on the senior registrar scale, and one of the FPCs thought that this had contributed to their difficulty in attracting people to the post. Moreover, an appointment on a hospital training grade usually meant that the person was accountable to a consultant, but, in fact, the project doctors were not clinically accountable to anybody. They were thought to have experienced professional isolation as a result. There was also the more general problem that those who were against the principle of a salaried doctor service were less supportive to the individuals concerned and to the projects as a whole. Another negative spin-off was thought to be the risk that, by giving this client group a salaried doctor, the project might encourage them not to integrate into existing services.

Individuals' views about the general issue of using salaried doctors for this client group were far from clear-cut, and were caught up with their views about the principle of a salaried GP service for all patients. They were also linked to the wider debate about whether special and separate services were needed for homeless people or whether resources should be directed at integrating them into mainstream services. A more specific question raised was whether it was reasonable to expect any doctor to do this job for more than two or three years. It was seen as a limited form of practice; the project doctors saw a skewed population and did not get the breadth of clinical experience necessary to further their own careers.

Strengths and weaknesses of the schemes
What did the chairmen and administrators of the managing FPCs think were the strengths and weaknesses of the pilot schemes in their area? Several major strengths were identified: some related to individual team members and the way they worked; others emphasised the importance of the projects in drawing attention to the problem of homelessness and health care.

There was a consensus about the valuable contribution made by team members, who were regarded as competent and conscientious and doing a good job. It was thought useful that they had flexibility and were not seen as too close to the establishment. It had been expected that this would aid them in striking up relationships with voluntary agencies. In one locality there was some disappointment that this had not happened to any great extent. The opportunities were thought to have been there, and it was considered unclear whether this failing had been a function of personalities, or whether the team had simply thought it inappropriate to develop this activity.

It was thought important that the projects had focused attention on the problem and had made people think about it in a more co-ordinated way. In particular, it was hoped that the projects would have a catalytic affect on local practices through team members contacting them. It was also believed that by managing the projects the FPCs had acquired a better understanding of the client group and had benefited in other ways too; they had become involved with other people and agencies with specialist interests who could put a different perspective on health service planning and provision for this and other disadvantaged client groups.

A diverse range of weaknesses were identified. In one locality a major weakness was thought to be the fact that the project had been under-managed, both strategically and operationally. This flaw was traced back to the way it had been set up. It was argued that insufficient thought had been given to what the project was trying to do and what resources it needed to do it with. There was a feeling that the initiative had been foisted upon the FPC without its being satisfied that these questions *could* be answered.

Another view was that whereas a strength lay in 'independence', the other side of the coin was 'separateness' and this could become a weakness. The project was separate from mainstream services and team members were professionally isolated from their peers. A number of practical weaknesses were also identified: for example, the projects could not provide 24 hour cover; and the teams were small relative to the size of the problem they were tapping into.

A wider concern in one locality was that the project had taken up a disproportionate amount of FPC time. Looking at this against the many needs of the areas in which the projects were located, the question was raised as to whether so much time spent on one relatively small client group could be justified. It was also thought that the schemes might have drawbacks in two other respects: first, that local providers would take the view that if there were a salaried doctor for the homeless there was less need for them to take responsibility to treat this client group; and second, that the projects might be raising expectations which mainstream services as currently organised might not be able to satisfy.

Success of the schemes

There were mixed feelings about how successful the pilot projects had been. No-one thought that they had been an unmitigated disaster and at the very least they were judged to have been successful in terms of direct care provision for homeless people. However, their major value was seen to lie in lessons learned.

One view was that if projects like these were to have a chance of success then they needed to have tightly focused and potentially achievable goals. Central initiatives were seen to be crucial in tackling difficult social problems but it was thought that unless they were set up with considerable care, they might well be counter-productive.

A disappointment expressed in one locality was that, while there had been measurable achievements in terms of direct care, the project had not given them the window to the problem that they had expected. As managers they were looking for solutions and the project had not been particularly successful in providing solutions. It had, however, made them realise that there was probably no one right way of tackling the problem.

Another view was that even the impact of the project on direct care for the client group was difficult to measure. Highlighting what he considered to be the extraordinary difficulty of getting hold of any reliable statistical base, one person commented, 'Many criteria are presentational; for example, Dr 'Y' treated 'X' number of people. But how many others are left untreated? You just don't know.'

Future provision

What did the chairmen and administrators of the managing FPCs think should happen to the projects when funding expired in March 1989? No-one recommended continuing the pilot schemes in their present form.

In one area we were told that the *financial commitment* needed to be retained but that it should be allocated in a different way. The argument here, and one that was shared by the project team members, was that the project base and team, apart from the doctor should be maintained and enhanced. But it was felt that the money spent on the salaried doctor could be better spent on sessional payments for local GPs to do the work. It was thought that this would have the advantage of enabling the homeless to be dealt with more as part of the general medical services. It was envisaged that local GPs could take over and develop the outreach work started by the project, with the aim of drawing as many homeless people as possible back into using ordinary general practice.

In the other area no clear view was expressed about what should happen next. The general opinion was that health care for the homeless was a problem which needed a many-pronged approach and that the pilot project had acted as just one safety-net. However, it was also thought that a more appropriate way of tackling the problem might be to fund specific sessions by local GPs. The 'hands on' outreach work currently done by the project team could then be transferred to existing services, providing these services could be encouraged to become more flexible. It was suggested that these sessions by local GPs would be more feasible if practices were allowed to employ more ancillary staff.

A variety of views were expressed about whether or not the pilot project as developed in their area could be transferred successfully to other areas to improve the provision of health care for homeless people. One opinion was that the current model definitely should not be replicated elsewhere, although the projects and their evaluation might well result in transferable ideas. The others agreed that under certain circumstances the approach developed by the pilot schemes might well be one possible option. However, first it was necessary to establish the nature of the problem *locally*, then the model could be considered along with the range of other options. In particular, a warning note was sounded that if the day centres through which the outreach work would be channelled were not available, then policy-makers should go back to the drawing board.

Looking at some of the wider aspects of the problem, to what extent did the chairmen and administrators think it was feasible to get homeless people to register with a local GP? It was generally acknowledged that this had been one of the objectives in setting up the projects but that little progress had been made. Opinion was divided on the extent to which uptake of existing services could be increased. One view was that there was a great deal more scope and potential for getting this client group to use mainstream services. For example, it was suggested that a link could be established between the local Accident and Emergency Department and the FPC, so that when a homeless person used casualty inappropriately they could be given advice and help regarding GP registration. In East London, it was also thought that local GPs were now more committed and willing to take on the homeless than they had been when the project started.

However, it was pointed out that, regardless of any specific primary health care initiatives, there would still be the problem of lack of motivation to use GP services on the part of some homeless people. Reflecting on this obstacle, one chairman commented that he had been struck by the comments of the team members that, for many, acceptance of chronic illness was part of their everyday existence. It was generally considered that there would always be the problem of some in this client group who did not want to register, and the question was raised as to how far they could be pushed. There was always the possibility that among the single homeless there were some who led that lifestyle because they chose to and would not welcome interference. Homeless families were thought to be a different issue. It was suggested that there was more of a case for searching out the children in homeless families because they were the next generation and, without intervention, they risked having 'a whole life of homelessness ahead of them', with all its attendant health care problems.

There were several suggestions as to what would make it easier for homeless people to register with local GPs. A major requirement was thought to be a relaxation of attitudes on the part of GPs, but a corollary to this was that GPs needed greater back-up in order to feel able and willing to give a commitment to homeless people. This was an argument for developing further the concept, and the practice, of primary health care teams whereby the GP was supported by the attachment of community psychiatric nurses, social workers and possibly clinical psychologists. There was also the suggestion that local surgeries would be less daunting to homeless people if they were open throughout the day and people could walk in and obtain advice from someone, not necessarily a GP. Another opinion was that if the intention was to reach disadvantaged groups in the community then policy-makers had to be prepared to finance vigorous outreach services, the details of which were less important than the commitment.

Given the role of FPCs vis-a-vis the independent contractors on their General Medical List, we wanted to know whether the chairmen and administrators thought that FPCs could take a stronger lead in securing access by homeless people to a good standard of general medical care. One view was that FPCs in general should be more flexible about registration and should make it clear to their GPs that they were prepared to accept as a basis for registration anything that could be remotely classed as an address. It was pointed out that FPCs actually had very limited scope, but they could become better informed themselves about the needs and circumstances of the homeless and share that knowledge with practitioners and with other agencies. The staffing and administrative structures of FPCs were thought to constrain them from taking much of an initiative themselves. For example, in one FPC we were told there were few staff currently available who could be effective in going round to GP practices to inform them about the needs of the homeless and persuade them to provide a service to this client group.

A more optimistic view was that FPCs had lots of potential to secure a good standard of care for homeless people, but they needed to be more imaginative in their procedures and more creative about their use of funds. One suggestion was that they should improve their recruitment policies. They should target their recruitment towards problem areas such as homeless people and ensure they engaged GPs who had the skills and commitment to take on these people. Our attention was also drawn to recommendations on ancillary staff reimbursement in the White Paper on Primary Health Care (DHSS, 1987). It was argued that if these recommendations were used creatively, they could provide the basis for building more effective primary health care teams.

7   Views of the Wardens

In Chapter 2 we discussed the outreach approach of the pilot schemes and described the hostels, day centres and night shelters visited by the two project teams. In particular, we concentrated on the centres where the project doctors had set up regular clinics. This chapter looks at the views and opinions of the wardens of these centres about the provision of primary health care for homeless people and about the pilot scheme in their area.

We conducted personal interviews with the wardens or co-ordinators of the five centres in East London where the project doctor held regular clinics during the twelve-month monitoring period and in Camden with the three centres involved. With the exception of one centre in Camden, where we interviewed staff shortly after the clinic was set up in the autumn of 1987, we interviewed twice in each centre: at the beginning and the end of the monitoring period.

The first interview was largely a fact-finding exercise about the centre, its philosophy and its facilities, and it also gave us the opportunity to find out the wardens' early impressions about the pilot schemes. The second interview covered some of the same ground so that we could see if their views had changed, but it also concentrated more on the achievements of the schemes and the pattern of provision for the future. In one of the Camden centres we lost this continuity because there was a change of warden during the monitoring period. Also, the regular clinic was discontinued in one of the East London centres during the period, but we went ahead with the second interview because we wanted to hear the warden's views about this loss of service.

Current provision of primary health care for homeless people

Health problems of users or residents

There was a consensus among wardens that addiction problems, particularly alcoholism and drug abuse, were major health hazards for the people using their centres, and they identified a number of complaints which they thought were often, but not always, alcohol-related: for example, stomach ulcers, epileptic fits and, in extreme cases, liver and kidney failure. Bad feet, malnutrition and the general debilitating effects of exposure were also seen to be part of the everyday existence of many of the users and residents. Respiratory problems ranging from TB to minor coughs and colds were thought to be common, and in one of the centres our attention was drawn to the fact that staff took the precaution of being immunised against TB. Hepatitis was also a worry for staff and there was also evidence of a growing concern about AIDS.

They were also very much aware of the mental health problems of their users or residents and the difficulties this created for their staff, as well as for the individuals involved. We were told by one warden - 'Psychiatric problems are a pain and create problems for us. The law doesn't help. It protects the freedom of individuals which is proper, but if the psychiatric patient doesn't want to co-operate there is nothing we can do. Involving psychiatric social workers and CPNs is a problem.' Although conscious of what they saw to be a high level of mental illness, particularly chronic mental ill-health, they were also concerned that they had no training to deal with this or even to recognise what type of psychiatric problem was involved.

Local provision of primary health care for users or residents

How much did the wardens know about the use of health care services by those attending their centres and what did they think about the level of local provision?

Getting them to focus on a nominated day in the week before the interview, we asked them to give us an idea of how many of their users were permanently registered with a local GP. The wardens in several of the East London centres found it difficult to comment on the registration status of their users. In one centre the warden knew of only one person who was permanently registered, but in another centre the proportion registered with a local GP was thought to be as high as 40 per cent.

In two of the centres in Camden the estimates were very low. One warden put the figure at about 8 per cent and the other said that he thought that only two of the people using the centre that day were registered with a GP, one of whom had been rehoused and had a flat in Paddington. In the third centre in West London the co-ordinator said that quite a few said they were registered, and more often than not it was with a particular GP in West London who was known to treat the homeless.

The wardens in East London knew of few local GPs who were willing to provide primary health care to homeless people. Only one of the centres had an arrangement with a local doctor who visited on a weekly basis. Two or three GPs' names were mentioned several times as being particularly co-operative and one was said to take on anyone who was homeless. However, as one warden observed - 'I know of two GPs who are willing to have these men on their lists, but whether this amounts to primary health care I don't know. They supply antibiotics and tranquillisers.' Another commented - 'I feel at least in mythical terms Dr.... is seen as the homeless persons' doctor around here. Good and bad things are said about him.' Talking about the same doctor, one warden told us that he would not refer to this doctor because he had heard that he prescribed too liberally - 'I have a very jaundiced view of the service provided at his surgery. I feel that the medical relationship he has with the homeless is ambiguous and who actually is doing the diagnosis and prescribing is sometimes open to question.' How much of this criticism was hearsay is open to question, but certainly a lot of mythology had grown up about his practice as this comment suggests - 'I have "heard" there is a hole in the wall you speak through'.

In West London the story was similar, and one of the wardens explained - 'They always get a rough deal. They don't get past the reception stage, and this includes hospitals.' None of the wardens knew of a GP who had particular responsibility for providing health care to people using their centre. In one case there was a practice very conveniently situated for day centre users, but they were said not to be welcomed by the elderly single-handed GP. Two of the centres were in the catchment areas of well-equipped health centres and we were told by the wardens that these were used by several of their clients, although the appointment system was thought to operate against their better use by homeless people. In both cases the doctors working at the health centres were willing to provide cover for the homeless if they visited the surgery, although we were told that one or two had been banned from the surgery, but the doctors would not visit the day centres without imposing an extra charge.

The wardens held similar views about why the majority of local GPs were not willing to provide services for homeless people, but these tended to be based on impressions or guesswork rather than tangible evidence. Most were concerned about the stigma of homelessness and we were told - 'GPs don't want them in their surgery'. The receptionists as well as other patients were singled out as being unsympathetic to the homeless in the surgery and it was questioned - 'Do we need to educate receptionists? They are often a major obstacle.' We were also reminded that the experience of stigma makes homeless people reluctant to use doctors' surgeries - 'Much has to do with "waiting". If a homeless person is sitting in a room and he is very different then he may find it intimidating.'

GPs in inner London were thought to be very busy and overloaded and were seen to prioritise. They were thought to be reluctant to take on homeless people because they assumed they moved around a lot, often had multiple problems and were time-consuming. It was also suggested that the problem of alcoholism was 'rampant' among the single homeless population and this was not something that every GP could handle.

We asked whether the wardens knew of any local initiatives, excluding the DHSS pilot schemes and any health facilities their centres provided, which were intended to improve provision for homeless people. In East London we were told that a doctor provided a surgery on a voluntary basis at one of the Missions, but this was the only initiative which involved general medical services. We also learned about several local agencies which dealt with alcohol problems and catered for the homeless as well as people who were housed. In Camden wardens were familiar with a separate drop-in centre for medical care which had been operating for several years.

Emergency care procedures for users or residents

Wardens found it difficult to get emergency care for users or residents who came to them with a serious health problem. We asked them to tell us about the most recent instance which had resulted in the person going to hospital, and checked whether this case was typical of their experiences with emergency cases. Some individual case-studies are described below. They indicate that a local GP was rarely involved in the admission and that the centres were thrown heavily on their own resources in terms of transporting people to hospital, getting them admitted and providing some type of support in cases where they became in-patients. However, since the DHSS pilot schemes had been set up, the wardens had begun to turn to project team members for assistance. The most common causes of referral to hospital were drug over-doses and psychiatric problems, along with trauma resulting from accidents or assaults. Where patients had not wanted to stay in hospital or had been refused admission, wardens often had little knowledge about whether or not they had received medical care:

Case 1: A day-centre in East London, situated near the London Hospital. One Sunday a user had been attacked by another man with a set of chinese clubs on a chain and received serious wounds to his hand and head. He had been taken by a member of staff straight to the casualty department of the London Hospital because this was thought to be the easiest and quickest method of getting medical attention. Staff at this centre would rarely call an ambulance because they wanted to avoid arousing any panic. The injured man had refused to stay overnight in hospital because he had a pathological fear of hospitals. The hospital would have admitted him had he been prepared to stay. Instead, he went back to his squat which he shared with several other men. This case was typical of most emergency cases at the centre in that the person had been taken by staff to the casualty department, but it was not necessarily typical of the medical problem involved. Other emergency cases had involved, for example, fits, suffering from exposure, and instances where individuals had collapsed in the centre or on the street.

Case 2: A night shelter in East London. The most recent case had concerned a woman who had arrived at a weekend and had exhibited bizarre and disruptive behaviour. Staff had contacted a CPN (who was then working for the DHSS pilot scheme) and he had taken her in a taxi to a psychiatric hospital. At the time of interview she was still in hospital in a psychiatric ward. On discharge she was likely to be homeless again and would no doubt go back to the night shelter where she could stay temporarily, so long as her behaviour did not become disruptive again. The warden commented that they had been fortunate in that the woman had agreed to go into hospital. In circumstances where they were unable to cope with a person's behaviour and they refused to go to hospital, then the shelter staff would have to ask them to leave. The centre had never had anybody sectioned under the Mental Health Act. This case was not untypical, but more often than not the cause of the emergency was a drug overdose.

Case 3: A day centre and evening centre in East London. The most recent emergency case at this centre had involved a woman with depression. The centre staff had contacted the project doctor working for HHELP and following this a member of staff had taken her to a hospital. She had been detained in hospital for about four weeks and had then been discharged back to a derelict caravan. This case was untypical because the admission to hospital had gone smoothly. Normally the centre found it difficult to get someone admitted. The warden thought it had helped that the woman had been referred from the centre by a doctor. Centre staff had been able to visit her while she was in hospital and although this on-going support stretched their resources, they considered it important.

Case 4: A day centre in East London. Here the last emergency case had been typical of those experienced at the centre in that it had involved a man taking a drug overdose. The project doctor had been available to deal with the problem and although he had thought that the tablets would not do much harm, he had been concerned about the person going back to a squat. He had rung for an ambulance, which had taken about 20 minutes to arrive, and had given a letter to the ambulance man to aid easy admission at the hospital. The man had had his stomach pumped out but had not been kept in overnight. If the project doctor had not been available, the centre staff would have contacted the hospital direct and would not have thought of contacting the patient's GP.

Case 5: A detoxification centre in East London. Their most recent admission to hospital concerned a man who had been unable to

165

get out of bed. Normally, those admitted to the centre would be out of bed within 24 hours of admission. He had been considered to be in need of nursing. The detoxification centre had contacted a local alcohol agency who in turn had contacted the project doctor attached to the DHSS pilot scheme. This doctor had arranged for the man to be admitted to the Mile End hospital. On discharge the man would be received back to the detoxification centre. This case was not atypical except in that the centre had in the first instance contacted a local alcohol agency which had recently been set up instead of troubling the project doctor.

Case 6: A day centre in Camden. The case that most readily came to the warden's mind was that of a young woman aged 39 with respiratory problems. The warden had rung a local doctor who knew the patient and had sent the patient to her by taxi. She was diagnosed as having bronchitis and was admitted to hospital where five weeks later she had a pulmonary embolism and died. This case was exceptional in terms of the age of the patient and the outcome. The warden also commented that a great difficulty with so many of the people using his centre was that they were frightened of hospitals and of those in positions of authority. He said - 'Unless you can take them by the hand and bolster their self-assurance, they won't go. They are petrified of the environment and won't stay in.' He thought that probably two users a month were admitted to hospital and as they often had no husband or wife or other relative, the day centre tried to fill the gap by providing a visiting service.

Case 7: A Drop-In centre in Camden. The staff at this centre had frequently experienced difficulties in getting their users admitted to hospital and the case they described typified this. It concerned a man who had felt giddy and was taken by the warden in a taxi to the casualty department of the nearest hospital. This was before the DHSS pilot scheme had started and the man had not been registered with a GP. He had not wanted to be taken to hospital by ambulance. The warden recalled that initially the hospital had been reluctant to admit him and the first thing they had asked the warden about him was, 'Does he drink?'. After they had examined him it was found that he needed by-pass heart surgery. After a couple of months in hospital he had been discharged to Arlington House.

Case 8: A shelter in Camden providing accommodation and outreach teamwork. The most recent serious health problem at this centre was considered by staff to be atypical because they were unable to get the person admitted to hospital. It had concerned a man who had needed help with a leg problem and was also severely incontinent. He had been regarded as a danger to himself and to others in the shelter. Initially they had not contacted a local GP and had taken the man to the local casualty department, who had apparently refused to see him because he was too dirty. The staff had then obtained a letter of referral to a different hospital from the project doctor working with the local DHSS pilot scheme. The man was not admitted to this hospital either but he was found hostel accommodation. They were unsure whether he had received any medical care.

Improvements in hospital care of homeless people
We asked the wardens whether there were any ways in which they thought that the hospital treatment of homeless people could be improved. There was general consensus that two major problem areas needed to be tackled: prejudice and ignorance about homelessness on the part of many hospital staff; and after-care following discharge from hospital. There was some sympathy concerning the inappropriateness of casualty departments being expected to solve some of the problems of homelessness, as the comment by this warden illustrates - 'I'm not sure hospital services regarding the homeless can be improved because hospitals are not there to treat homelessness, but to treat medical problems'. And another observed - 'Hospitals are not a housing department'.

We were told by one warden in Camden that the situation would only improve if 'Homeless people were treated like those who aren't homeless'. He argued that they were not treated the same because hospital staff realised that, unlike someone with an address, they could not be discharged home. He said he was frequently contacted by medical social workers who say - ' "XYZ" is being discharged tomorrow, can you find him somewhere to go?'. A criticism was that hospitals often discharged people who would be ready to return to their *home* if they had one, but were not strong enough to be sent out onto the *streets* again. One suggestion was that some sort of convalescent facility needed to be provided for homeless people after discharge.

According to one of the wardens we spoke to, 'Prejudice starts on the reception desk', and we were told by another who had generally good relations with the local casualty department - 'There are occasions when ambulance men, police and reception people at the hospital will not respond to a homeless person's needs unless there is strong advocacy by a day centre worker on their behalf. My experience is that once you get through these barriers the nurses and doctors are sympathetic.' It was suggested that staff training aimed at developing a better understanding of the various health care needs and problems of homeless people, in particular alcohol abuse, would be helpful. However, there was some pessimism about the extent to which attitudes towards the homeless could be improved, and one person we spoke to observed - 'Some of it is only human nature. If two people are waiting and one is clean and one is not, the natural tendency is to avoid the one who is stinking.'

The DHSS pilot schemes: assessment of current practice

We asked the wardens what they thought about the services provided by the two pilot schemes and how, by the end of the twelve-month monitoring period, they viewed their strengths and weaknesses.

There was some consensus about the objectives of the projects, but there were also some unique perspectives. Wardens were agreed that project team members were aiming to provide effective, good quality health care to local homeless people in places where they congregated. They were thought to be plugging a gap in mainstream services and giving a service to people who would ordinarily not get assistance on health issues. As one warden in East London observed - 'Their objective is to provide effective health care for individuals who live on the fringes of society and to do so in the situation where these individuals are most in contact with society'. Another warden in the same area developed this point further. She knew that they wanted to provide a service for *homeless* people, but she hoped they would also offer a service for *other* people locally because this would fit in with the aim of the day centre to try to stretch out into the community locally.

There was general agreement that the projects had a role to play in helping people use mainstream health care services, but there was some doubt as to whether this aim was being fulfilled in either locality. We were told by one warden in East London - 'I know they want to get people on GPs' lists and have had difficulties'. And another told us - 'Its role should be to help people use other health services, but I don't think this has been achieved. People still come back looking for the project doctor.'

It was also suggested that another objective of the projects was to encourage people to take more of an interest in looking after their health. A co-ordinator in one of the Camden shelters told us - 'It should be rehabilitative. It does a lot to restore the worth of people. It does a lot for their self-respect and makes street life more bearable. If people have medical problems they can get them seen to. Health problems on the streets are not just minor problems.' In addition to educating potential users, the schemes were also thought to provide valuable support to centre staff, as this warden in East London commented - 'The team support and educate staff in situations where health care is so clearly a problem'. Another of the wardens in East London speculated that perhaps team members in his area should perhaps channel their experience into a more campaigning role for better and more co-ordinated health care facilities for homeless people.

Strengths of the schemes

We asked the wardens both at the beginning and at the end of the monitoring period what they thought were the strengths of the pilot schemes. In early 1987 wardens in both East London and Camden were agreed that a major strength of the scheme in their area was that it provided a regular service to the homeless, in a familiar environment in which they felt comfortable. There was also consensus that by regularly providing the service the team members would develop a more understanding approach than those who provided it casually. We were told by the warden of an East London day centre - 'It is a service provided on the ground at the level where the homeless are and because of that it is bound to derive a specialised knowledge and understanding of the medical needs of the homeless'.

The warden of another centre in East London emphasised the stability of the service and the fact that it provided the first step for people who ordinarily would not bother to use health services. He explained - 'It helps them over their fears of using health services and encourages them to feel entitled to health care'. He also thought that by extending the facilities offered by the day centre, the presence of the scheme enhanced the image and philosophy of the centre. A similar point was made by one of the wardens in Camden who told us that the scheme was becoming known among homeless people and some were visiting his day centre specifically to see the project doctor - 'Word is spreading around "cardboard city" that it is here. We are getting travellers asking about the service and coming in specifically for the doctor.'

Another perceived strength of both pilot schemes was that project team members were flexible and informal in their approach, and would have more time to build up relationships with users and with the centre staff. We were told by the co-ordinator of one of the Camden centres that the service offered was '...a lot more informal than the health centre and they won't be frowned at'. It was hoped that another strength would lie in project workers operating as a cohesive team which would not work in isolation but in conjunction with other agencies in the area, including voluntary agencies. The shelter in Camden that undertook outreach work on the streets as well as providing accommodation was impressed at the way the pilot scheme had integrated with their own project. The co-ordinator commented - 'We have people who are here at night and can see the doctor in the morning. Also we do street work and people can come in just to use the service. The project doctor has been out on a tea run to see people.'

By the end of the monitoring period wardens liked the regularity and continuity of the services and thought that it was important that team members came to the centres, rather than being office-based. One of the wardens in East London speculated that one of the reasons why the CPN role had *not* developed successfully was because the person involved had wanted to be office-based. It was generally agreed that the flexible approach was suitable for the client population, and one of the wardens in Camden commented - 'We are talking about a group who are quick to complain if they don't like something'. Most of the wardens in both projects were also appreciative of the help and support provided by team members to staff. We were told by one - 'A strength is the access to advice and consultation that the staff have. It is not just a question of the doctor coming to see residents. He is also here for staff to consult about residents.'

There was consensus that the personalities of project team members were an important strength, and we were told about the project doctor in East London - 'You have confidence in him, you get results. I'm talking about personality more than anything else. He has had an impact.' Similar comments were made about the Camden project team. In one centre, where a nurse employed by the centre worked alongside the project doctor, we were told - 'A strength is the quality of the staff operating the service. Because the nurse is part of the staff team here she can contribute to the overall aims of the centre, not just the medical service.' And in another centre the warden complimented the doctor's judgment regarding his prescribing policy - 'The project doctor doesn't overly prescribe drugs. Lots hope to get drugs and he's wise to that.'

There were also more individualistic views. One warden in East London liked the balance between involvement and objectivity that the team had achieved in his centre - 'The project has direct contact through the centres with the day-to-day problems of the clients. And yet at the same time they're not involved in the running of the centres or involved in policy decisions and control. Therefore, they're more impartial and objective in saying what can be done.' An associated strength identified by this warden was that the HHELP team had helped centre staff evaluate the content of their jobs and the services they offered. He said - 'There is also a tendency to scrutinise the centre's processes with the assistance of the HHELP team. This has not affected clients directly. But it is raising consciousness and a sense of possibilities *within* the centre.' He illustrated this by explaining how the project social worker had helped him set up a Thursday afternoon club for those people who were being or had been resettled, who lived alone and who needed support. He said this idea had been on the centre's agenda, but the social worker had been supportive and instrumental in getting it translated into action.

Another warden in East London told us that the pilot scheme in his area had helped to promote the credibility of local day centres and

171

hostels by raising the profile of the homeless. It had also made it easier for them to obtain health care for their clients because it had a standing with statutory agencies, for example social services, which voluntary bodies often did not have. He explained - 'The service has given us credibility in the sense of taking the needs of the single homeless seriously. It has given us clout when referring people on for psychiatric treatment, hospital treatment, housing etc... It has given us more confidence as an agency. It has felt better staffed, better equipped to deal with people's overall wellbeing, catering for the whole person, not just a part.' He also thought that his centre had benefited from the fact that the project team visited several other agencies. Before the scheme had been set up, his centre had been overcrowded on the one evening each week when a doctor visited on a voluntary basis. This had become less of a problem since the pilot scheme was introduced because people were able to get medical care at a number of other local centres.

Weaknesses of the schemes

We also asked the wardens to identify any weaknesses they associated with the pilot projects. In early 1987 there was some concern that as they were special schemes they would not be seen as an integrated part of the medical provision. There was also some speculation about the drawbacks of having such small teams to tackle what was considered to be an extensive problem. It was thought to be a problem that team members were not able to provide cover every day of the week. In Camden one of the wardens told us - 'They are not here enough. I would like to see them here all day. Yesterday we had someone using oedema drugs. He should have been hospitalised. The project doctor would have had the clout to do this.'

A further weakness identified early on by several wardens was that the design of the schemes meant that the services would not reach all those who needed them. As one of the wardens in East London explained - 'A weakness in the outreach work is that day centres are the feeder for the service and not everyone who is homeless uses the day centres. They could only be reached by someone tramping the streets. As the service becomes more widely known by local statutory and voluntary agencies it will pick up these people. It takes time.'

Women and ethnic minorities were two groups of homeless people who we were told rarely used the day centres and therefore had poor access to the project teams' services. One warden in East London informed us that about 12 per cent of those attending his centre were from ethnic minority groups but that they were all loners. He said that if any 'group' attempted to use the centre there would be a problem of racial discrimination by the other users. He also reflected on the problem of hidden homelessness among women. He said - 'This centre is a dangerous place for women unless they are eccentric or tough. They get used. They always take a back seat.' To try and combat this problem, the centre had set up a women's session one day a week.

There was also concern in another day centre in East London that the DHSS and others may be taking too narrow a definition of homelessness. Bearing in mind that some of those who attended the day centre and used the pilot scheme services were housed, albeit it inadequately, the warden commented - 'It is important there is an understanding of what homelessness is and what it is not. Our interpretation of homelessness is broad. We will see anyone who is in "housing need" which includes those who may have been homeless or have moved into a flat but don't feel part of the borough because of lack of support.'

Although most of the centres had established good relationships with the project teams, there was an initial feeling in one day centre in East London that 'we are standing on each other's toes'. The co-ordinator told us that there were problems in defining roles and recognising boundaries. Centre staff appreciated the input of the team, but they felt they had few rights as regards the services provided - 'They are professionals coming into our centre, but what rights do we have?'. She would have liked the CPN to visit the day centre, but she had felt unable to tell him to do this. She felt that part of the problem was that they did not see enough of team members to establish a rapport with them. She also thought it was a failing that there was no one person to whom team members were accountable and who could ensure good practice.

At the end of the monitoring period the wardens felt more able to comment about the weaknesses of the pilot schemes, but generally speaking these were seen to be far outweighed by their strengths. In

East London we were told that the lack of an emergency out-of-hours service was a main drawback. It was particularly noticeable because local GPs were loath to come to the centres. We were also told about the lack of specialist psychiatric help. One of the wardens in East London commented - 'Health care issues don't just mean physical health, they include mental health. Among the homeless there are a lot of psychiatric problems. There doesn't seem to have been anything provided for that. Perhaps because the problem is so large, it is difficult to tackle.' Another warden in the same area said - 'The mental health dimension is weak and in terms of health care that is an important dimension for the centres. Mental illness is a high profile problem for us. We could have done with more education, information, support and counselling in that area.' Making a similar point another warden compared his experiences in Tower Hamlets with his previous job - 'Before here I worked in South London where there was a community psychiatric service and the counsellor came out on call'.

There was also some concern expressed in one of the East London centres that there was sometimes a problem in trying to contact the project doctor. The warden explained - 'If you are ringing HHELP, which is just around the corner, you often meet the answering machine. This is no good in an emergency.' And the centre warden who had earlier expressed concern about the issue of their rights vis-a-vis the pilot scheme restated her unease about the lack of consultation with the centres - 'It is up to the team in the end to decide what to do. The day centres have no real say about what happens or not. The centres may feel insecure. We were going to meet the Steering Group of HHELP but this has never happened.'

In Camden our attention was drawn to a number of other weaknesses, some of which were peculiar to individual centres rather than the general design of the pilot scheme. The warden of one day centre told us - 'I'm not sure that we have the medical room and waiting room sited in the best place... There is currently a lot going on around the medical room and there is not sufficient privacy. There also needs to be a physical update in terms of furniture because it is run down. Also, it is up several flights of stairs.' In another centre in Camden the warden emphasised the sensitive issue of confidentiality surrounding patient data. He was unhappy that project team members were unwilling to share information about clients with centre staff. He argued - 'We feel we are all part of a team. Any information that would help us help clients should be shared.'

Success of the schemes

The wardens found it difficult to be specific about the criteria they would use for assessing the success or otherwise of the pilot schemes. Much depended on how wardens viewed the aims of the schemes and, as this comment illustrates, they were not always sure themselves - 'I see it as providing a service to our residents and I haven't thought of it as having aims'. There was general agreement on two issues: that the schemes would have achieved some success if they reached people who had not seen a doctor before, and if they had networked people into local community services. But there was also agreement that these indicators were very difficult to turn into reliable outcome measures.

We were told - 'A measure of success has got to be whether someone continues to use that service on a regular basis and becomes more stable in linking with established medical services'. But there was concern about the ambiguity of attendance figures. It was pointed out that you could measure success, 'Statistically by the number of people who use it, but this could also indicate failure!'. We were also reminded that the quality of the service provided was as important as the volume of people using it, as this warden explained - 'I would use the number of individuals who use the services as a measure of success, but not simply the volume but also the quality of the service derived by them. The response the service manages to evoke from clients in terms of caring for their own health is important.'

And a warden in Camden made the point that, while the team in his area were providing a good *medical* service, it was not altogether clear whether this was the best way of tackling the major health hazards experienced by his clients:

> What problems have been dealt with? What I suspect intuitively is that for quite a number who have used the medical service, the medical problem is not the reason for coming. I suspect a good 60 or 70 per cent of users of this day centre have drinking problems and this is something that is not being tackled realistically. When they come to the

medical service they are asking for more than help with medical problems but also want help with drink and drug problems. I'm not sure whether we are, or should be, doing anything about this. I think we should provide more preventative health care and counselling.

In Camden another warden commented that the pilot project had proved successful in his centre because it had saved a few people's lives by identifying major illnesses such as strokes.

We had been told that the personalities of project team members were an important asset to the pilot schemes, yet in East London there was also concern that the success of the schemes might be inappropriately judged by the performance of team members. This comment related specifically to the mental health aspect of the project which had lapsed after the project CPN had resigned. One of the East London wardens commented - 'Lack of success might be because someone has not got to grips with their role. I don't want the project to be judged as a failure because people have not come to grips with roles because of lack of support, training or money. The project is valuable.'

Factors hindering success

We asked wardens to tell us whether they had been disappointed with any aspects of the pilot scheme in their locality and to identify any factors which they thought had hindered its success. In several East London centres there was concern that the CPN had resigned early on and that the project had not systematically tackled mental health problems. We were told - 'The whole mental health area was under-served by the project. It needs a lot of development. I don't think that was entirely the fault of the CPN. He came in with hospital assumptions. It needed a different approach and his job should have been researched and defined *before* a worker was appointed.' And another warden commented - 'There was a lack of psychiatric input, which I see as one of the main needs of homeless people'. He added that some of the day centre clients objected strongly to the presence of others in the centre who had psychiatric problems, and had asked for a group discussion to air their views.

Several of the wardens thought that the project team members themselves had not been given enough support. We were told by a warden in East London - 'There seems to be a certain degree of demoralisation due to the way it is funded and managed. But the workers have largely managed to surmount this.' Our attention was also drawn to the temporary nature of the schemes - 'In the background there is the sense that this is a temporary arrangement and we can't rely on this help long-term. There is a fear that there will be a big gap when and if it goes.' The warden of one of the centres in East London had already experienced the withdrawal of the project doctor's services and remarked - 'We would still have liked to have developed our own surgery time here with the doctor. The clients are well served but as far as our Mission and its perceived approach is concerned, we would have liked to have retained the GP services.'

Another of the wardens in East London thought that a lack of clarity surrounding some of the team members' roles had initially hindered the success of the scheme. In particular, it was pointed out that the doctor provided both immediate medical care and referrals to the local GPs, and it was thought that there was a contradiction between these two roles. We were also told that the changes in team members had at times been disruptive. Referring to the doctor from America who had been attached temporarily to the project, one of the wardens commented - 'We were slightly disappointed when this doctor came on the scene. We felt lumbered with a stranger who was unaware of UK procedures. But it has worked out very well. At the changeover it was difficult to re-adjust. This was also true when the current project doctor took over from the original project doctor.'

There was some disappointment that there were still groups of homeless people that the projects had not reached, as this co-ordinator in East London explained - 'The team have got out to day centres as far as possible but even the team are aware there are areas yet to be addressed. For example, those homeless people on the streets who do not use day centres. If the accident and emergency departments are aware of the project and link homeless people in, this would be one way of bridging the gap.' This point was also developed in one of the Camden centres where we were told - 'Someone using the day centre may be banned because of their behaviour and that could deny them access to the medical service'. Another warden in Camden thought that the timing of the surgeries in his centre had worked against successful take-up of the scheme. The project doctor visited in the mornings, but the centre was at its busiest in the afternoons.

Having been frank about the weaknesses of the schemes, the wardens were keen to remind us that the pilot schemes had definitely improved the local provision of health care for people using their centres. This comment by the warden of a day centre in East London summed up the general tenor of their views - 'It has vastly improved access to a doctor on the part of a large number of homeless people; it has improved the quality of care available to them because of its regularity and seriousness; and because of that it has improved the quality of the clients' *own response* to their health problems'. The important role the schemes had played in raising the awareness and expectations of homeless people about health care was emphasised in several centres in both project sites. And the haven it provided for those people who could not or would not use mainstream services was highlighted by this warden in West London - 'It has improved provision for people like 'XYZ', who is mentally unstable and is banned from the Health Centre. They won't give him the medication any more which he still needs. They had no suggestions as to what should be done with him. The project doctor has taken him on.'

Need for additional health care services
We asked the wardens whether there were any additional health care services not already provided by the pilot project which they would like to have seen provided at their centres. Two types of service were most commonly desired:

- some form of psychiatric care and counselling;
- a greater emphasis on preventative health care, health education and information on diet and nutrition.

Other services which were frequently mentioned included:

- chiropody;
- dental treatment;
- health care specifically directed to women using the centres and, in particular, provided by a female doctor;
- help and advice concerning drug addiction to cut down on the number of referrals to specialist agencies;

- a delousing facility nearby or on site to help improve hygiene;
- an occupational therapist to help people with physical difficulties;
- more detoxification facilities, including day beds in hospitals.

While some of the wardens thought these services could be provided as part of a special service for homeless people, others, like this warden of a short-stay hostel in East London, were uneasy about extending special and separate provision - 'Generally I would be unhappy about us providing more on-site facilities. I would rather they plugged into existing services.' Similarly, in Camden one of the day centre wardens expressed indignation at his centre having to pay for a district nurse. He said - 'What she is doing should be what everyone can receive on the NHS. We are supplementing the NHS. Just as other sections of the population can receive district nursing services paid for by the NHS, so should the homeless here.'

Future provision of primary health care for homeless people

To get some idea of the impact of the pilot schemes on the pattern of use of health care services by homeless people using the centres, we asked the wardens where their clients had sought primary health care before the local pilot project had been set up. We also asked them where they thought these people would seek care if the project team's services were no longer available.

Previous use of primary health care

The situation in each centre depended on a number of factors. These included whether or not the centre had a history of providing some sort of medical cover; the availability of other local facilities; and the pattern of use of health care services by the clientele in individual centres. The particular circumstances of the centres are described on a case-study basis below. However, several common factors did emerge. In East London, homeless people had relied heavily on one particular doctor before the pilot scheme had been set up, and there was some concern among wardens about the type and quality of care they had received. In both project localities there seemed to be little optimism that homeless people would of their own accord make more use of local GPs if the special services were discontinued without an effort being made to arrange a handover to local practices. In the absence of such action to achieve continuity it was thought more likely that they would slip back into their earlier patterns of use. There was also general concern that, without the availability of the pilot schemes, there would once again be a pool of homeless people who would not bother to seek medical care until they were seriously ill.

Case 1. A day centre in East London where volunteer nurses provided a service both before the pilot scheme was set up, and alongside the project team. Here the warden said that, before the project team started visiting, clients wanting medical care might have bumped into one of the volunteer nurses on a casual basis. He added that it was 'awful looking back and nine times out of ten we provided nothing'. He was aware that some people had used a particular doctor in East London who was known to take on the homeless, but that since the project doctor had been available this local doctor's name had not been mentioned by clients. As to what he thought would happen if the pilot scheme was withdrawn, he said - 'They would probably fall back into their old ways of not bothering or perhaps expecting us to carry on providing some kind of health care'. He did not think many people in his centre would use the local accident and emergency department.

Case 2. A day centre in East London where no medical service had been provided before the inception of the pilot scheme. The co-ordinator said that, before the HHELP project, day centre users had obtained health care from three main sources: the local accident and emergency department; a nursing sister, who had provided a form of nurse practitioner service for the homeless; and the same local doctor that we had been told about in other centres. She speculated that if the pilot scheme were withdrawn, the majority would be forced to rely on the local casualty department.

Case 3. A short-stay hostel in East London. A local doctor had provided a weekly surgery here, but the co-ordinator told us that the centre had stopped using his services before the pilot project had been set up because 'we didn't like the level and type of service he provided'. He said that those who had become dependent on drugs would still use this doctor rather than, or as well as, the project doctor because he was more likely to prescribe drugs. He thought that if the scheme was withdrawn word would travel fast and residents would return to using this other GP.

Case 4. A day centre in East London. Before the introduction of the pilot service, people attending this centre had either sought help from the nurse practitioner mentioned above, who then held a clinic in another local day centre, or from two local GPs. They had occasionally used the medical service provided on a voluntary basis at a nearby Mission. The regular clinic provided by the project doctor at this day centre had been discontinued during the monitoring period. The warden thought that the reason for the withdrawal was because the project doctor had thought that take-up had been low, but he regretted this decision. He said, 'the service needs time to be built up. There is no tradition of medical service here and that explains why take-up is low at the moment.'

He conceded that there was a big overlap (perhaps 80-90 per cent) of clients between the centres attended by the doctor and other team members and that there was a long tradition of medical care at one of these centres which people habitually used. He said that users would now see the project doctor at this or other local day centres. Asked whether he thought it mattered that the doctor's services were no longer available at his centre he commented - 'I think it will strike them, the clients, inasmuch as they will not have a complete service available to them as homeless people... There will be repercussions in terms of the ethos and professionalism of the centre ... In the long run it will weaken the quality of the service.' Concerning the impact of the doctor's decision on the centre he added - 'Within his priorities he's got reason... his priorities don't include us as a centre, and that's our priority'.

Case 5. A detoxification centre in East London. Before the project doctor started visiting this centre on a regular basis, they had the services of two local doctors. One of these doctors was now in practice elsewhere, but the other continued to provided a weekly session on Saturdays. Staff in this centre were already having discussions about what would happen after March 1989, when the initial funding for the pilot scheme expired. If the project's services were no longer available, they would consider the feasibility of making greater use of the resources provided by one of the local alcohol agencies.

Case 6. A day centre in Camden. The warden in this centre had only recently been appointed and was unsure where users had sought medical help in the past. He said that if the project team's services were discontinued, he hoped day centre users would seek medical care from 'the new Marylebone Centre in the crypt'. He was very much committed to collaborating with other local agencies and hoped to set up a joint group with this new medical centre to see how they could help each other. He also told us that a new CPN had been appointed by Bloomsbury Health Authority and the day centre had offered him the opportunity to run groups on the premises for users.

Case 7. A Drop-in Centre in Camden. The warden told us that before the project doctor and nurse had started holding regular clinics, most of the users had gone to the local accident and emergency department. Often they would only go if they felt very ill and minor illnesses had been neglected. If the project doctor and nurse were withdrawn he suspected that, as in the past, some of the people attending his centre would not bother to seek help and others would revert to using the accident and emergency department.

Case 8. A shelter in Camden providing accommodation and outreach teamwork. The pilot scheme's services had not been available at this centre until late in the monitoring period. The co-ordinator thought that people who before had limited or no access to a doctor were now getting seen. If the scheme were to be discontinued, many of these would not get medical care at all.

Need for special provision of primary health care services?

Did the wardens think that homeless people in their locality needed special and separate provision of primary health care services? We asked them this both at the beginning and end of the monitoring period. Early in 1987, six out of the seven wardens we spoke to thought that special and separate services were necessary, but their views on this were heavily qualified. Several drew the distinction between what they would ideally like to see and what they thought was appropriate given the reality of homelessness. As one of the day centre wardens told us - 'Yes, given the circumstances but ideally no'. He felt that the fundamental problem was housing and that 'there needs to be specialist provision because there is no point dealing with psychiatric and health problems if they have nowhere to live. Ideally it would be best if people could use ordinary systems, but given current circumstances specialist services are necessary.'

Another distinction was made between what was appropriate in the short term and what should the long-term aim. One of the wardens in East London said - '*Initially* a good proportion of homeless people need specialised care. Perhaps some of the individuals in hostels are capable of registering with a local GP and receiving proper medical care but many of the homeless, especially those on the street, find their only effective contact with society is through places like day centres. Therefore there should be a medical service for them *at* the day centres.'

The observation that some but not all homeless people needed special provision was also made by one of the co-ordinators at the short-stay hostel in East London:

> Some of them do need special services. We get so many different kinds. Some would register with a local GP like anybody else if possible. Some are reluctant to go to a local GP of their own accord. It is safer and easier to see a GP in this room. The pilot scheme is a first step, but not for ever. We would like to see the end of special schemes but for that to happen the NHS would have to adapt and change and we can't see it is likely to. While it isn't coping with their needs, they need something else. People who use the project doctor are getting a better service than most people.

A number of other reasons were given to explain why integration into mainstream services was unrealistic for all homeless people. The warden from the detoxification centre explained that people in his centre often needed special services because the combination of alcohol abuse and homelessness led to problems which could not be easily accommodated within mainstream provision. He thought that, having become homeless, it was often difficult then to settle in stable circumstances, yet medical services were generally geared to a stable environment.

A warden in Camden told us that integration into mainstream services would not work for two main reasons: first, because of the way the system was organised; and second, because GPs and other health care professionals were only human and there would always be intolerant as well as tolerant ones among them. In another day centre in the same locality, which was regularly used by some of the most disturbed and unkempt people we met during the client interviews, the warden commented - 'A lot of them are aware of their appearance and they are embarrassed about it. They also tend to be loners, so to try and get them into a normal health centre setting is unrealistic. They don't want to go.'

The one person who argued against special provision said she was keenly aware that homeless people and those in bad or insecure housing had difficulty in being accepted into the normal system, but that these difficulties did not just apply to the homeless. She felt that the services offered by the pilot scheme should be extended to people in different circumstances. They should be integrated into existing NHS provision but this provision should be more informal and community-based.

When we interviewed the wardens again towards the end of 1987 their views had hardly changed, although in most cases they had been reinforced. Referring specifically to what he saw as the invaluable role of the pilot scheme one person told us - 'The aim of the programme was to try and route people into the services available. But there has been no abatement in homelessness. The East End is a magnet. You have to provide special provison. There are other projects trying to help but having a special team is invaluable. It is an incredible resource and we couldn't do without it.' Another warden argued that it was too soon to withdraw special provision - 'We do still need special provision because contact and education is necessary for them to be registered with and accepted by local GPs. We have not progressed far enough in this area. More work needs to be done and in the meantime, HHELP's services are useful.'

The one person who had been uneasy early in 1987 about special provision was more inclined to support it after several months' experience of the pilot scheme. She said - 'I have seen the take-up which seems to be large. There is a need. But I still have ambivalence over "special needs". I feel the service has valuable elements that could be extended to others in the community; for example, women and ethnic minorities who have difficulty in getting primary health care.'

In Camden the project team extended their services to another centre in the autumn and the coordinators we spoke to here was in two minds about special provision - 'I'm not sure. They should have better access to health care, but I'm not sure that setting up separate provision doesn't isolate them more. Ideally they should use a normal GP but as society is today, it is not easy.'

Feasibility of permanent GP registration

Approaching the issue of special provision or integrated services from a different angle, we also asked the wardens how far they thought the objective of getting homeless people to register permanently with a local GP was feasible. Opinion in the short-stay hostel was that from the point of view of the residents it was feasible, but from the GP's point of view perhaps it would not be. We were told it would be simple for the hostel staff to make it part of their administrative procedures that residents registered with a local GP and brought proof back. However, it was thought that GPs would be unlikely to accept them because of their lack of long-term residence.

A diversity of views were expressed by the day centre wardens. We were told by one in East London that if the centre conducted a registration drive they could perhaps put 20-25 per cent of their attenders on the list of a GP. However, he qualified the value of this by saying - 'But again the quality of care they get is questionable. I would tend to think the main problem is the awareness of GPs. If they were more sensitised to the issues it would be easier and more plausible to conduct a registration drive.' He admitted that a reason why the centre had not campaigned harder about health care issues and encouraged clients to register and make contact with local GPs was because 'we've relied on the project doctors'.

In another day centre in East London it had been estimated that perhaps 90 per cent of users could be registered with a GP, but towards the end of the monitoring period the warden admitted that this figure had been over-ambitious - 'We had high hopes that the project doctor's role would be to slot people onto GPs' lists. Now we think this is not realitic because GPs' lists are full. Initially we were against primary health care being done by a special team because we wanted people to go on to GPs' lists. Having had the team here has changed our view. I

185

have seen what is done and how, and what is being offered is not a second class service.'

The pilot scheme was seen by another East London warden as a first step towards encouraging people to register with local GPs and he thought that for a large percentage this aim was realistic. He suggested that a useful development of the initiative would be to use local GPs on a sessional basis within the day centres. These GPs could initially see people at the centres, but once they had built up a relationship with them they could then encourage them to visit the surgery. But a more pessimistic view was expressed by this warden - 'There will always be a number of homeless people who choose not to register and such people are exploiters of anything and everything'.

There were also conflicting views in Camden about the feasibility of getting homeless people to register with a local GP and this may in part be explained by the different mix of homeless people attending the centres. One warden told us - 'It would prove very difficult because of client attitudes and the attitudes of GPs and other health workers. If one or two get a bad experience, word travels like wild fire.' He drew a parallel between trying to get clients registered with GPs and trying to integrate them into the community in other ways - 'We get tutors from the Camden Institute coming in to teach with the aim of getting individuals to join the institute. Only a few will join and it is the same with GPs.' He added that it could be done if the centre arranged transport to take them to a GP for mass registration, but they would then be intimidated. He explained - 'They are conscious of their dirty and smelly appearance. We would have to go with them. Historically it doesn't work.'

The newly appointed warden of another centre in Camden was more optimistic and said - 'I would have thought for a sizeable percentage of users here it is possible. But there is a core of people in the forties age group and above who would be difficult to attract into the system. But the younger ones, who have not been homeless so long and are used to using ordinary medical services, could be persuaded back into the health service proper.' His predecessor had been less positive - 'I don't think it is feasible for the vast majority. If you are not concerned that your lifestyle is detrimental to your health and lifespan then it is unlikely you will register with a GP. A large problem is their motivation which is so low. Motivation, or lack of it, is a central problem in homelessness. After years of it, people are debilitated.'

Transferability of model to other areas

All the wardens agreed that as a way of improving the provision of primary health care services to homeless people the pilot project as developed in their locality could be transferred successfully to other areas. One told us - 'I have no direct experience of homelessness in other cities but there is a national problem and the same needs would be apparent and the same response would be necessary'. But others were more circumspect in their recommendations. In one East London centre we were told - 'It could be transferred, but whether or not it is advisable I don't know. Many workers with the homeless are against special schemes so there would be practical problems.'

Another view was that, although it was very important to transfer the approach developed by the pilot scheme to areas where there was demonstrable need, these areas would have to be selected carefully so that there were a cluster of local agencies to participate in the scheme. This point was reinforced by one of the day centre wardens in Camden who was in favour of developing the model elsewhere, but said - 'It would have to be in the right place; for example, where there were centres like this, night shelters with a high turnover, and outreach work'. One of the wardens in Camden argued that the model might only work if were sited in established day centres where it could be seen as just one of the facilities provided. He said - 'If you opened a special surgery for the homeless it might not work. Here it is part of the general service offered, along with the workshop, telly, canteen etc. It is part of the total wholeness of the individual. We get more use than Great Chapel Street centre. It is more likely to be used because it is part of their own environment. Just as mum, dad, husband or wife would advise on health, the staff fulfil this role. Therefore I favour this arrangement to a separate drop-in centre for medical care.'

Several of the wardens stressed the importance of taking local needs into account and we were also told in two of the Camden centres that the model could be improved by extending the outreach work to street work, with doctors and nurses identifying and helping the homeless on the street. One of the co-ordinators explained - 'In some respects it could be transferred successfully if it were put in centres with grass roots contact on the streets. But if it is put in places which are solely day centres these exclude those people who are more isolated and don't want to be in a group.'

Future of the pilot schemes

So what did the wardens think should happen to the pilot scheme in their locality once the initial period of funding expired? In East London centres there was general consensus that the local pilot scheme should be continued, either in its current form or with some modifications. Depressed by what he saw to be the ever growing problem of homelessness, one co-ordinator told us - 'If the present climate continues I feel the team could continue for ever. It depends on what happens elsewhere in the NHS. If it is on the cards that St. Clement's Hospital will close, I can only see gloom and woe ... I can't see an alternative at the present time.' And an equally strong position was taken by the warden who said - 'I think it should be maintained. It would leave an enormous vacuum if it were taken away.'

Another could see no advantage in permanent registration with local GPs and took the view that - 'The way the project is operating at present is the best. I'm not necessarily in favour of encouraging or forcing people to register with local GPs. I'm not sure of the advantages. The project services are provided by people who *want* to help the homeless and that is preferable.' Even those, like this warden, who ideally favoured integrating homeless people into mainstream GP services did not think that this was realistic at this point in time - 'Potentially the doctor's services could be taken up by local GPs but as yet I'm not aware that there is sufficient sympathy among local GPs for that to happen. Until it does, it would be dangerous to lose the GP.'

A number of suggestions were made about how the pilot scheme in East London could be improved if it were to be retained. In one centre we were told that it was important for the team to provide a more supportive role to staff working in the centres, not just direct service provision. This day centre also wanted to be consulted more about the project team's activities. Strong arguments were made in favour of retaining the specialities where there was under-servicing for the homeless, particularly in the fields of mental health, social work support, general counselling and women's needs. Emphasis was placed on the importance of the social worker's role and we were told - 'There is no point having a team if it is only medical with no housing back-up'. The social worker was also thought to contribute valuable expertise in resettlement work and on welfare rights issues.

But it was suggested by several wardens that the medical input could be better provided by *local* GPs, who would need to be willing to liaise with other agencies working with the homeless. As one person told us - 'The doctor's role could be a community facility in that GPs could do sessions here but have their own local practices. They could entice people to their practices. But this would take time.' From the doctor's point of view this approach was thought to be more satisfactory than using a salaried doctor designated for the homeless because the local GPs would not be dealing solely with homeless people.

In Camden, where the project team was smaller and more medically based than in East London, one of the wardens made a case for retaining the scheme, but expanding the team to include a CPN and an alcohol counsellor. He thought that a bigger team would be able to go to other day centres and night shelters and could begin to do outreach work on the streets with those homeless people who for one reason or another chose not to use these centres.

Linking the future of the pilot scheme to the way he wanted to develop the practice and philosophy of his day centre, another warden we spoke to in Camden supported the continuation of the scheme with the proviso that it should become part of the overall service offered by the centre. He explained that the funding implications for the project team were that they would be contracted to the centre and not set up and funded separately from the other services on offer. The budgetary implications for the centre were that to make this a reality it would need to raise funds and attract grants to be able to contract these staff.

Throughout this chapter it has become clear that in weighing up the impact of the pilot schemes the wardens were looking to improve the services available to their users both directly through improved service provision, and indirectly through enhancing the facilities offered by their centres. They were concerned about improving the quality of health care services used by homeless people and their access to these services. They were also interested in what was good for the practice and philosophy of their centres.

A clear message emerging from the centres was that the wardens were supportive of the schemes. They rated them as highly successful in terms of improving health care provision and, in East London, ancillary services for homeless people using their centres. They also valued the support that individual team members had given to centre staff.

8 Views of Professionals and Voluntary Workers

How appropriate are mainstream primary health care services to the needs and circumstances of homeless people? Do health care professionals who provide these services think that homeless people can be integrated into mainstream provision or do they favour special provision of primary care services for the single homeless? How far do their views coincide or conflict with the views of those working in the voluntary sector who have an interest in the health care of homeless people? We interviewed health care professionals working in the localities of the two pilot schemes to explore these and related issues, and to find out what they knew and thought about the DHSS pilot schemes. An explanation of our sampling procedure, with a list of all the authorities and agencies contacted and a discussion of the response rate, is included in Appendix 1. We also covered the same ground in interviews with representatives of local organisations concerned with the health and housing needs of homeless people.

The sample
We spoke to a total of 76 professionals providing care in the community. These included 34 local GPs, 17 district nurses, 20 community psychiatric nurses and 5 social workers. Concern about the use of hospital accident and emergency departments by homeless people is documented in the literature review and as homeless people often use these departments instead of going to a GP, we also interviewed 15 professionals either working in or taking referrals from the departments

191

of two large London teaching hospitals; one in East London and the other in West London. These included six senior house officers (SHOs), six nurses and three social workers. We also talked to the consultant in accident and emergency in each hospital. The views of the voluntary sector were provided by representatives from 14 local organisations; most of these were voluntary bodies, but two were council-run centres used by homeless people. In East London we also held a group discussion with Salvation Army officers.

General medical practitioners

We interviewed a total of 34 GPs: 18 had practices in the vicinity of the City and East London project and were selected at random from the City and East London FPC's list of general medical practitioners; and 16 were in the locality of the Camden project and were selected from the lists supplied by Camden and Islington FPC and Kensington, Chelsea and Westminster FPC. Twenty-six of the GPs were male and eight were female. They were broadly spread in terms of age: nine per cent were in their twenties, 24 per cent in their thirties, 33 per cent in their forties, and 34 per cent were over 50. Almost half the GPs had worked in the same locality for more than ten years and 36 per cent had been there for between five and ten years.

In both areas the practice arrangements of the 34 GPs we spoke to were varied: a total of 26 GPs (76 per cent) worked in a group practice with more than half based in health centres; five were single-handed GPs and three were each involved in a partnership with one other GP. Although we were interested in list size as one indicator of work-load, the information we collected from GPs was not comparable. Single-handed GPs were able to give us an indication of their list size, which averaged around 2,100 patients, but those working in a partnership or group practice did not distinguish the number of patients on their own list from the total number of patients registered with the practice.

Nature and extent of involvement in service provision for homeless people

The overwhelming majority of GPs in our sample said there was one or more hostel, night shelter or day centre used by homeless people within a one mile radius of their surgery, but *none* of the GPs provided regular sessions at any of these centres. One of the doctors in East London described himself as a visiting medical officer to a large hostel for homeless men, but said that the small retainer paid to his practice by the local authority was not to cover regular sessions. It was simply a nominal payment to ensure that the hostel had a GP on call, and he said that he would provide this cover anyway because the hostel was on his doorstep.

Almost half the GPs reported that although they did not provide regular sessions at centres catering for homeless people, they had been called out in the previous year to provide emergency services to a user or resident at one of these places. However, for many of these doctors such visits had been infrequent; just under half had been called out in these circumstances five times or less during the previous year. One GP working in a health centre in East London said that he was regularly called out once or twice a week by centres used by homeless people. He was an exceptional case and argued that all GPs had to 'muck in' and that their responsibility to provide care for people in their locality included looking after their share of homeless people.

We also asked all the GPs in our sample whether or not they had treated any homeless people at their practice surgery, as opposed to visiting them in hostels, night shelters or day centres. All but two said that they did see homeless people at their practices. But further questioning made it clear that several were talking hypothetically about what they would do if a homeless person turned up at their surgery. So far this had not happened, but they insisted that they would provide treatment to any homeless person who did attend. We do not know the extent to which this intention would be translated into actual behaviour.

Registration policy: practice and problems
As noted frequently throughout this study, the reluctance of GPs to treat homeless people is often cited as the main reason behind the difficulties of access to primary health care by single homeless people (Liverpool CHC). We have already heard the consumers' view of services provided by GPs, but if the integration of homeless people into present general practice provision is going to be considered as a serious option then it is also important to understand the problem as perceived by the

providers of these services. We therefore asked the GPs about their registration policy with regard to homeless patients. In particular, we wanted to know what problems they associated with permanently registering homeless people, and whether for the purposes of *permanent registration* it made a difference to them if the person was a hostel resident or of no fixed abode.

The GPs used a variety of types of registration or claims forms when treating homeless people. Temporary resident registration was the most common form of registration and was mentioned by just over 90 per cent of our sample. Just over half said they might take some homeless people on their lists on a permanent basis, but several took the same view as the East London GP who said that 'the more efficient the FPC is at taking people off the lists the more reluctant GPs are to permanently register them'. Almost half said they sometimes used immediately necessary treatment forms and a couple recalled claiming the emergency treatment fee for a patient who was homeless. While the majority were familiar with the different ways in which they could treat homeless people, a few, like this GP in Camden who had not actually seen anyone who said they were homeless, were not entirely clear about the regulations: 'It would depend on how long they are in the area. I have only just discovered the form that can be used for immediately necessarily treatment. I would probably use this if the person was not staying in the area. Do GPs know about this form? I didn't.'

A minority said there were no particular difficulties involved in registering the homeless, but the majority (28 GPs) described a range of problems which they had either experienced or anticipated. The fundamental problem which was identified by more than half these GPs, and which was seen as giving rise to a myriad of other obstacles to continuing care, was the *mobility* of homeless people. In the words of one West London GP:

> The problem is their mobility which creates extra work for us all. They can't guarantee staying in this area and they may go and see another GP if they are unwell. It is purely a difficulty of them not staying in the same place. There is no point beginning a long investigation if they are not going to

be here long. You don't want to start unnecessary investigations at one hospital and then again at another.

We were frequently told that the problem was primarily a bureaucratic one. It was said that the FPC did not allow a GP to register permanently a patient who did not have an address. But often the problems created by mobility were closely associated with financial as well as bureaucratic disincentives. One GP in East London explained the financial disadvantage involved in permanently registering a patient who, within the same quarter year period, moves on and registers with another GP: 'The problem is a logistical one. If we sign someone on to claim the capitation fee and they've disappeared by the end of that quarter and registered with another GP, no matter how many times we have seen them we don't receive a penny. The hassle would be financial as well as administrative.' Another GP in East London stated the problem more bluntly - 'It's a money problem. If people come and go in a quarter they don't stay on our books long enough to allow us to get paid, so the system isn't conducive to looking after homeless people.'

Another common theme was the difficulty of fulfilling their contract to provide 24 hour care to patients who lived in hostels or night shelters or were on the streets. As one GP in NW1 pointed out - 'You can't pin them down. Hostels are often night shelters and you cannot visit them in the day. It is difficult to get messages to them. You don't have time to go into the places as a routine thing. If we had more money we would at least be able to do that.' And another GP in the same area asked - 'If he is of no fixed abode how can I visit him? What am I supposed to do? I'll give him immediate treatment. If he is registered on a permanent basis and the same week he is moving I don't get paid a penny. It's better for me to register them for immediate treatment and then I'm paid.'

Almost three-quarters of the GPs said that for the purposes of permanent registration with them it *did* make a difference whether the person was a hostel resident or on the streets. Of these, just over two-thirds referred to the registration policy of the FPC, which most understood to mean that they could not permanently register someone who did not have an address. For one GP in this group the question was perceived as 'quite ludicrous' because it was his view that 'A doctor who registers NFAs as permanent would be in breach of contract'. For another GP in East London the situation was much less clear cut - 'I don't know if you can register them permanently if they are of no fixed abode. I'd check. If you could perhaps it would not make a difference. I'd register them and I suppose they'd disappear, but so do other people.'

People living in hostels were not necessarily viewed as homeless by the GPs, in contrast to those living on the streets. Just over a quarter of the GPs who said the difference in accommodation status was relevant to registration were prepared to register hostel residents permanently, but not people of no fixed abode. As one GP in East London explained, this was partly because they were seen as less transitory and they did have a current address where the GP could visit them - 'I'd prefer to register hostel people. They are more permanent and some stay in hostels for a time and we know where to go if they need home visits. It is impossible to follow others up as they keep moving on.' But another GP questioned the basis of this distinction - 'The problem is that you can't visit them if they are NFA. They have to come and see you. My instant reaction is to say I would rather have them in a hostel but there is actually no difference whatsoever. To say there is a difference is an emotional reaction rather than a logical reaction.'

Another commonly given reason for not wanting to register people of no fixed abode was the difficulty of obtaining medical records. This comment by a GP in a group practice in Camden was typical - 'We're not keen on no fixed abode because of the difficulty of acquiring medical records. And again their mobility and the fact that they tend to be single. We prefer families if we can. People in hostels seem to be fine.' As with this young GP in NW1, many GPs were also more generally critical of the way the medical record system worked, or rather did not work - 'It is impossible to give adequate care without records. The present system of getting records is anachronistic, outdated and appalling like a double decker bus being pushed backwards across the Sahara.'

Problems in providing medical care for homeless people

Although we initially got GPs to focus on the difficulties they associated with *permanently registering* homeless people, we also asked them whether there were any other problems which made it difficult for them to provide care for homeless people at their practice surgeries. Well over a third of the GPs in our sample said there were no other difficulties, and those who did perceive other difficulties in caring for homeless people at their surgeries tended to distinguish between different groups: for example, single homeless people, homeless families in bed and breakfast accommodation, alcoholics, drug addicts and those with chronic mental health problems.

A common belief was that homeless people tended to use a number of doctors and that this made continuity of care exceptionally difficult. As one GP in West London told us - 'We've no previous records on them with the result that we've no communication and there is nothing to stop these people from seeing me one day and going round the corner to another doctor the next day'. There was particular concern about prescribing drugs for homeless people, both because of the difficulty of checking the past medical history of the patient and because they could not be sure that the patient was not already getting drugs from another GP.

We heard from the consumers that they found it difficult to cope with appointment systems, and a complaint made by several GPs was that homeless patients were more likely not to turn up for appointments. This had made several GPs sceptical about the value of referring homeless people for investigation or treatment, as with this GP in West London - 'Even if you refer them they don't attend hospital and their appointment could have been given to a genuine patient'.

Homeless people were also commonly thought to make high demands on both time and resources. The point was made forcibly by one GP in NW1 that they were often seen as an unwelcome burden on the work-load of already over-stretched GPs - 'Some are abusive and a higher proportion are deceitful. A high proportion look for drugs through deceitful means. It's more time-consuming dealing with people from these complicated social backgrounds who have multiple physical and emotional problems, time-consuming and emotionally draining on me.' The burden was seen to fall on the receptionists as well as the GP - 'They are also a tremendous extra burden on the receptionists, who have to sort out all the accompanying problems they bring'.

Then there was the problem of the reaction of their other patients towards homeless people using the surgery. Several GPs, like this doctor in East London, were concerned about - 'The reaction of our other patients, it's their appreciation of it. They are going to have to be in the same waiting room and there are certain anti-social aspects of them, both behavioural and olfactory.' And as a female GP in West London observed - 'The receptionist gets upset and so do the patients. The receptionist likes to keep the surgery smart and tidy.' This view of homeless people was common but certainly not universal among the GPs who perceived difficulties in treating homeless people at their practice surgery. In several cases GPs were critical of themselves and their colleagues for holding on to this stereotype - 'These are the GPs' problems and perceptions. For example, a belief that homeless are likely to be aggressive, hostile and dirty. They are perceptions and might not necessarily hold water as not all homeless people are like that.'

However, even GPs who were particularly sympathetic to the health needs and circumstances of homeless people were concerned about not having sufficient time available to meet these needs, as with this GP in W1 - 'Basically we just don't have the time available. I'm a psychiatrist in general practice and I know what's needed but it can't be done. It takes a lot of time.' And another concerned GP in East London explained that it was not just a problem of time, but also one of trying to do the job without adequate support services and often from unsatisfactory practice premises - 'We really don't have enough back-up services to cater for the social, emotional and physical problems that they have. We need lots of social workers whom we don't have and also don't have the room for.'

A problem identified by GPs who were prepared to take on homeless people was that too many of their colleagues were not willing to share the burden. As one GP in a health centre in NW5 told us - 'The only difference in treating homeless people is in terms of numbers. By coincidence homeless families present a variety of social problems. It would be unreasonable for us to take on too many. It wouldn't be good from anyone's point of view if the numbers exceeded five per cent of the practice.' And another West London GP argued - 'If there is only one doctor in the locality prepared to treat them, it puts all the burden on him, whereas it should be on a patch basis with each GP obliged to treat those in his area.'

Health care problems of homeless people

The most commonly mentioned health problem of single homeless people was alcohol abuse. In both areas just over three-quarters of the GPs we spoke to thought that the health problems of the single homeless were often alcohol-related. A similar proportion of GPs in West London also mentioned the problem of drug abuse, but in East London fewer GPs mentioned it. In East London, however, respiratory problems seemed to be more common. Nearly half the GPs in this area perceived respiratory complaints as a major health problem of the single homeless whereas no GPs did in Camden. Psychiatric illness was identified as a major problem by over half the GPs in both project sites. GPs also mentioned gastrointestinal conditions, dermatological complaints, poor nutrition, smoking, poor hygiene, general debilitation and poor living conditions. In addition, the homeless were thought by several GPs to be more vulnerable to everyday infections and ailments.

The health needs and problems of homeless families were perceived to be rather different from those of the single homeless, as this GP in NW1 pointed out - 'The health needs of homeless families are different: overcrowding, social deprivation, lots of problems, highly stressed and often language problems, and poor user knowledge of services. Overcrowding increases the incidence of minor problems. They are disadvantaged in every way. Very basic things like vaccination schedules which require organisation are difficult to organise. They are a group with a high degree of medical problems.'

According to almost half the GPs in both localities, homeless families have an exceptionally high degree of social as well as medical problems. And like this GP in East London, most GPs felt ill-equipped to cope with the the fundamental social problems - 'Basically I am a doctor and have to accept there are basic social problems that no matter what the NHS can do, until you can actually provide the basic home, hot water etc. that they need, a few tranquillizers aren't going to solve the problem. It's basically a social problem initially, rather than a medical one.'

In both areas stress was perceived as a major health hazard for homeless families and psychiatric illness was thought to be common. We were told by one doctor in West London - 'Stress is a major problem. It's mostly the families who don't know the system. They don't speak the language so they've got cultural isolation. A lot of young children and wives are not able to take time to rest and recuperate and are in a situation of being away from family support.' GPs often referred to the specific vulnerability of children, particularly their susceptibility to infections.

Several GPs were scathingly sceptical about the problem of homelessness per se, as in the case of this GP in W1 who said - 'Why are they homeless? It's their lifestyle. These people are sure the world owes them a living and Camden is a soft touch and we're near Euston and Kings Cross. Camden owns 70 per cent of housing so there shouldn't be any homeless.' Another commented - 'They go homeless on occasion in order to improve their chances of better housing. This leads to difficulties in primary health care provision as addresses are often falsified or become inaccurate before recall letters arrive. We can never find them.'

And a tiny minority, like this doctor in East London, commented on the personal inadequacy of homeless people - 'Some of the major problems are poverty, wife beating, smoking, eating the wrong food. They are inadequate people, bad ancestry, bad parents, bad upbringing, less brain. They are more likely to be homeless, more stupid and get into debt.' A similar observation was made by a GP in NW1 - 'They must be psychologically inadequate or why are they homeless? There is no need for it. I don't think they want to settle anywhere. They like to keep moving.' Faced with views such as these, perhaps it is not surprising that some homeless people feel doubtful about the welcome they will receive at GPs' surgeries.

Around half the GPs we spoke to thought that the health problems of homeless people differed from those of the general population in the area, and this tendency was more marked in West London. In particular homeless people were thought to have a higher incidence of alcohol-related problems, personality problems, drug-related problems and psychiatric illness. The homeless were also thought to have lower expectations about their health than the general population. As this GP commented - 'The general population seeks medical advice earlier, takes treatment more seriously. The homeless put off going to doctors and rely on treatment advised by friends, which is not always the best for them.' And like this GP in East London, several observed that it was actually the lack of accommodation that differentiated the health problems of homeless people from those of the general population - 'It's the context of the problem, the homelessness, which makes the difference.'

Present provision of primary health care services for homeless people

Just under a quarter of all GPs interviewed thought that existing provision of primary health care services for homeless people was satisfactory. Referring to the policy of his own practice one GP in East London insisted:

I think there was perfectly good provision before the pilot project started. Our surgery is open 9 - 6.30 every day. We don't discriminate between people in any way, whether based on gender, colour, creed or domestic situation. We treat many homeless people who are free to consult us whether registered with us or not. I myself am the visiting medical officer to the largest hostel for homeless men. My senior partner for many years has had large numbers of NFAs under his wing. No one has been turned away on account of their social circumstances and it is for this reason that I do not think the pilot service is necessary.

However, although these GPs thought that existing facilities were adequate, it did not necessarily mean that they thought that homeless people were able or willing to make good use of primary health care services. As another GP in East London observed - 'I think the facilities are there but it is a question of the consumer getting together with the resources. In this area, we are well endowed with various organisations to help the under-privileged. It's a question of co-ordination so that the goodwill available can be organised to the best benefit of those who need it. It would be difficult for someone who didn't know their way about the administrative jungle to find their way to the care'.

In direct contrast, a similar proportion of GPs explicitly said that existing provision of health care for homeless people, excluding the pilot schemes, was generally poor. One GP in East London said - 'Provision is poor apart from the project. There is scattered charitable provision. Not much change since Dickensian London.' And another told us:

We don't provide primary health care for the homeless at all... We don't cater properly for people who are made homeless and put into hostels where they are out of sight. They tend to traipse back to us all the way from Kensington because they can't be seen locally. I don't think this is a deliberate end. It's part of the NHS that those out of the sphere of the NHS find it difficult to enter. Perhaps our system has too much rigidity. There is also the separate issue of how much the State should take responsibility and how much should be left to the individual, though some cannot take responsibility for themselves.

In West London existing provision was condemned by one GP as 'Abysmal!'.

Several GPs admitted that their comments were based on impressions and gut feeling rather than on firm evidence - 'A lot of people slip through the net. It's purely a feeling that a lot of people are not registered and not known. I've no evidence.' In addition, several had had no experience of providing health care for homeless people but had been influenced by what they had read about the issue - 'I assume from what I read it is substandard. People find it difficult to register and doctors are reluctant to take them on. The homeless are tending to be taken into hostels. Health care is reflecting marginalisation instead of integration.'

But one East London GP in particular argued that he had plenty of evidence to suggest that the majority of his colleagues were not prepared to take on homeless people:

As far as I understand, and I've been treating homeless people for 17 years and have an open door policy, I'm seeing more and more. I have to ask, why are more coming to see me? Why do voluntary agencies ring me up for help? I think the vast majority of GPs won't see these patients. This is borne out by conversations I have had with voluntary workers. This is at cross purposes to what GPs will say. They will indicate they do, but they don't act. No one wants to take the medical profession on and accuse them openly of not seeing these people.

Around half the GPs we spoke to were non-committal about whether or not they thought that existing services were adequate. Several said they felt unable to comment because they had had no direct experience of the problem. A few speculated that it would be difficult to integrate homeless people into existing GP services for all the reasons they had given when discussing their registration policy. Almost a quarter of answered the question by making positive reference to the pilot schemes, and this could be interpreted as indirect criticism of existing provision.

The pilot schemes

Knowledge of the schemes

Just over three-quarters of the GPs in both areas said they knew about the pilot schemes. They had heard about them from a number of sources: several had found out about them through contact with a project team member; others had been informed about them by the local FPC or had read about them in the medical press or literature about the project; and a few had learned about them through professional or academic contact at conferences or meetings. In weighing up the impact of the pilot schemes on local providers of services, it is important to note than a total of eight GPs, four in East London and four in West London, said they had heard nothing at all about the schemes. After further questioning, it also became clear that several of the GPs who said they had heard about the inception of the schemes knew nothing about their objectives or progress.

Objectives of the schemes

There was no clear consensus about the objectives of the pilot schemes, other than the general observation that they had been set up to improve the local provision of primary health care for homeless people. Just under a third of GPs who knew about the schemes thought they had been set up to plug the gap in current provision created by the reluctance of ordinary GPs to take on the homeless. As one GP in NW1 explained - 'Since local GPs were not keen to look after these people a scheme had to be formulated and the DHSS hasn't got provision in the normal way of looking after people who are not registered. They had to find an alternative scheme to give the homeless the medical care they need.'

However, this additional form of service provision was seen as totally unnecessary by one or two GPs, like this doctor in W1 - 'It is creating a second tier of primary health care and quite unnecessary in this age when cuts have to be made everywhere. I think it's a waste of resources and money ... there are adequate GPs in this area who cater for them. I resent any need for a special doctor and special nurse.'

Several GPs thought that the main objective was to take health care to places where homeless people congregate, thus making it more accessible, a view expressed by this doctor in East London - 'The purpose is to bring health care to that section of the community which is not able to get it through their own volition either through their own ignorance or inability or inclination'. An alternative understanding, put forward by another GP in East London, was that the scheme provided 'a separate walk-in clinic for homeless people'.

Encouraging homeless people to register with GPs was singled out as the main objective by several GPs in both areas but, as with this GP in East London, some were unclear about the current status of this objective:

> The pilot project was set up not so much to provide medical care but to make it easier for homeless people to be registered and to find out who would see them. If that is the case then they have failed abysmally. The project know I see homeless people, temporary or permanent, but they have never rung me to ask me to take someone on my books. Therefore I presume what they had as their remit has changed. Either the DHSS has changed the remit or they have themselves.

And as this comment by a GP in West London illustrates, some were unsure whether the project was temporary or permanent - 'I'm not totally clear if it's permanent or a way of getting established GPs to look after homeless people in the future. I think the centre is probably permanent.'

A number of other objectives were identified by individual GPs. These included: encouraging homeless people to register with GPs; identifying homeless people who needed a GP; assessing the primary health care needs of the homeless; experimenting with and evaluating a specific model of health care provision; educating professionals about the problems of homelessness; and liaising with other health service providers and agencies.

Interaction between local GPs and the project teams

We found little evidence of interaction between local GPs and the project teams. In particular, in both project sites referrals between the local GPs we interviewed and the schemes were almost non-existent. In West London *none* of the GPs had received a referral from the Camden Project team and only one doctor said he had referred a homeless patient to the pilot scheme; and in East London two GPs said that they had received referrals from the project team and one had made a referral to the scheme.

Apart from referrals, a handful of GPs said that they had had some sort of contact with project team members. This was usually through attendance at meetings or some other form of professional or academic contact, but very occasionally involved case-meetings about a particular patient. We understand that in East London there has been a flurry of activity since we conducted these interviews because the project team have been canvassing local GPs and others about the future of the pilot scheme in that area.

Strengths and weaknesses of the schemes

GPs who said they knew about the schemes gave us their views about the strengths and weaknesses of the schemes as an initiative to improve the provision of primary health care to homeless people. Several said they did not know enough about the way the projects operated to be able to comment, and among the others there were as many views as there were people.

A number of the strengths which were identified concerned the *acceptability* and *accessibility* of the services provided. As this GP commented - 'They are getting to a section of the population who are at greater risk than ordinary members of the population and hopefully picking them up and referring them for treatment for conditions that otherwise may be left until too late for treatment'. They were described as plugging a gap in existing provision, and helping in screening and prevention, and were thought to be respected by hospital services. Another perceived strength was that the project team was mobile and took health care to centres used by homeless people. GPs commented favourably on the experimental and research aspects of the pilot schemes, and also that they educated other service providers about the health care needs and problems of homeless people and provided a link between statutory provision and voluntary agencies.

Another cluster of strengths concerned the *commitment* and *effectiveness* of the team members involved in the pilot schemes. Highlighting the importance of the personality of the project doctor, one GP in West London told us - 'The personality of the doctor who does it is important because it has to be a labour of love. His availability, adaptability, amiability and accessibility are important. The main thing is the doctor. It's he who can make it succeed or fall down dead.' A good many of the GPs thought that it had been the right decision to employ salaried doctors to run the pilot schemes. Explaining why he supported this approach, one West London GP told us - 'A definite person for a definite job. No changing or backing out. A definite contract. And because the person involved would become a specialist with the "know how" about their lifestyle.'

A handful of GPs in both areas thought that the schemes had no strengths and should not have been set up in the first place. Not wanting to dismiss the the efforts of fellow professionals, one GP nevertheless argued - 'We are talking about politics not medicine. I don't think there are any strengths except the goodwill and energy of those involved. In fairness to them this has to be said.' A colleague in East London was equally blunt - 'It is a completely useless, pointless exercise pushed by people with vested interests who want to push the myth of the special needs of the homeless. In my opinion it is completely unnecessary, borne out by the fact that we have never had a referral and did not know that the first project doctor had been replaced. And we have people daily from that category in our surgery anyway.'

There was no consensus of opinion about the weaknesses of the schemes, but some strong views were expressed. A number of GPs thought that a major weakness was the insufficient contact the project teams had with other professionals, and as this NW1 GP said - 'A weakness is probably that they're not part of the GP set-up in a way. It's set up as an independent situation, no links into general practice so that when they've stabilised people they could pass them on to GPs. It would be better done with something like Kentish Town Health Centre, together with a doctor who already had links. No professional links are being built up.' A similar observation was made about the East London project - 'It is fairly isolated from general practice. They wouldn't come and use the health centre clinics as they would use the project. It is providing an extra service for a special group.'

The issue of salaried GPs is clearly key to the structure of the schemes. The fact that the schemes operated with salaried doctors was seen to isolate them further from general practice, as this GP observed - 'Whoever provides this service needs to be well bonded into local services and support. An imposed, salaried GP in general is not.' Insufficient contact with other professionals also included lack of feedback about the scheme. As this GP in East London told us - 'The obvious weakness is that we get no feedback of what they are doing and what they have done so I am unaware of how their work impinges on ours or assists it.'

Some GPs thought that the project teams would inevitably provide a second-class service compared to general practice. They pointed to the drawbacks of using salaried doctors who worked from nine to five with no night or weekend commitment and no locum cover during holidays. One GP in a health centre in NW1 explained - 'It can't provide the same level of care as a practice like this - 24 hour care and other services. It approaches the problem the wrong way. It isolates them more by giving them a doctor who is nine to five, a second-class service. It may be our fault rather than theirs though.'

There was also some concern expressed about the schemes having had insufficient publicity, a lack of resources and support and also organisational and management weaknesses. Additionally, problems connected with continuity of care beyond the life of the schemes were identified. One GP in East London was worried that because of these drawbacks the project had insufficient clout -'Coming at a time when services are contracting, it's a Cinderella group and will have trouble taking off unless they shout loud. It is going largely unrecognised and it is isolated.'

Several GPs thought that the fundamental weakness of the schemes was that the service was simply not needed. As one GP in East London explained - 'I have worked for the past 28 years in Tower Hamlets, a district where there are people who would be considered to be "homeless" (although the term is used to mean several different categories) ... My partners and I have surgeries from 9.30 until 6.30 pm. No appointments are needed - the door is open to anyone. We *never* turn anyone away who needs help. In my opinion, there is no problem of the homeless as far as medical care is concerned. People, homeless or not, are people who have access to the NHS. It is wrong and unnecessary to discriminate in this way.'

But none were as forceful in their arguments against the special schemes as this GP in East London who told us - 'It is an attempt to set up a service for which the need does not exist and it thus a waste of money. Also, it is an attempt by the State to erode the freedom of people to choose when and where they seek medical care and to patronise and exploit a disadvantaged group of people for the sake of social theory.' He was concerned about what he saw as ,'the political implications of reverse discrimination in this way' and said, 'It's only a small step to go further to say you will have a medical service whether you like it or not'.

Success of the schemes

What criteria did the GPs use for assessing the success or otherwise of the schemes? Again there were as many views as there were people, but *consumer satisfaction* emerged as a distinctive theme, linked with an assessment of how far the pilot schemes were meeting the medical needs of the homeless. In the words of one GP in East London - 'Consumer satisfaction is important. I don't think one should look at medical outcomes. There is a bottomless pit of need and this would not be a relevant measure. We don't know enough about the natural history of the medical problems of the homeless. We do not have an adequate base-line to make that kind of assessment.' And according to another

GP in that area the criteria for measuring success were - 'Acceptance by the consumer, the ability of the team to relate to and with the people being treated. And if they can pick something up it proves worthwhile if one assumes you are dealing with people who wouldn't find their way into the NHS otherwise.'

Like this GP in W1, several thought we should collect the opinions of consumers of the services and hostel and day centre supervisors, as well as project team members, which of course we did. 'You would have to interview a representative section of the clients and the doctor concerned. I don't think you would get more accurate than that. The project doctor does keep statistics, but I don't know what they mean. I don't know if he does either.'

However, several GPs thought that a measure of the take-up of services provided by the pilot schemes was an important indicator of success, and statistics on attendance and referrals to local service providers were thought to be an essential part of this. In particular, it was suggested that information collected about the patients treated by the project teams should include a count of those who were not registered with a local GP. There was also some interest in morbidity measures to see whether or not the pilot scheme was contributing to the diminution of morbidity among the homeless population. A number of GPs linked take-up of the project teams' services to a welcome reduction of demand on hospital accident and emergency departments, like this GP in W1 - 'I would think them successful if they saw people who would otherwise go without medical treatment. And if the homeless stopped crowding out casualty departments of local hospitals.'

A handful of GPs argued that the essential data about health care for homeless people were already known, reinforcing their view that since mainstream services were adequate the projects were unnecessary.

Transferability of the schemes

In both East London and Camden about half the GPs we spoke to thought that the pilot schemes could be transferred successfully to other areas. About a quarter were unsure about this and the rest were strongly of the view that this model of service delivery in its current form should not be developed elsewhere. Among those who thought the initiative should not be transferred several, like this GP in W1, thought that special projects for homeless people were unnecessary and that the money involved could be better spent - 'I don't agree that money should be spent on special projects when often these people have everything they need'. There was also the view that special projects actually stigmatised homeless people and isolated them further from mainstream services. We were told by a GP in East London who was sympathetic to the needs of homeless people - 'They have a right to use a GP with a "normal" practice of people who are not homeless'.

Community services: district nurses, community psychiatric nurses and social workers

We interviewed a total of 42 district nurses, community psychiatric nurses and social workers. The majority of nurses were based in health authority health centres or clinics. Of the others, two community nurses working for Bloomsbury Health Authority had an office base in a local hospital and one worked in a rehabilitation centre. Two of the CPNs in East London were based in a psychiatric hospital and one CPN in West London worked in a day hospital. The community social workers in East London were all members of a fieldwork team in Tower Hamlets. We also talked to the Director of Social Services in City and East London about social work provision for the homeless in her catchment area in the City.

Around half the CPNs we spoke to were male but all the district nurses and all but one of the social workers were female. They were spread across a wide age range. Although the length of time they had worked in the area varied, just over two-thirds of all the district nurses, CPNs and social workers had worked in the same locality for more than a year.

Nature and extent of involvement in service provision for homeless people

Only a tiny proportion of the 37 nurses in our sample said that they provided regular sessions at hostels, night shelters or day centres used by homeless people. In West London this included two district nurses and three CPNs. The district nurses provided cover at two centres; one centre was visited on a twice-weekly basis and the other monthly. The CPNs provided services at seven centres, three of which were visited on a weekly basis and the others fortnightly. In East London only two CPNs provided regular sessions at centres for the homeless. These centres included two large Salvation Army hostels and two day centres, all of which were visited weekly by a CPN. A weekly service was also provided for the women's group at another local day centre.

In West London the CPN service employed by Bloomsbury Health Authority was conducting an 'in-service pilot' to explore ways of improving its response to the mental health needs of single homeless people, and one of the CPNs who said they provided regular sessions had been appointed to a specialist post to meet the needs of this group. None of the social workers provided regular sessions in centres used by homeless people.

Sessional work by CPNs in centres in both areas was varied. One CPN in West London said - 'I provide support to staff, I have a consultancy role and discuss individuals' problems without necessarily seeing them. In terms of client contact I provide counselling, administer medication, refer to other agencies, help with practical problems and refer on accommodation.' Typically, direct work with clients involved administering medication and injections, providing counselling and advice, arranging admissions to hospital and, at one centre, taking part in the women's group activities. Support for staff in the centres was largely through advice on mental health issues, discussion of possible new clients and helping staff to liaise with appropriate agencies.

There was no clear pattern as to where the initiative came from for providing general nursing or community psychiatric nursing services to these centres. In some instances the centres had asked for general or psychiatric nursing assistance, but on other occasions the health authority involved had offered its services. Excluding these regular sessions, almost two-thirds of all the nurses, CPNs and social workers in our sample had been called out on an ad hoc basis to provide services at centres used by homeless people, but very few had been called out more than about five times during the previous year.

Just over a third of all the nurses and social workers had provided services to homeless people in other contexts as part of their job. In some cases homeless people had been referred to them from hostels or from hotels. Some were long-standing clients who had previously been housed and had since become homeless. A few were families or single-parent mothers. Some of these clients were seen at the professional's work base, but others were visited at their own base, which included hostels, bed and breakfast places and squats. The services provided directly to these clients by district nurses and CPNs were similar to those given during the regular sessions in centres used by the homeless. The social workers provided counselling and advice and they frequently had to tackle serious housing or financial problems, as well as more routine tasks like dealing with applications for bus passes.

Five of the professionals in our sample (three social workers, one district nurse and one CPN) also provided services to homeless people on a voluntary basis in their own time. The CPN provided counselling and information to residents of a local hostel, while the others gave practical help along the lines of food, clothing and outings to homeless people in hostel or church-owned sheltered accommodation. One of the social workers in Tower Hamlets was involved in helping homeless Bengali families.

Health care problems of homeless people

How did these professionals view the health problems of homeless people? The list of major health problems associated with the homeless was long. However, a marked difference from the GPs was that the nurses and social workers were more likely to express the view that *housing* difficulties were at the root of most of the health care problems experienced by homeless people. As one district nurse in West London argued - 'More housing needs to be provided here. It's the basic need for housing that is not being satisfied. They have to sort out the housing first.'

In general, the nurses and social workers were less likely than the GPs to stress the major morbidity characteristics of homeless people, but were more likely to identify the social problems or health hazards caused by living rough or, in the case of families, in bed and breakfast accommodation. One district nurse in East London summarised these problems as - 'Everything that goes with homelessness. Sleeping rough in winter time, hypothermia, exposure. You can't claim benefits so readily so you can't eat properly or you rely on fast foods so it affects diet and general health. And alienation from society as well, just drifting down the scale.'

The circumstances of living rough were thought to make the homeless more susceptible to infections and also intolerant of people trying to help them, as this CPN observed:

Being homeless they are prone to more disease. Because of their living conditions they are more prone to infection. The area they live in and the people they meet are more likely to be a health hazard. Being single homeless is a problem on its own and leads to alcohol abuse and drugs, so their mental state will be poor and aggravated causing criticism of the people who try to help and lack of tolerance of carers.

For families in bed and breakfast accommodation, poor nutrition and poor hygiene were seen as major health hazards and, as with GPs, specific reference was made to the vulnerability of children living in these cramped and highly stressful conditions.

It was commonly thought that many of the health problems experienced by the single homeless were alcohol, drug or diet-related. One CPN in East London told us - 'Alcohol is at the top of the list. They tend to drift into excesses of alcohol and other drugs so consequently their mental health must be of prime concern. They are inclined to stay in groups of drinkers to the detriment of their general health. They are prone to depression because of isolation. They are often cut off from their families.' And another CPN in East London observed:

Obvious things are a major problem like physical health deterioration because of eating cafe food, not having enough money or somewhere proper to sleep. Being homeless you cannot support yourself nutritionally well, and even if you are in a hostel they aren't particularly sanitary and long-term lack of privacy takes a toll on even the most stalwart characters. Turning to drugs and alcohol is a temptation a lot can't resist which is harmful to health too.

Not surprisingly CPNs placed particular emphasis on the mental health problems common among homeless people. This comment in Tower Hamlets was typical - 'Their mental health is affected as well as their physical condition. They are often schizophrenics who haven't been recognised as such and have become withdrawn in a world of their own.' We were told by one CPN that her experience had convinced her that depression was particularly common among homeless women:

> Women tend to be very depressed and go into clinical depression. I did a survey a couple of years ago of about 20 women in the community and 20 who were homeless in hotels and you could see a marked difference with depression, taking tranquillizers and so on. There is that helplessness of not knowing what is happening to them, taken from one place to another. Uncertainty about where you will end up and now the policy with housing is they are only offered one place and it's that or nothing. So they can end up housed but in appalling conditions.

Another CPN drew our attention to the problems of institutionalisation and how this could make it difficult for homeless people to be drawn into mainstream service provision - 'The effects of continual deprivation, drug abuse and the violence of street life is an institutionalisation of itself, and for every one year, it takes ten to undo. The answer to that is more provision of homes, better support of those about to become homeless, who are on the eviction list, and those who are homeless should not be for more than a few days.'

Just under two-thirds of these professionals thought that the health problems of the single homeless differed from those in the local general population and, as with the GPs we interviewed, this was more marked in West London. In East London a high proportion of the housed population were thought to have their own share of problems too, as this CPN observed - 'There are problems which are specific to the inner city in that there are very few places where there is cheap property available. Most places are built on prime land and Councils haven't got the money. There is a very high ethnic minority population historically in this area and it's hard for those who have homes as well.'

The way in which the health problems of the homeless were seen to differ from those of the general population was largely one of degree rather than substance. Homeless people were thought less likely to seek health care at an early stage in their illness as this social worker commented - 'They don't receive regular medical checks. I'm sure a lot is missed because things are left until they are more serious in nature and probably need hospitalisation. I've never heard a homeless person say, "I'm off to see my doctor".'

One of the most revealing comments about the consequences of living rough or in squalid conditions was made by another social worker in Tower Hamlets - 'When you talk to someone who seems chronologically ten years older than they are you get some idea of the wear and tear on the body'. This observation was also commonly made by our interviewers.

Present provision of primary health care services for homeless people

All but one of the district nurses in East London said they could not comment on the present provision of primary health care for homeless people as they had no experience of the problem, and this was also true of several nurses in West London. The comment by this district nurse in Tower Hamlets was typical: 'I haven't come across any homeless people at all so I don't know what provision there is'.

The CPNs and social workers were more forthcoming in their views about the appropriateness of mainstream services for homeless people, but they also admitted to a lack of knowlege about what services were available, like this social worker in Tower Hamlets who expressed concern over her access to information - 'There isn't a co-ordinated response to user needs. There just doesn't seem to be any information. I feel myself uninformed over what exists and what is available. What I have learned comes from clients and not from the Health Authority. So I know by default what exists; for example, which GPs are seeing homeless people, what sessions are held in hostels, centres, missions. I only know through personal contact rather than through planned information.' It seemed that few had yet addressed the problem either in their basic training or through subsequent in-service training, as this CPN in East London explained - 'We are only just beginning to talk about it and recognise the problems and look at how social aspects like homelessness can affect people's health. It is something that wasn't mentioned in our training at all.'

Around half the CPNs and social workers we spoke to thought that existing statutory provision of health care for homeless people was poor. One of the social workers in East London told us - 'It is certainly not as good as the services available to established residents. There have been some interesting innovations to compensate. For example, St. Botolph's where they have a volunteer doctor and nurses who provide a supplementary service in lieu of the usual primary health care and also have a chiropodist there.'

One of her colleagues in Tower Hamlets illustrated what she thought was the inadequacy of existing provision in that area by describing some of the experiences of her homeless clients:

> I've had a lot of homeless clients and most aren't registered so it's hard to get help. And if they go into casualty they wait for three to four hours. They do tend to go to casualty rather than a GP. It's almost as if they don't count because they are homeless and rootless and also there is stigma to going into a GP's surgery. I'm just thinking of some of my clients. If they are known to be dossers they don't get seen and are turned away. I had one girl who was alcoholic and mentally ill but never had health care. She was just sent from hostel to hostel. They kept pushing her out. She eventually fell in front of a bus and ended up as an in-patient and so was ultimately seen and treated. She also had a baby with no ante-natal care whatsoever. And there is nowhere where they can go for alcohol treatment or anything else.

Another of the social workers raised the question as to whether the problems of homeless women were being neglected - 'The hostels seem all male. I wonder if there are problems for women. There are a lot of difficulties to get women on detox. The only place I've been able to use is Greenwich... They seem very vulnerable because they are women. There are issues of children in care, termination of pregnancy, lack of facilities geared to women. These places are very much male domains.'

Not surprisingly, the CPNs thought that the mental health needs of the homeless in their locality were not being met. As one CPN in East London told us, without being registered with a GP it can be difficult to get access to psychiatric help:

I understand GPs are very reluctant to take them on because of a lack of an address. CPNs do have a direct referral service but most tend to go through GPs so I feel they just don't get seen. I feel virtually every other primary health care service has the same system so as far as the homeless are concerned I think primary health care is pretty awful. People who are homeless tend to be those who don't trust authority. They are people who have pride and don't like to see psychiatrists but they do have needs but often they get stepped over. Their need is psychological rather than psychiatric.

Those professionals who thought that existing provision was adequate were not complacent about the use of these services by homeless people. We were told that homeless people were difficult to integrate into existing GP services, that GPs' attitudes were sometimes unhelpful and that there were registration problems. We were also reminded by this CPN and others that some homeless people were simply not motivated to use health care services and it would be very difficult to re-educate them - 'Once a person goes into a homeless state they don't look on things in the same way. It is important to me to have a doctor, clothes, food and warmth but it isn't to these people and how can you get them interested again?'

The pilot schemes

Knowledge of the schemes

Overall about half of these professionals knew about the pilot schemes. The numbers involved were small, but there seemed to be marked differences between the project sites. In East London only one of the district nurses and less than half of the CPNs knew about the scheme in their area, whereas in West London most of the district nurses and CPNs were at least aware of the scheme. Like the GPs, they had heard about the schemes from a variety of sources: through contact with project team members; from literature about the projects; through the media; and from clients who had used the services provided by the pilot schemes.

Objectives of the schemes

There was a lack of consensus about the objectives of the schemes, other than the general observation that they had been set up to provide primary health care specifically for the homeless. Few were as familiar with the scheme in their area as this CPN in Tower Hamlets, whose detailed description of the purpose of the East London project summarised most of the objectives put to us individually by other professionals:

> To research into the present homeless situation which obviously isn't being dealt with. I see it very much as an experimental project which I think is good because I think these things should be on an experimental basis. To provide a choice for the homeless so that they can go and see a GP, a counsellor etc. So whether they use it or not at least they have the choice which without being on a GP's list they don't have at present. To provide a centre for other professionals in the area to find out how to deal with the homeless they come across, which is very important to me. It helps me to do my job properly. And also to provide some sort of treatment for people asking for help.

These nurses and social workers had had minimal interaction with the pilot schemes. Only one person, a CPN in East London, had received a referral from the project team and only three people had made referrals to one of the pilot schemes; these were a CPN and a social worker in East London, and a CPN in West London. Apart from referrals, several people in both project sites had had some professional contact with project team members and had found this helpful.

Strengths and weaknesses of the schemes

There was a wide range of views about the strengths and weaknesses of the schemes among those professionals who knew about them, but nobody argued that they had no strengths and should not have been set up. The most commonly mentioned strength was that the project teams provided a multidisciplinary team approach to the problem. As this district nurse in East London told us - 'They've got a team of mixed professionals which is a good thing to start with. You can draw from one another's expertise. You definitely need a doctor for health care, a nurse for treatment and a social worker for other problems. You need a full team.'

Another cluster of strengths concerned the commitment and effectiveness of team members, and this comment by a CPN in West London was typical - 'Their strength is the personalities of the people and their political awareness. They take a wider view of the issues related to homelessness. I feel the project doctor is about the most approachable GP I've ever met. I really get the sense it is a multidisciplinary team.' The flexibility of provision and the fact that team members took the service to the users was also identified as a strength, as this CPN said - 'My understanding is that it is to be flexible and responsive to the client's needs rather than being rigid. That impresses me a lot.'

Several of the professionals, like this CPN in Tower Hamlets, thought it important that the schemes were making them and their colleagues more aware of the health care problems and needs of homeless people - 'A strength is the fact that they are researching the problem first. It is a problem no one has really tackled in the past. They tried to absorb them into hostels whereas now someone is saying this is a problem. There are a lot of homeless people in the borough.' In this respect the experimental nature of the schemes was singled out by another CPN as one of their strengths - 'A strength is that it is a pilot project and hasn't shown itself to be anything else. It's a thorn in your side because it makes you think of the homeless and being a pilot doesn't make you think that it is not my problem any more. The team seems to have a very professional approach which means they are not dismissed as a load of cranks.'

Few weaknesses were identified, but it was thought that there was insufficient publicity or feedback about the schemes and not enough interaction with local service providers. One district nurse in West London complained - 'We don't learn anything about it. I once asked a senior nurse,"This homeless sister, what does she actually do?" We don't know. I expect it's general nursing ... some can be infected so it will be easier for them to be treated there without the risk of infection spreading.'

A CPN in the same area also told us - 'They are not very well publicised. It would be useful if they made people aware of it. I don't know how they liaise with other agencies but if there was close liaison between them and CPNs this would be useful. I think it would be mutually beneficial because I'm sure they see a lot of people with mental health problems and we have a lot of expertise to offer them and could offer them education and help them to plug into existing psychiatric services.' And in Tower Hamlets we heard a similar story from the CPNs who also wanted to know more about what the team members were doing, so that they could learn from their experience and expertise.

Other weaknesses which were identified included the smallness of the teams and the problems of continuity beyond the life of the project. As this CPN in East London speculated - 'A weakness is its temporariness. The scale of commitment is such that the limitations of the scheme make it too awe-inspiring to think about. The smallness of the team too. The homeless have so little trust that you need a lot of patience and I feel the scheme will run out before they realise what a useful thing it is.' There were also a handful of people, like this CPN in East London, who thought that the schemes were not multi-disciplinary enough - 'It is still seen as a medically dominated team. The doctor is seen as the focus. The focus has changed with the change of doctor. He used to be seen as the "doctor for the homeless". Now the doctor is less of a focus and it is more of a team and all the better for that.' Our attention was also drawn to the risk that a special scheme for the homeless might allow local service providers to avoid their responsibilities to this group and would stigmatise them further.

Success of the schemes
As with the GPs, there was little consensus among these professionals about the criteria for assessing the success of the schemes. Criteria that were suggested included: a count of attendances to indicate the level of take-up; consumer satisfaction; how far the medical needs of the homeless were met; and how far links were established with hostels and with local service providers. However, the one thing that most of the professionals were agreed on was that all of these measures would be difficult to pin down.

As one of the CPNs commented - 'This is a really tricky one! Obvious things are attendance because at the moment that is going to be dramatically low because of the homeless's lack of trust of anyone in authority. I think it's one of those things unassessable on paper, but only by intuition, and perhaps only those who run it can answer that to say if they feel they are being useful.' And another CPN observed:

> It is difficult. It would be interesting to know how many people they've managed to reach, identify and help. Also to know if they've managed to prevent any ill-health using preventative measures. Though how you'd quantify that I don't know. Also, of those people they did talk to, how many wanted to be rehoused and how many had successfully been rehoused. Perhaps even a questionnaire of the homeless people would be helpful to see if they had found it useful and if any more could have been done.

Another criterion suggested for measuring the success of the schemes was the extent to which they were known about locally. It was put to us by one of the social workers that - 'We don't know much about it so the outreach part of it is not reaching us. Not me at any rate. It has certainly never been discussed in the team when I've been there. I haven't had any feed-back on the project and how it is developing. The management may have but it certainly hasn't reached field work level and I haven't heard it discussed outside the department by other professionals working in the area. In other words, it doesn't seem to have a very high profile. Whether it's had any impact on our service or not I wouldn't be in a position to say.'

Transferability of the schemes

Roughly two-thirds of those who knew something about the schemes thought that the model as developed in their locality could be transferred successfully to other areas, so long as it was not adopted too rigidly. This comment by a CPN in Tower Hamlets was typical - 'Yes, I don't see why not as long as they are prepared to be flexible and adapt to particular needs. But the basic philosophy feels right.' Only one person argued strongly against the model being reproduced elsewhere in its current form, and this was because she thought that the underlying philosophy was unsound. She thought that the team in her area were doing 'contradictory work'. She argued that the project in West London needed to decide whether to have an entirely advocacy role or a purely clinical input. She did not think it was possible for them to have both and illustrated her point about mixed messages by saying, 'If they go into a day centre I can't see how they can then encourage people to go and register with a local GP, as they themselves are so nice and it is so easy'.

Hospital accident and emergency staff

We spoke to six junior casualty officers (SHOs), six nurses and three hospital social workers. At the time of the interviews they were either working in or, in the case of the social workers, taking referrals from the casualty departments of two large London teaching hospitals.

All the doctors had been qualified for a minimum of one year, and were all aged under 30 years. Three of the nurses were sisters and three were staff nurses. Around half the hospital staff we interviewed had worked in the area for less than a year, but five had worked in the locality for five years or more.

Nature and extent of service provision for homeless people

The majority of the hospital staff had had recent experience of providing care for homeless people who had attended casualty. The doctors had provided general treatment for illness and for trauma resulting from accidents or assault, and in some cases had admitted homeless people as in-patients, as this casualty officer described - 'I've treated those who have been assaulted, examined those who come to the department drunk, directed some towards alcohol support groups and a handful towards drug crisis places'. In addition to making referrals to other agencies, in certain cases they had also directed homeless people to local GPs if they were intending to stay in the area.

They had also dealt with depression and drug overdoses and were concerned that in these cases the precipitating factors were often social rather than medical, and were not capable of being tackled in casualty. One doctor in West London gave the example of a family with a baby where the partners were only sixteen or seventeen years old. In her view there was no real medical problem but 'they interpreted their social problems in a medical way'. She commented - 'With the large numbers of people coming to casualty all we can do is sort out the medical problems and it is difficult if they haven't got one'.

The nurses' involvement with homeless people was largely one of cleaning them up and arranging for hostel accommodation. A sister in the West London hospital told us - ' I've been involved in telephoning hostels for beds, washing their feet in the sink, delousing and keeping them under general observation'.

The social workers had provided a range of services including counselling and making referrals to other agencies and projects. Recalling her contact with homeless people over the last six months one of the social workers commented that she had - 'Arranged accommodation for them in hostels, bed and breakfast or whatever, made referrals to other agencies and in some instances with young people encouraged and enabled them to go home'. She had also referred people to the DHSS pilot scheme in East London.

We found that almost all the hospital staff had encountered difficulties in providing services for the homeless. In particular, they referred to the general problems of follow-up and after-care, and specifically mentioned inadequate psychiatric support and lack of social work back-up. As this doctor in East London explained - 'Often I like to write to the GP and ask the people to call in or explain what I've done. You can't do that. You have to ask the homeless patients to come back here. Also, if it's something where you want someone to watch them or be with them when it's not so severe like a minor head injury or someone there to watch if they have difficulties, you feel you are sending them out into a vacuum where there is no one who is really interested.' A similar comment was made by a doctor in the West London hospital - 'You see them and then throw them back onto the street when treated. You know they haven't got anywhere to go but there is nothing you can do.'

In common with many of the community-based health care professionals we interviewed, the accident and emergency staff we spoke to emphasised the point that lack of accommodation was the fundamental problem that needed to be tackled, not simply the health care problems associated with homelessness.

A range of problems were associated with lack of accommodation and as one of the social workers in East London observed: 'This problem is going to get worse as three hostels are closing down and there is no alternative provision'. In particular, there were the problems of providing treatment for someone who lived rough, as illustrated by this nurse - 'I had a man in with an ulcer on his leg. He was given antibiotics and told to elevate the limb! Of course it was unsuitable treatment. Where could he elevate it? Consequently he eventually came back and had to be admitted with a condition that if you or I had had, might have given us a couple of days off work at most.'

Doctors and nurses alike would have preferred to have less of a counselling role and thought it was inappropriate for them to be 'saddled' with finding accommodation for homeless people. As one of the doctors explained - 'I'm not particularly good at counselling and finding homes. I know the names of a few hostels but that's all.' She thought that these should be community-based services. There was also general agreement among the hospital social workers that much of what they were doing was superficial and did not get to the root of the main problem, which they perceived to be lack of housing. A typical comment was - 'In many ways we are only plastering over the cracks. The services we provide are only very basic. Housing needs to be provided, then income can be stabilised and everything can improve.'

Several of the doctors and nurses reported instances where they had encountered homeless people in casualty who had been abusive and anti-social and these exceptional experiences had had a marked influence in shaping their image of homeless people. We were told by one of the casualty officers in West London - 'They are sometimes so dirty. You stand back with your rubber gloves on. You don't think of them as people. You think, Oh God, there goes another one.'

The majority of hospital staff thought that the work they had carried out for homeless people could have been more appropriately done by someone else. Like this doctor, several of the casualty officers thought that they were providing services to the homeless which could be done more effectively by local GPs, with adequate support services - 'I'm a great believer in a properly run GP service. The most important aspect is that they can have immediate free access and follow-up. Somewhere where they know where they are and can follow them up and contact other agencies like social workers and district nurses and all the things tied into general practice.' But there was also a consensus among casualty officers that some people would never learn to use GPs.

As one of them observed - 'the hard core down and outs will come back here regardless'.

Health care problems of homeless people
The hospital staff were more familiar with the health problems of the single homeless than with those of homeless families. Just over half said they did not know enough about the health problems of homeless families to be able to comment about this group. Two issues concerning the single homeless were highlighted: first, it was commonly believed that many of their health problems were alcohol-related; and second, around half thought that respiratory problems were a major health problem for the single homeless.

The hospital staff in West London found it more difficult than their colleagues in East London to comment on whether the health problems of homeless people in their area differed markedly from those of the general population living nearby. As one doctor explained - 'It is impossible to answer this question. We don't have as large an indigenous population here as in East London.' However, homeless people were thought to have a greater incidence of TB and other respiratory problems than was found in the general population. The homeless were also thought to be more likely to have medical and social problems arising from poor accommodation and a lack of primary health care.

Present provision of primary health care services for homeless people
Most of the casualty officers and nurses we spoke to knew little about primary health care provision outside the hospital setting. The comment by this doctor in West London was typical - 'I've got little experience of the community. But a lot of the problems cannot be tackled in accident and emergency. We can sort out medical problems, but not other problems; for example, depression.' However, a handful had strong views about problems confronting homeless people who wanted health care, like this social worker who told us - 'Provision is dismal. When I say dismal I'm excluding the HHELP project. All health care is difficult because of the stigma of vagrants. People are not necessarily vagrants who are admitted with no fixed abode. There is

immediately an assumption they are the same with the same lifestyle. It is not always the case.'

All the hospital staff we spoke to believed that single homeless people tended to use the accident and emergency department inappropriately as an alternative first point of contact with the health service, instead of going to see a GP. However, as one of the doctors in West London acknowledged, she and her colleagues viewed the problem 'with the jaundiced eye of a casualty officer' and, while they thought they got all the homeless, GPs would probably have a very different view. Our attention was also drawn to the fact that inappropriate use of casualty was also thought to be common among the general population in these areas.

The examples we were given of inappropriate use by *homeless* people can be summarised as: attending casualty for minor complaints and problems that a GP could deal with; presenting with long-term chronic problems; coming in to get prescriptions or wanting help with alcohol or drug-related problems; and simply trying to get a bed or warm place to stay for the night. However, their comments about inappropriate use tell their version of the story more graphically.

A female casualty officer in East London talked of homeless people - 'Asking for admission because they have nowhere else to go. Presenting with chronic problems, chest complaints going on for years. Asking for HIV tests. We don't either counsel or cater for that. And asking for homes really. Some use the waiting room to sleep overnight.' A male colleague also thought that homeless people abused casualty by treating it as somewhere to get a bed - 'They use casualty as a place to sleep in at night. A casualty department should be here for people involved in trauma or who suddenly become very ill or require immediate attention.' Similar points were made by a hospital social worker who took referrals from the staff in the accident and emergency department - 'Homeless people come in with a variety of physical problems that could have been dealt with by a GP. All manner of minor things, from a sprained ankle to feeling generally unwell...and being realistic a number will come because it's warm and they're hoping to be admitted to get a roof over their head, or as a cry for help basically.'

In West London the complaints were similar. One of the nurses commented - 'A lot of the time they are alcoholics found in heaps at stations. They come along because they have injured themselves. Often trivial, angling after a warm bed for the night. We often provide a mattress for them in rooms around the side of the casualty department ... some appear regularly and are well known.' Alcoholics were seen to be a particular nuisance, as this doctor explained - 'Sometimes ambulance men, alerted by the public, bring in a person off the streets. There is nothing wrong except alcohol and they sleep it off here. This is inappropriate and timewasting. We have to examine them top to toe and they are too drunk to talk about what might be wrong with them.'

We asked why they thought that homeless people often chose to use accident and emergency departments rather than go to a local GP. They were not short on answers but, as with this doctor in West London, most insisted that we should put this question in the context of misuse of facilities by the general population - 'The general population, especially in central London, are using A and E inappropriately. Especially the commuters who work in London.'

Homeless people were commonly thought to use accident and emergency departments because hospitals were seen to be more accessible and treatment was available at all hours. In the words of one of the doctors - 'They think we are more accessible because they can just walk in day or night. We are opposite the tube. GPs are difficult to get hold of. I should think a lot would turn up their noses at the homeless. The wait tends to be longer. It's warm and they can be here for three or four hours and quite often we just let them stay.' The fact that there was no appointment system to negotiate in casualty was also thought to be attractive to homeless people, as this doctor in East London recognised - 'It is immediately accessible. There is no appointment system so they see a doctor straight away. And because they've got, or feel they've got, no other option.'

Hospitals were also thought to afford people more anonymity and it was suggested by several of the staff we spoke to that homeless people might actually prefer this anonymity, rather than the more personal service offered by a GP. And staff also thought homeless people used casualty departments because they were not registered with a GP.

The hospital staff had a number of ideas about how to reduce inappropriate use of accident and emergency departments by homeless people. Their main recommendation was to improve GP services to the homeless. Some thought that special clinics might be necessary and most thought that more education and information about using health services was essential, like this doctor - 'Inappropriate use of our services could be reduced by providing a different service either by letting them register with a GP even if they are homeless, or by setting up special clinics for them. And by patient education when they come here, telling them about other services and how to register with a GP.' Another idea was to have 'a number of local GP practices especially committed to providing care for homeless people'.

Even if GP services were improved and made more flexible there would still be the problem of motivating homeless people to use them, as this nurse in East London recognised - 'You could educate them on their health and where to go. You could provide an alternative, like a GP especially for them ... but how would you get them to go though, that's the problem.' But as another nurse in East London speculated, some would always prefer to use the accident and emergency department - 'We will never train them...they're very often second generation. They know that mum always brought them here. It's just the tradition in this area. They won't be deflected.'

The pilot schemes

Only three of the hospital staff we interviewed in East London, a casualty officer and two social workers, had heard of the East London Homeless Health Project and they admitted they knew very little about it. One of the social workers commented - 'I don't think they have done enough in the way of publicity. Lots of people don't know of their existence and the services they can provide and where they can be found.' In West London, *none* of the hospital staff we interviewed knew about their local pilot scheme.

Voluntary bodies

What did the local voluntary bodies with an interest in homeless people think about the present provision of health care to this group and how did they view the DHSS pilot schemes?

To find out, in each project area we interviewed representatives of the main co-ordinating agency for local organisations concerned with the homeless; in East London the umbrella organisation was No Fixed

Abode (NFA), and in West London it was West End Co-ordinated Voluntary Services (WECVS). We also spoke to representatives of 12 local agencies. These were mainly project directors, co-ordinators or leaders and hostel managers, but we also spoke to a handful of specialist advisers concerned with aspects of housing or community care. Their ages ranged from 25 to over 50 and half were female. Only one had worked in the locality for less than a year, and more than half had worked in the same area for five years or more.

In East London we also held a group discussion with representatives of the Salvation Army and this was attended by 17 officers, including the Provincial Officer and all Officers in Charge and nurses working in Salvation Army Hostels in the Central and North London Province.

Nature and extent of involvement in service provision for homeless people
Eight of the local organisations or projects we spoke to provided accommodation for homeless people; three were daycentres (two in West London and one in East London) and five were hostels (two in West London and three in East London). Most of the hostels provided short-term or medium-term accommodation for men only. One offered medium-term rehabilitation and resettlement facilities for people recovering from mental ill-health. A number of these centres provided health care services for homeless people. In one of the hostels a doctor provided two surgeries a week on a voluntary basis. At another a nurse was available every day, a doctor visited twice a week and a chiropodist every two weeks on a voluntary basis. In the large hostel for men in East London a nurse employed by the district health authority was available on week-day mornings. One of the daycentres also offered a range of health care facilities, including a doctor, a nurse and a chiropodist twice a week.

In addition to the two co-ordinating agencies already mentioned, the other organisations we spoke to included: an agency working with people with alcohol problems, a large proportion of whom were homeless; a project providing outreach teamwork with people on the streets; a campaigning self-help group set up by homeless people; and an organisation which offered advice to voluntary bodies about the

229

development and management of special needs housing projects for single homeless people.

Health care problems of homeless people

There was some agreement among the representatives of voluntary bodies that the single homeless were particularly susceptible to respiratory, psychiatric and alcohol-related problems, but, more importantly, they found it difficult to generalise because they tended to differentiate much more between the various groups of homeless people than the health care professionals had done. They drew our attention to what they saw as limiting misconceptions about homelessness and homeless people. As one community care adviser explained - 'It is difficult to say because they are a very varied group. Obviously they may have special problems of alcohol and drug abuse. But the stereotype has changed significantly. There are now new single homeless people who are young, black or female and stereotypes have broken down. There is also a group with mental ill-health.' There was also agreement that homeless people tended to have lower expectations about their health status than the general population, as this voluntary worker in East London explained - 'There is a general problem of people's self-perception of health mixed with the difficulty of maintaining good health. Health is not seen as a priority.'

Present provision of primary health care services for homeless people

The representatives from agencies in the voluntary sector and those working in the council-run centres tended to have a more negative view than the health care professionals about the appropriateness of mainstream health care services for homeless people. The majority thought that provision was poor and needed improvement. In particular, they commented about the difficulty of integrating homeless people into existing GP services and the lack of knowledge among GPs about the needs of homeless people. As one community care adviser explained:

> I think it is very poor for two reasons. Many single homeless people don't have access to primary health care, both those who sleep rough and those in specialist housing projects with

special housing needs. The problem is finding a GP prepared to take them on to his list. Many GPs have very little knowledge of the needs of homeless people. The stereotype is of elderly white men, alcoholics, who have bugs and lice. They've no realistic picture of single homeless people and their needs.

The hostels had had mixed experiences in acquiring health care for their residents. The warden of one hostel in East London told us - 'I can only speak from my experience of people here. There is excellent service from local GPs and follow-up from hospitals. Very often it is the men who choose not to get treatment. They might have difficulty getting chiropody and dental treatment but, apart from that, I often say they are treated better than private patients.' But in another hostel in the same area the warden was less confident about the quality of care given to residents:

People in this hostel are a special case because we have an arrangement with a local GP and there has been a nurse here since the GLC took over. Many homeless people are registered with other GPs perhaps we'd prefer them not be to be registered with. We wonder about the quality of service they provide. Sometimes we have problems registering people when we rehouse them. GPs are very wary about taking them on. They think all homeless people are psychopathic alcoholics.

Many of the workers in hostels and day centres were concerned that homeless people had difficulty in obtaining psychiatric care. We were told - 'There is a lack of psychological provision. People are not being dealt with by the statutory services. It's left to organisations like us who haven't got the right training.' And another warden commented - 'Mental health is often overlooked. The general depression of living in this area adds to their problem. It has a snowball affect. Homelessness may be the last straw. I don't know how they cope. There is not much outreach work from psychiatric workers and no preventative work at all.'

The problems encountered by homeless people who were chronically mentally ill were also highlighted in the group discussion with Salvation Army Officers. With the increasing threat of hospital closures, the question was raised as to what would happen to these people if hospital care were replaced with short care treatment facilities. As one officer observed - 'It was said to be bad for these people to be in large institutions called psychiatric hospitals, but it is equally bad for them to be in large institutions called Salvation Army Hostels'.

Homeless people were also seen to be at a disadvantage in obtaining dental or optical services and, as the warden of a day centre in West London argued, the level of statutory social work support was thought to be unsatisfactory - 'Statutory social workers are just there to help families or those who are a danger to others. There is no preventative action. Once people have been rehoused they're left to cope on their own. We need to focus on low-level support for those who have been resettled and to relate this to medical services. Basically, we need a more holistic approach to health care.'

The pilot schemes
All but two of the organisations we spoke to knew about the DHSS pilot scheme in their locality; the two exceptions were a day centre in West London and a hostel catering for the mentally ill in East London. Information about the schemes had reached the voluntary workers largely through contact with a project team member or through some other professional contact.

There was little consensus about the objectives of the schemes and a fair amount of confusion. As one worker commented - 'I think it is to provide separate health care services to the single homeless via a salaried GP. But I'm fairly confused as to whether the aim was initially to link people with the existing GP service.' There was also a feeling that there had not been enough consultation or discussion with local organisations when the schemes had first been thought of and set up.

We asked the day centres and hostels whether they used the services provided by the project teams. Although none hosted a regular clinic by either of the project doctors, six of them had called upon the services provided by one or more team member. In West London the project nurse regularly visited two of the hostels and the nurse unofficially attached to the project provided nursing services at one of the daycentres. In the three hostels in East London the alcohol counsellor, the social worker and the project doctor provided support and information for staff, and made their services available to residents whenever they were needed. In East London, the agency working with people with alcohol problems had received referrals *from* the project team but had not made referrals *to* the scheme, although occasionally it did confer with them about individual clients.

Strengths and weaknesses of the schemes
Those working in agencies in the voluntary sector provided us with a long and varied list of strengths that they associated with the pilot schemes, and by and large these were similar to those already described by the GPs and other health care professionals. As one of the local co-ordinating agencies confirmed, even if they were unsure about the philosophy behind the projects they recognised the commitment and effectiveness of team members - 'They are working directly with people who are homeless. With their sleeves rolled up in there. Not just talking about attitudes and perceptions.' The one aspect they emphasised which had not been mentioned by the professionals was that it was important that the schemes were *statutory* because this was an indication that the government was taking the health care problems of homeless people seriously. This point was illustrated by one of the daycentre wardens who told us - 'The fact that the DHSS are taking an interest is very important, rather than ignoring the subject as in the past. It shows that they are concerned.'

However, there was also some criticism of what they saw as a top-down solution to the problem by the government, and in identifying weaknesses of the schemes they emphasised the lack of discussion with local agencies about the objectives and design of the projects before they were introduced. The co-ordinating body in West London told us - 'There was a lack of consultation and joint planning beforehand. The project does not feel rooted into other services going on.' A specific criticism made by one of the workers in West London was that the approach to improving the health care of homeless people had not been linked with initiatives to tackle their housing needs. She told us - 'There is little co-ordination between the DHSS projects and little consultation between housing agencies as to what is needed...there is a lack of knowledge among housing workers about the health care structure and about the policies of health care...The DHSS needs to start co-ordinating its projects with people in the housing field.'

Another criticism was that the life of the projects was too limited. The representative of the umbrella agency in East London said - 'It's too short. It should have been at least five years. While we appreciate its nationally experimental nature, it has not tried to plug into or see itself as a local service... They have been devolved down into the locality and when they have had to deal with local services, they haven't had the clout.' Like most of those we spoke to in the voluntary sector, he was also concerned about what would happen when the funding for the pilot scheme in his area ran out - 'I think there is enough there for it not to be wrapped up. If you inject that resource into day centres and whip it away, what happens to them, to their agenda?' This issue was also raised by the community care adviser attached to one of the West London agencies - 'Ideally single homeless people should have access to the rest of the system. I don't know how far the aim is to try to integrate their case-load into GP practices. They need to make arrangements for this if the project ends. Not just dump people.'

There was also considerable concern and frustration among local organisations that the aims and design of the pilot schemes were based on stereotyped views of the homeless that were outdated, and that their services were therefore not reaching some in this group who had difficulty in obtaining primary health care. The co-ordinator of the campaigning self-help group argued - 'The project so far has focused almost entirely on day centres. This comes from the homeless and rootless conception in the DHSS. Day centres are important street agencies but many do not use them. The project is aimed at a stereotype definition of who the homeless are.' This observation was also made by a community care adviser for an agency in West London who said - 'I'm concerned that the existing projects just deal with the tip of the iceberg because they deal with the traditional stereotype of the single homeless person, not with the true picture'.

Success of the schemes

Many voluntary sector representatives were unsure about the objectives of the projects and therefore found it difficult to comment about criteria for assessing success. However, a co-ordinator in East London said he would consider the scheme in his area a step forward 'if it has raised health as an issue for people and chipped away at homeless people's perception of good health'.

Generally speaking, they were much less concerned about statistics recording the level of take-up of services, and more concerned with the fact that the projects had at the very least reached some people who would otherwise have gone without health care. The co-ordinator of the self-help group in West London told us - 'Statistics are meaningless. To me it is encouraging that first of all it has started. Secondly, it is beginning to get to men and women who were previously ignored. It is just a small blip on a radar screen but it is a start.'

The clear message that came from our interviews with representatives from agencies in the voluntary sector was that the *experience* of the pilot schemes should be shared, even though there was no consensus about whether the *approach* as developed locally by the pilot schemes could or should be transferred to other areas. There was a reluctance to generalise about the schemes in terms of success or failure, and the co-ordinator of one of the East London agencies advised us -'As a conscious positive lesson there is much to be learnt from it. Part of learning is about mistakes. Often projects are wrongly judged as a success or failure.'

Special or integrated services?

We asked the health care professionals and voluntary bodies about the pattern of provision in the future. How did they think that primary health care for single homeless people in their locality could best be provided? In particular, taking into account the pilot schemes, were they in favour of this type of special and separate provision of health care for homeless people, or did they think that the homeless could and should be integrated into mainstream services?

Just over two-thirds of all the health care professionals and representatives of voluntary bodies thought that single homeless people in their locality needed special provision (Table 8.1, p.242). The numbers involved were small, but the GPs and CPNs were marginally less in favour of this approach than the other professional disciplines, particularly those who were working in hospital accident and emergency departments. Among those representing local voluntary organisations just over three-quarters said they thought that the single homeless needed some kind of special service.

Many of these responses were heavily qualified and the figures would be misleading without taking into account respondents' comments and recommendations. Around a third of those who said that special and separate provision was necessary for homeless people thought that the lifestyle and particular problems of the homeless could not be accommodated within existing mainstream services. One of the GPs told us -'This is a very contentious issue. One school of thought is that they should have access to mainstream services and that access should be improved. But services are geared to people with a residence and a settled way of life. There is a mismatch, and therefore there does need to be special provision.'

Those favouring special services commonly thought that the social problems of homeless people overshadowed and were inseparable from their medical problems. One of the casualty officers said, 'Their problems tend to be different and when they get sick, they tend to be much sicker and they seem to have nowhere to go where they can see someone they know regularly'. And one of the social workers sharing this view remarked - 'Existing services are not geared to provide them with the health care they need. Also, because of their particular problems they do need a special approach. Somewhere where they can go ... an environment where the person feels comfortable and is seen with dignity, where they know they will be treated sympathetically and seriously. They know if they go to GPs they are not wanted and they do have particular needs.'

Because of these needs, it was also suggested that more emphasis needed to be placed on multidisciplinary teamwork with homeless people. One of the casualty officers advised us - 'There would need to be open clinics, warm and cosy with provision for drinks. And a multidisciplinary team. Not just doctors. Also nurses and social workers, working alongside the hostels.' Similarly we were told by one of the CPNs in West London - 'Just the sheer magnitude of the problems they present necessitates a team effort. It needs a united approach with many professionals involved to deal with the many problems they bring.'

It was commonly argued by those in favour of special services that particular skills and training were required to meet the exceptional needs of homeless people. One GP said - 'You need specialist skills, you need people trained to care for the homeless. The homeless have particular stresses - physical and emotional. Ordinary GPs would be capable, but there are problems of social isolation, broken homes etc. and people geared to these problems can help them more.' In particular, specialist carers were thought to be necessary to tackle alcohol and drug problems. We were told by one of the GPs in East London - 'You need people specially trained to help drug addicts and social casualties who have good links with all specialist agencies'. And another commented from experience that 'the one specialist service which is missing badly is emergency detoxification centres'. Regardless of the expertise required, we were assured that caring for the homeless required a special kind of commitment and interest because, as this CPN observed from experience - 'They are very needy but often throw it back in your face. Just when you feel you've done a piece of work or just started it they'll leave and you never see them again.'

A handful of GPs who were in favour of special provision gave reasons which had more to do with taking the pressure off general practice than with improving health care provision for homeless people. Worried that 'dirty, smelly itinerants' would upset the other patients attending the surgery and turn some of them away, one GP in West London commented - 'After all, we are running a business and we need to keep our numbers up'. She had not actually seen a homeless person in her surgery but nonetheless had strong views - 'The homeless are likely to be dirty, aren't they? I'm sure most are unsavoury characters. They wouldn't be homeless unless they had chosen that path.' And another told us - 'They need somewhere to go where other patients won't object, as some are very dirty and unpleasant'. To try and break down these stereotypes, another GP suggested - 'Maybe there could be more education of doctors about homeless people. It's interesting to listen to people involved in the project about their work. We could all benefit from knowing how they attack it.'

It is important to take into account the fact that many of those who said special provision was necessary believed this to be the case in the *short term*, but not in the *long term*. One of the health professionals explained why:

> I would say in the long term 'no' because of alienation. You want to get people rehabilitated. In the short term? It's very hard. I suppose if there wasn't Great Chapel Street there would be a lot more ill-health. They wouldn't need it if people's attitudes were different but at the moment you need places like that and it is very well used. A lot of homeless people are not motivated to register. They don't put a priority on health. So if there is not a positive attitude and encouragement they are less likely to use the services. If GPs accepted homelessness in their locality and took people on and visited hostels there might not even be a need for Great Chapel Street.

It was suggested that special projects, like the DHSS pilot schemes, could be useful pump-priming exercises. They could be used to help change the attitudes of GPs and other health care professionals towards taking on homeless people and one worker from the voluntary sector told us - 'It would help if we could pull doctors out of mainstream services into specialist centres so they could become aware and then take ideas back to other mainstream workers'. They could also inject the extra effort and commitment that was necessary to tackle the problems of low self-esteem and self-image which were thought to get in the way of homeless people seeking help.

An ambivalence towards special provision was particularly marked among those working in the voluntary sector. The community care adviser attached to one West London agency said - 'I think there has to be provision in the same way that health care is provided to the rest of the population, not contrived to separate people. Voluntary bodies have spoken out against special projects, but recently we've realised that we are not able to say what we do want instead.'

It was suggested by the co-ordinator of one of the voluntary agencies in East London that it was perhaps incorrect to attempt to draw a clear demarcation line between special provision and integration into mainstream services. He did not like separate provision, but thought that special projects were useful as a temporary expedient if they became another entry point into mainstream provision. He told us -

'There is a need for building bridges between existing services and those not willing to use them. People who have been homeless for a long time get detached from health services and perceptions of their own health. Therefore you can't just assume that if all GPs said "we welcome the homeless" they would go. To bridge the gaps you may need to provide interim special provision.'

A similar feeling was evident at the group meeting with Salvation Army officers, where we were told - 'The need is frequently not for *more* services but for *better access* to those that we have got already'. Officers were agreed that - 'It would, therefore, seem best if both options were available - the ultimate aim should be that help be forthcoming through the mainstream services, but that projects like HHELP would assist in linking up those outside such a service at present'.

Almost a quarter of the health care professionals and several of the workers from the voluntary sector were strongly against the introduction of special and separate services in their locality. A common theme among the GPs in this group was that existing GP provision was either satisfactory, or could be improved, and it would be an unnecessary expense to introduce special services for the homeless. Permanent registration was seen as problematic for all the reasons they had given us, but they tended to share the view of this GP - '...Registration is not the central point. Treatment is the central point and they can get that if they are registered or not.'

A number of GPs had ideas on how mainstream provision could be extended or adapted to accommodate homeless people. Some argued for more ancillary staff and better support services. Others thought that the solution lay in financial incentives - 'My inclination is to use the existing set-up then look for inducements to take people on. Money has to be the only inducement really. They could be a special capitation category. You could also use special salaried GPs in specialist set-ups recommended for areas where there are high concentrations of homeless.' Another West London GP told us - 'Better payment would enable one to take on fewer patients and give them more time. That is what is needed, not money wasted on special projects.' Several, like this GP, also thought it impractical to treat the homeless as a special client group - 'Frankly I haven't isolated them in my mind.

We have about 15 per cent of patients who come from all kinds of chaotic backgrounds. Once you start providing specialist care for groups where do you stop?'

The debate about how to adapt the existing system to meet the needs of the homeless population is largely a question of service delivery. The stereotype of the single-handed, elderly, lock-up-shop GP is becoming increasingly outmoded and the energy and drive of some GPs was typified by a GP in West London who had a well-thought-out plan as to how some kind of outreach approach to service delivery for homeless people could be developed within the framework of existing services. He described a proposal he had submitted to his local Health Authority:

> I have proposed...the formation of a primary health care centre based at the Hospital for Women in Soho Square to offer a wide variety of primary health care services including conventional GP practice, but also chiropody, dentistry, pharmacy, alcohol and drug services, CPNs, health visitors, social workers and short-term beds for the treatment of acute illnesses. This would also have outreach workers to go and treat people in situ, underneath the arches and so on, but would be based at the centre so they would have a place to come back to. I would have no objection to prescribing and treating someone with, say, TB on the Embankment or prescribing through a nurse for someone I haven't seen. The alternative is to put them in very expensive hospital beds.

Suggested improvements to existing mainstream services were not restricted to GP services. One of the GPs in West London suggested - 'Why not have a larger nursing service? The pilot project has broken down...we'd be far better off putting proper nursing services into hostels.' And a measure suggested by one of the casualty officers in the West London hospital to reduce inappropriate use of casualty by homeless people was to appoint a liaison officer, both to improve communication between hospitals and community services and to provide some kind of follow-up service. He told us - 'It might be useful to have a person we could contact about the homeless and who could follow them up in the community. Not necessarily working 24 hours a day in the accident and emergency department. We have a liaison officer for the elderly. Is this a good model to copy? The "homeless" person officer would not need to be here 24 hours a day but would be a key person to contact. A lot of the people who they could help might already have social workers or health visitors.'

A powerful argument against special provision was that this would further isolate homeless people from society. We were told by the co-ordinator of the self-help group for homeless people in West London - 'Special services would marginalise the homeless further. We are not special. We are being denied the right of a house. This in turn denies us medicine and education.' As one of the CPNs explained, the underlying philosophical argument here was that homeless people should have the same rights to mainstream health care as anyone else - 'They should be entitled to use the same as everyone else. They have problems registering with GPs which is a hindrance, but they should have the same entitlement as anyone else. Specialist agencies should be provided to look at the problem of homelessness, but they should have equal access to everything that is going on.' And one of the GPs in West London argued against the appointment of salaried doctors to provide health care for homeless people on similar grounds - 'Homeless people have a right to see a GP with a "normal" practice of people who are not homeless'.

Another concern among those who were against special projects or health care schemes was what would happen when the funding for them ran out. A manager of CPN services who was an advocate of improved mainstream provision argued - 'The danger of special services is if the money runs out they may go. With integrated services you can prioritise from time to time.'

There are thus many different views about the potential forms of provision in the future. In the face of this diversity of expert opinion, anecdotal evidence and prejudice, perhaps we should pose the question: is it possible or even appropriate to attempt to develop an all-embracing solution to the problem of health care provision for homeless people, who after all do not constitute a homogeneous group for policy-makers to focus on? As this casualty officer at the sharp end of the problem summed up: 'I think the homeless must be divided into different groups. You can't put all the homeless into one category and create one solution.

Among the homeless there are some who can be helped and are retrievable. But some want to be left alone.'

Table 8.1   **Views on whether single homeless need special and separate provision of primary health care services**

column percentages

	Total	GPs	Community Nurses	Community Psychiatric Nurses	Social Workers	Hospital accident & emergency staff	Local voluntary organisations
						Profession	
Yes	67	59	65	55	80	87	79
No	24	32	29	30	20	-	14
DK	10	9	6	15	-	13	7
(Base=all)	*105*	*34*	*17*	*20*	*5*	*15*	*14*

9   Discussion of Findings

The evaluation

The Department of Health and Social Security funded the two pilot projects providing primary health care with the objectives of identifying and contacting as many homeless people as practicable within the locality of the FPCs concerned, gaining their confidence, diagnosing and treating their morbidity and, wherever possible, securing their admission to the list of a general medical practitioner. The research was commissioned to evaluate the two pilot schemes, with the aim of testing the objectives set out above. It was recognised that the evaluation would be essentially a descriptive study, looking at the organising and functioning of the two schemes, referral patterns into and out of the schemes, the incidence of morbidity and mortality of consumers, and assessing the views both of professionals and voluntary workers as well as the clients themselves on the delivery of primary health care to homeless people. It was hoped to develop measures of outcome to test the effectiveness of the schemes on the health and wellbeing of the consumers - the homeless people. The schemes were designed as 'pilot' schemes, and there was an assumption that they were being assessed as 'model' schemes. It was hoped that lessons learned from the way in which they functioned could be applied elsewhere.

The question to be asked is to what extent the schemes fulfilled the objectives laid down by the Department. The first thing which must be said is that the schemes were different from each other. They were set up in different ways and the composition of the teams was different. The East London scheme was based on a service offered by a doctor which was already up and running in a number of centres, while the

Camden scheme started from scratch. The areas in which they were working were different in terms of the history of health care which was on offer to homeless people.

It is fundamental to any assessment of the schemes to point out that neither of them was operating in a historical vacuum, and some of the problems encountered by both teams in setting up and developing services were undoubtedly caused by a legacy in the areas of differing approaches to the provision of health care to homeless people. Homeless people have always attracted a lot of attention from voluntary workers and dedicated professionals. The two pilot schemes, particularly because of their centrally 'imposed' nature and their central funding, were not unnaturally regarded with some suspicion and even resentment by a number of groups and individuals, some of whom felt that they had been providing a good service for years. It was not surprising that new teams with no apparent track record in this curiously closed world of service to single homeless people might find it difficult to break into the magic circle without undergoing some very close scrutiny, and indeed, meeting hostility. It must be stressed too that many of the day centres and hostels visited had had varying experience of health care provision under their roofs over a number of years, not all of which was of a high standard.

These factors must be taken into account when the schemes are assessed. It is one of the clear messages from the research that schemes of this kind take time to establish themselves. However attractive the idea may be of setting up pilot schemes of this nature de novo and seeing how they work and hoping that they may act as models, this is simply ignoring the way in which innovations work. The history of innovations shows that the most 'successful' are established by 'pioneers' who act as the inspiration and driving force. They see a need, they strive to satisfy it and they make the service work. They may well demonstrate 'success' in a very short period of time. When and if they depart, the scheme or service often falls apart because it has lost its designer, organiser and driving force. The actual success of the organisation is very difficult to measure since very often so much has depended on the initiative and ability of one person.

These schemes did not have the attributes described above. This is not to say that they did not have enthusiastic and dedicated staff, but neither of them was led by a 'personality' with the burning desire to provide a new and different service to homeless people. What the teams were being asked to do in a very short period of time must be recognised. They were charged with providing a service, establishing a multi-disciplinary team, setting up new outlets, developing outreach work, nurturing and developing contacts within the local voluntary and professional community, and monitoring their activities in a way to which they were unaccustomed. They were expected to do all this while struggling with administrative matters which often appeared to be trivial, but which severely affected the way in which they could operate. For example, the difficulty of simply getting supplies preoccupied one of the doctors initially to a quite disproportionate extent, thus depriving the service of his other more relevant skills.

Team management is one of the most difficult skills of all, and multidisciplinary teams create particular problems. The pilot teams both suffered from a lack of clear management advice on how they should operate. There were certain problems inherent in the multidisciplinary composition of the teams which should have been tackled before they started work. There were no clear lines of accountability. The team members were employed by different authorities and there was no precise definition of responsibility. Both teams struggled in their own ways to work through the difficulties of group dynamics while providing a service and developing new outlets. They were not always successful, which is not surprising. Again, the stresses of starting a new service with a new team while under close scrutiny and constrained by a limited time scale clearly compounded all the problems commonly encountered by people working together.

Against this background, how should the schemes be judged? They did provide a service, which the consumers appeared to like and to use. Whether it was a service which was very different from the services provided by other professionals or voluntary workers in the areas was very difficult to judge, since these other services were not being examined by the research team. We could only assess the general provision by what other people said about the other services, and a rather hazy picture was presented.

In evaluating the schemes it was always necessary to bear in mind that the criteria used for judging them varied widely among the providers and consumers we interviewed, not only because of the different perspectives from which the schemes were viewed, but also because they might be considered successful on one count, but not on another. It was not uncommon for respondents to disagree about the relative weight which should be given to the twin objectives, and this was marked among the team members themselves. Evaluative research of this kind is always complicated, even where the objectives are clear and simple. In this study the objectives were not clear and simple, and indeed it could be argued that not only were the objectives incompatible, they actually ran counter to each other. This lack of clarity on the main purpose of the schemes must be borne in mind in the following discussion.

We broke new ground in that we collected the views of the consumers themselves, the homeless people, as well as interviewing health care professionals and representatives from voluntary agencies offering health or social services to homeless people in the two areas. We also recorded what day centre or hostel wardens had to say about the health care experiences of their clients. We were left in no doubt that there is a problem in ensuring that homeless people can obtain primary health care when they need it, but found that strikingly different interpretations of the problem existed among those providing or seeking care.

How the pilot schemes worked and were used

The pilot schemes

What was the service that was actually being provided? It was different from general practice and from most other primary health care initiatives directed at homeless people. In both areas small multidisciplinary teams of professionals visited a limited number of day centres, night shelters and hostels, providing primary health care to homeless people who attended these centres. They did not treat homeless people at their administrative base and, as they did not treat homeless people on the streets either, they did not reach those who did not use the centres. The lack of facilities in some of the centres sometimes restricted the type and standard of service the teams were able to provide. But it appeared to be largely the differences between the schemes and general practice that made the service attractive and acceptable to the homeless people who used them.

Each team employed a *salaried doctor* instead of using local GPs. The service provided by these doctors was more limited than that offered by local GPs to the general population in that they were not able to register patients, they could not offer 24 hour cover and they visited each centre only once, twice, or at the most, three times a week. On the other hand, because they went into the centres they reached homeless people who might otherwise not see a GP at all and they were able to give patients more time than they would get in general practice. The Camden scheme had a nurse who undertook some health promotion work as well as offering general nursing services. The East London scheme had the expertise of an alcohol counsellor and a social worker and initially it also had a community psychiatric nurse.

It is important to take into account that in each area the actual service provided by the team was enhanced by an additional nurse who was not officially a team member, but whose contribution became inseparable from that of the pilot scheme. In East London just over a quarter of all consultations with the team were with the health authority nurse who worked part-time at Cable Street Day Centre. Similarly a quarter of all the consultations recorded by the Camden team during the monitoring period were actually made with the nurse employed by West London Day Centre. Any judgment of the services provided by the schemes must take into account the fact that these nurses provided an enormous input which was not actually part of the original design of the schemes.

Essentially the service provided by both project teams was very unlike that provided by a conventional primary health care team. It was provided by the doctors on a sessional basis in different centres. Other team members also established regular sessions, but not necessarily in the same centres as the doctors, and they also visited a number of other local centres on a more ad hoc basis. No team member provided care outside 'office hours', except in very exceptional circumstances.

Who used the pilot schemes?

Who actually used the services? The decision to channel services through day centres, hostels and night shelters clearly excluded those who did not use these traditional street agencies. We can only speculate on how the health care needs and problems of these people may have differed from those using the centres. We do know, however, from talking to the wardens and the users of these centres that they were predominantly male domains and also that they were rarely used by people from ethnic minority groups. It was not surprising therefore that the pilot schemes' services did not reach many homeless women or those among the ethnic minorities who were homeless.

The overwhelming majority of users of the schemes were male, living as single persons and likely to be unemployed. Most were either living on the streets, squatting or staying in temporary hostel accommodation, but in East London a good number were more settled and living in long-stay hostels. As other studies included in the literature review suggest, homeless does not necessarily mean rootless. As many as a quarter of those we interviewed at the centres - both users and non-users of the schemes - said they had their own accommodation. They could not therefore strictly be called homeless. However, the wardens we interviewed argued strongly that initiatives directed towards the homeless needed to take a broad definition of 'homelessness' which would cover anyone in 'housing need'. For them, this included those who had moved into independent accommodation, but continued to use day centres because they lacked the emotional, practical or financial support necessary to cope on their own.

It was not apparent from the use of the schemes or from our interviews with homeless people that it was necessarily general medical services that were needed. Many people did consult the doctor because they had respiratory problems, skin complaints or injuries sustained in fights, assaults or falls. But a high proportion had mental health problems, and the wardens singled out the need for directing more effort and resources towards tackling the mental health problems of their clients as a priority. The wardens themselves rarely had the training to deal with these problems or even to recognise what type of psychiatric problem was involved. A lot of consultations were for problems which were alcohol-related and again the wardens confirmed that alcohol abuse was widespread among their clients. Few facilities were available in either project area for people with serious alcohol problems who wanted to undergo detoxification.

It is also important to realise that many of those using the pilot schemes wanted advice about a social or medical problem rather than actual treatment. Some simply wanted to chat with someone who was friendly and sympathetic to their circumstances and for this purpose in both project areas they would often seek out the nurse, where one was available. Users often commented that they liked the service because team members treated them as human beings. A common complaint about local GPs was that they tended to treat homeless people as 'morons'.

Myth and reality of registration

Our study threw light on the myth and reality of homeless people's experiences regarding GP registration, and raised questions about what registration actually means for homeless people. It was sometimes difficult to see what benefits homeless people got from registration. Registration with a GP is one indicator of whether or not a person has access to a GP through the usual channels, but it says nothing about the quality of care that individuals receive or indeed whether they actually get care at all when they need it. There is also no guarantee that people who are registered will necessarily go to that GP when they want health care.

We found that more homeless people were registered with a GP than was perhaps realised. Almost half the 885 people who used the East London scheme and just over one third of the 576 individuals who used the Camden scheme during the calendar year 1987 said that they were registered with a GP. The proportion of those who said they were registered was even higher among the homeless people we interviewed, who included users and non-users of the schemes. Nearly two-thirds of the overall sample said that they were registered with a doctor, with the proportion lower in Camden than in East London.

Our study also suggests that the commonly held assumption that many single homeless people *do* want to register with GPs but are frequently turned away by doctors when they seek medical care, is unfounded. Looking first at the motivation of homeless people, we did not find that those we interviewed were clamouring to register with GPs. As we have seen, around a third of the people in our sample, which included both users and non-users of the schemes, were not registered with a GP and most of these had made no attempt to get themselves registered. Did they want to register? Was it important to them? The clear message that emerged was that for many homeless people, as indeed for many *housed* people, registering with a GP is not a priority. Many felt they had no need of medical care and could see no reason for registering with a GP unless and until they were sick. Others thought that registration was a waste of time given their mobility and the uncertainty of where they would be next week or next month. Lack of motivation to register with a GP also stemmed from low expectations about their health or from a previous unhappy or humiliating experience with health care professionals.

If homeless people were to make greater use of GP services, what sort of reception would they be likely to get? The literature review shows that stereotypical images of homeless people change slowly and we found that misconceptions and lack of understanding about homeless people were still prevalent among many GPs. While a good number indicated a willingness to treat individuals who were homeless, in practice it came down to a very few who took on substantial numbers of homeless people. The overwhelming majority of GPs interviewed for this study were concerned about creating an additional burden on their workload and they thought that homeless people might be disruptive and unacceptable to other patients using their surgeries. Some spoke from experience, but others who had had little or no contact with homeless people at their surgeries anticipated problems based on stereotypical images concerning the appearance and behaviour of single homeless people.

It was clear that the GPs in our sample would be far more likely to treat homeless people as *temporary residents* than to give them permanent registration. It was also apparent that those living in hostels were not necessarily regarded as homeless by GPs, who argued that it was easier to fulfil their contract to provide 24 hour care to a hostel resident than to someone living on the streets.

The mobility of homeless people was the fundamental problem which the GPs saw as giving rise to the numerous obstacles to continuing care and which could also create a financial disadvantage to their practice. If they permanently registered a patient who, within the same quarter year period, moved on and registered with another GP, they would not receive the capitation fee. GPs often claimed that registering homeless people was largely a bureaucratic problem, in that their FPC would not allow them to register a patient who did not have an address. It was conceivable, however, that insisting on a home address was a convenient way for GPs to avoid having to face up to the problem.

It would be wrong to attribute GPs' reluctance to registering homeless people simply to intolerant attitudes. Even among the minority of the GPs in our sample who were particularly sympathetic to the health needs and circumstances of homeless people there was recognition that among the homeless population there were many who would be demanding and time-consuming patients and that this created very real problems for over-stretched inner-city GPs. The problem for GPs in taking on single homeless people was also one of lack of time, facilities and back-up from ancillary staff, particularly for single-handed GPs in smaller practices.

Assessment of the pilot schemes
The pilot schemes were set up to offer a better quality of service to homeless people than they were currently getting and, wherever possible, to get them on to GPs' lists. How far were they successful in achieving these aims? And what criteria should be used in judging the success or lack of success in what they did? To what extent is it realistic to talk about 'success' in any case?

Users' views of the schemes
Why had people chosen to use the scheme rather than use another sort of medical care? Was it primarily because they were not registered with a GP? As we have seen, on the whole this was not the case, since a relatively high proportion said they were registered with a GP. Some who were already registered had moved away from the area where they were registered and their registration was irrelevant to their current circumstances. But most of those who were registered used the project doctor because it was convenient. They only used the project doctor when they had a minor problem - for a dressing, or for attention for a cough or cold. For more serious complaints they would go to their own doctor.

In both areas the majority of users of the schemes were highly satisfied with the services they received. This may genuinely reflect the fact that the teams were providing exceptionally good quality care. However, we have to bear in mind that it is difficult to assess the comments of homeless people on the quality of service they received, either from the pilot schemes or from other sources of primary health care, largely because so many of them had low expectations about health care and their own health. If people are uncertain about getting any care at all, then they may not be too fussy or critical about what they do receive.

The things users liked about the services provided by the schemes largely reflected their reasons for using them in the first place. The convenience of the schemes was attractive; there was no need to make an appointment and users thought there would be less 'form filling' involved than they would have to contend with in general practice. It appears also that users thought that the project doctor would be more likely to give them a thorough examination than an ordinary GP or a doctor in an accident and emergency department and to give them more time. Team members were liked because they treated homeless people with respect and it was often difficult to disentangle what users felt about personalities from what they liked about the service. This is very common where health services are being discussed. More generally, whereas general practice was geared towards people with a structured and stable lifestyle, the pilot schemes were liked because they appeared to be willing to approach homeless people more on their terms and on their territory. The nurses were very popular. Not everyone wanted to discuss their personal business with a doctor and not all problems were strictly medical.

Consumers had few criticisms about the structure or organisation of the services provided by the pilot schemes except that the non-availability of the doctor on certain days could be frustrating. Extreme dissatisfaction with the services provided was rare and tended to come from people with pronounced alcohol or drug problems, who felt that the project doctor had not given them the tablets or treatment that they had wanted. Whether or not they should have been treated differently is a largely a matter of professional judgment.

Professionals' views of the schemes

The team members themselves had strong views on the strengths and weaknesses of the schemes. They agreed that some sort of specialist care team was necessary but had different ideas about the ideal composition of such a team and the extent to which it should be integrated into mainstream services.

The wardens of the centres where the schemes operated were particularly supportive of the schemes and rated them as 'successful' both in terms of improving access to primary health care for their clients, and in terms of the valuable support and back-up they provided for centre staff.

Feelings about the schemes were very mixed among the health care professionals we interviewed. Many, particularly those who worked in accident and emergency departments, knew nothing about them. Very few ever referred patients to them or received referrals from them. Some had very clear ideas on how to provide good quality care to homeless people and tended to think that using multidisciplinary teams was the right approach, but others had had no experience of treating homeless people and had given the matter little thought.

The voluntary sector workers tended to be ambivalent towards the general concept of setting up special services for homeless people but were encouraged that the schemes had reached homeless people who had previously been overlooked. They were inclined to think of the schemes as useful alternative 'entry points' into mainstream services for those who had become so detached from health services and thinking positively about their health that they would be unable or unwilling to find a GP on their own.

But what criteria were they using for judging the schemes? They certainly did not share common criteria. Some looked only at the type of care provided, some were concerned with the way it was delivered, others judged it by the level of expertise, commitment and enthusiasm of those who were delivering the care, while others were concerned with the ability of schemes to raise the profile of the problem and also to contribute to raising homeless people's expectations of health care and their rights in this respect. The following discussion looks at the main issues.

Salaried doctors

Opinions were divided among the health care professionals and voluntary sector workers about whether or not it had been a good idea to use *salaried doctors* instead of involving local GPs. Individuals could often see both advantages and disadvantages in this arrangement, and GPs in particular found it difficult to separate their views about using salaried doctors for this client group from their views about a salaried service in general. On the whole the disadvantages were thought to be greater than the advantages.

Employing doctors to work specifically with homeless people may have increased the likelihood that they would be committed to improving health care provision for this client group, but the service they offered was often seen to be more limited than that offered by local GPs to the general population, particularly as regards the hours in which it was available. Using salaried doctors instead of local GPs on a sessional basis also meant that the schemes were seen to be rather detached from mainstream services. The amount of contact and referral activity between the teams and those working in mainstream services was not extensive and it could be argued that more work should have been done in the early stages by the teams in trying to increase liaison with other professionals.

Appointing salaried doctors specifically for homeless people was also seen to carry a risk of isolation, both for the users of the service and for team members. Some respondents thought there was a danger that homeless people would thus be stigmatised further and isolated even more from society. The wardens and the voluntary sector workers we interviewed were particularly concerned about this. It was also apparent that the project doctors, and other team members, had experienced professional isolation from their peers, and that this had stemmed largely from the way the schemes had been set up and from the confused management and accountability arrangements for the staff who came from a variety of disciplines. For the doctors, the problems were in some respects similar to those faced by single-handed GPs, but as they were dealing with a skewed caseload of patients, they also had to keep in mind their career prospects and ensure that their full range of clinical skills did not atrophy.

Outreach work

Our study showed that many homeless people have difficulty fitting into mainstream primary health care services which are geared towards people with a stable and structured lifestyle, so it is perhaps not surprising that many of the professionals and voluntary sector workers we interviewed thought that a major strength of the schemes lay in their commitment to outreach work. Taking the service to homeless people, instead of expecting them to visit a GP's surgery, avoided common problems such as missed appointments and the stigma often experienced by homeless people on occasions when they were made to feel unwelcome in GPs' waiting rooms. It also meant that the service reached those who were unwilling or simply not motivated to seek help from an ordinary GP.

From the wardens' point of view, the schemes' success was not limited to providing services direct to clients. The teams' style of outreach work meant that they gave a lot of support and back-up to staff and volunteers in the centres they visited. The non-medical members of the East London team were particularly active in providing support and training for centre staff, as was the nurse employed by the Camden scheme. This support was highly valued by the wardens, who were interested in what was good for the practice and philosophy of their centres, as well as in improving direct service provision for their clients. There can be no doubt that this 'networking' by team members was one of the most successful aspects of the schemes. The teams were small and by sharing expertise with other workers they could indirectly help a greater number of homeless people. This is of particular value in a 'pilot' project of limited duration. It increases the possibility that the services and knowledge base developed by professionals with expertise will continue and spread.

Multidisciplinary teams

Professionals and voluntary sector workers often stressed that homeless people have a wide range of interrelated social as well as medical problems. One of the major strengths of the schemes was believed to be their use of multidisciplinary teams of workers. Team members were frequently described as committed individuals, flexible and responsive to homeless people's needs and able to draw on one

255

another's expertise. However, the reality of the multidisciplinary nature of the schemes should not be overestimated. While the scheme in East London included an alcohol counsellor and a social worker working alongside the project doctor, the smaller team in Camden was firmly medically based, comprising a doctor and nurse. During the monitoring period neither team was able to provide the specialist expertise needed to deal with the mental health problems of homeless people using the centres, and it was these problems that particularly concerned the centre staff. The East London team originally had a CPN, but great difficulty was encountered in integrating him into the team.

Although it was widely believed that using a multidisciplinary team was an appropriate response to the problem, there were also lessons to be learned about using and managing such teams. There did not appear to be enough real thought given to the composition of the teams, or the interaction of team members, or much guidance given on their roles. The teams sometimes appeared to have been put together and told to get on with it. More specifically, there were a number of crucial weaknesses in the infrastructure and management of the schemes. It was questionable whether sufficient thought had been given as to how the teams would operate and where they would get their supplies. The fact that team members were appointed incrementally, were employed by different authorities and had different lines of accountability adversely affected the functioning of the teams. And the working relationships and dynamics of small teams are not always easy, as the Camden 'trio' discovered. These difficulties were compounded by their feelings of professional and geographical isolation which stemmed from the design of the schemes.

Take-up figures

It was widely held to be inappropriate to judge the schemes simply on the basis of the number of people who had used them, and it is clear in any case that figures on take-up should be interpreted with caution. A high level of use might be said to indicate success in providing a service which was attractive and acceptable to homeless people. But it might also suggest that the schemes were failing to encourage those they treated to go and register with a local GP. It is also very difficult to judge the schemes on the basis of take-up figures alone because we have no idea of the size of the potential demand. The take-up might represent only a fraction of what is really needed. We have no base-line to work from and no figures of health care provision for homeless people by mainstream services with which to compare the take-up figures.

However, we know that 885 people used the East London scheme during the calendar year 1987 and that between them they made a total of 3,198 consultations. Just over half of these users consulted once only during the calendar year. In Camden, where there were fewer regular surgeries, 576 people used the scheme during the monitoring period and during these twelve months they made a total of 2,022 consultations. Around 58 per cent of these people used the scheme once only during the period.

What emerges from the figures is that the services provided by the schemes were used by single homeless people. The statistics show quite clearly that a high proportion of the consultations were for alcohol-related or mental health problems. There was also clear evidence that many of the consultations, especially with the nurses, were for problems which might have appeared relatively trivial. And it must not be forgotten that a quarter of the consultations in each area were with a nurse who was not part of the team and who would have been employed at the centres seeing clients whether the pilot schemes had been set up or not.

Health status
It is difficult to comment on the extent to which the schemes were successful in improving the health status of individuals. We were able to look at outcomes defined as the 'terminating actions' to consultations, but to go beyond this and measure outcomes concerning the morbidity of homeless people using the schemes, proved impossible both for us and for the team members. Outcomes in general practice are known to be hard to measure, and with this client group there were the added problems that they were not a stable population, it was often difficult for the doctors to obtain reliable information about their medical history, and patients were often impossible to follow up.

Central government initiatives

These schemes were seen as top-down solutions to the problem by central government. There are advantages and disadvantages in centrally imposed initiatives to tackle difficult social problems. One advantage identified by voluntary sector workers, but interestingly not mentioned by the health care professionals we interviewed, was that the schemes were statutory, because this signified that the government were taking the health care problems of homeless people seriously. Another argument was that in the short term they could have a pump-priming effect, raising general awareness of the problem and getting more GPs interested in and willing to take on their share of homeless people. However, we were also warned that, unless such schemes were set up with considerable care, and with objectives which were tightly focused and potentially achievable, they might well be counter-productive.

A common criticism in the voluntary sector was that the schemes had been centrally imposed with a lack of previous consultation with local agencies. As a result the schemes were not seen as rooted into existing local services. As we have seen, most of the accident and emergency staff and quite a few of the GPs, nurses and CPNs we interviewed for this study had not even heard of the schemes. It was widely thought that the schemes had not been publicised well enough, that there was too little feedback about them and that there was not enough interaction with local service providers.

There was a big question mark over whether the health care needs of homeless people can be tackled without addressing their housing problems. The consensus view among the voluntary sector workers we interviewed was that they could not, and that a major flaw of the schemes was they had not been linked into initiatives to tackle the housing needs of homeless people. The need to address housing problems before much of an impact could be made on the health care front was also emphasised by the nurses, CPNs and social workers we interviewed, in contrast to the GPs who were more likely to be concerned specifically with what they saw as the health needs of homeless people, irrespective of their social or housing conditions.

Overall assessment

So what did the schemes actually achieve? As the foregoing discussion has shown, much of course depends upon whose perspective you view them from. For the consumers they provided a good standard of health care, better in some ways than the care they received from GPs or from accident and emergency departments. They plugged a gap in health care provision in that they reached some homeless people who had not seen a doctor before. They raised the profile of the problem of health care provision for homeless people and they also provided the wardens and their staff at the various centres and hostels with valuable support and back-up.

On the other hand, there were a number of drawbacks to the schemes. The care they provided was only available on certain days. The schemes were channelled through day centres, night shelters and hostels and therefore did not reach homeless people on the streets who did not use these agencies. And some people who were already registered with a local GP apparently used the project doctor as an alternative to their own GP for relatively trivial complaints.

How far was it an advantage to have a multidisciplinary 'team' employed specifically to provide care for homeless people? Both teams had problems with team management and to some extent the difficulties experienced in trying to operate as a team, separate from mainstream services, actually seemed to get in the way of service provision. Our findings support the need for retaining some form of special service operating on an outreach basis to improve the provision and take-up of health care services by homeless people, but it does not follow that a special team, separate from mainstream services, is the best option.

The question which also arises is whether many of the problems which were in fact treated by a doctor simply because one was available could not have been better treated by other professionals. It looked as though a service which gave more prominence to nursing care, psychiatric care, health education, counselling and support might possibly have been more appropriate to the needs of this client group, given the nature of the presenting problems.

To what extent were the schemes successful in achieving the long-term objective of getting people registered with local GPs? Neither project appeared to have made much progress in getting people registered who did not already have a GP. For the project doctors, the task of getting homeless people registered with GPs seemed incompatible with the other main objective, of providing them with a good standard of primary health care. They found it difficult to treat homeless people at the centres and at the same time tell them they should go and find a GP. They felt that in doing this they were sending out 'mixed messages' about their commitment to providing care. More generally, the fact that the team provided a service which proved attractive and accessible to homeless people may actually have militated against their getting patients to register with GPs.

How far was the objective of getting homeless people permanently registered with local GPs achievable universally in any case? There was a consensus among all the health care professionals and voluntary sector workers we interviewed that among homeless people there were many who could be encouraged to register with GPs, but that there would always be some who would never be willing or able to use the system or be considered 'acceptable' in general practice. This observation was borne out by our interviews with homeless people.

The next step?

The questions now arise of whether the schemes should be continued, and to what extent the model of primary health care developed in each of the pilot sites is an appropriate one to use elsewhere to improve the access of homeless people to primary health care services. We do not recommend that the pilot schemes should be continued or transferred elsewhere in their *current* format. The value of the schemes for future policy lies predominantly in lessons learned about several key issues: the composition and management of such schemes; the types of services homeless people actually want or apparently need; and the extent to which services for homeless people need to be integrated into mainstream services and linked with local agencies dealing not just with health care, but with housing as well.

However, in deciding what to do next in the two project areas it is important to take into account the concern expressed by team members and wardens about what would happen to the homeless people using the schemes if these services were stopped abruptly when the funding for the schemes came to an end. The decision about what to do next is all the more complicated because, as our findings suggest, there is perhaps no one all-embracing solution which will ensure that all homeless people get primary health care when they need it. This is because homeless people do not belong to a homogeneous group for policy-makers to focus on. Some are already registered with GPs and some could be encouraged to do so, providing these services are made more flexible to accommodate their needs and that GPs are given greater back-up in terms of ancillary staff in order to feel able and willing to take on homeless people.

But there are other homeless people who for one reason or another cannot or will not be able to negotiate the system, or are unlikely to be regarded as 'acceptable' in general practice. There are grounds for providing some kind of specialist service aimed at this group, but whether it has to be a full primary health care team service is a matter for considerable discussion. There is also the possibility that among the single homeless there are some individuals who lead that lifestyle because they choose to and who would not welcome being pushed towards the 'commitment' of registering with a GP. The reason they live the way they do may have much to do with the rejection of a settled lifestyle and all that this entails.

There appear to be three main options open for the future: (i) the schemes fold up completely and special services of this kind for homeless people are discontinued; (ii) the schemes continue in their present format; (iii) special services for homeless people continue, but in a different format.

If the first option were taken and the schemes were closed down then the situation would not be much different from what existed before the pilot exercise was set up. Homeless people would have to seek primary health care through the usual channels unless any special health care services were made available to them through the voluntary sector, or by professionals offering their services in an ad hoc way in the centres on a voluntary basis. There are strong arguments against this option. We have shown that there are many homeless people who are not able or willing to use mainstream services and, even if they were, access to these services would not necessarily be meaningful unless these services became more flexible and GPs' attitudes towards homeless people changed. What would happen to the people currently using the schemes if they were closed down? It appears that some would try a casualty department or go to their own GP, but many were less confident about their ability to find an alternative source of care and others would simply not bother to look for a doctor.

But there are also strong arguments against retaining the schemes as they currently operate, in particular the use of salaried doctors to provide care specifically for homeless people. It was generally agreed that the project doctors were energetic and committed medical practitioners and that they provided a good medical service, bearing in mind the lack of facilities in some of the centres and the managerial and administrative tasks which took up so much of their time. They were liked and respected by the users of the schemes and their expertise and the regularity of their visits were valued by the wardens. Nevertheless, they provided a more limited service than local GPs in that they could not provide 24 hour cover and were not obliged to do 'home' visits. They were supposed to encourage people to register with local GPs, but were hindered by the problem of 'mixed messages', and their detachment from mainstream services added to their problems of professional isolation. The extent to which services to the homeless should be the only job of professionals and depend on these individuals is also questionable. Working exclusively with homeless people is demanding work and at the same time does not use the full range of a doctor's skills. It is unlikely that any one doctor, or any other health professional, would want to do this work for more than a couple of years and the continuation of the schemes would depend on regularly recruiting committed individuals.

The case for a special service within more flexible mainstream provision

Our study points to the third option outlined above: that special services for homeless people should continue, but delivered in a different way. A multi-pronged approach to improving the provision and take-up of health care services by homeless people is necessary and there is a strong case for a special service for homeless people within more flexible mainstream provision. There can be no doubt that some homeless people could be encouraged to use mainstream services if these services were made more responsive to their needs, but it seems likely that there will always be some who will remain unable or unwilling to do so. For these people , a special *service* operating on an outreach basis is needed, but not a special and separate *team*.

We recommend a multidisciplinary specialist service because the pilot schemes have shown that homeless people often have a multiplicity of social as well as medical problems which are often difficult to disentangle one from another. However, the study has indicated that the general medical services element of this service is not best provided by a separate salaried doctor for homeless people, as under the existing schemes. There would in fact be a number of advantages in local GPs taking over the surgeries already set up in the centres by the project doctors.

If the new approach to providing a special service retained the twin objectives of the existing schemes, of providing good quality care and encouraging people to register with a GP, using local GPs in the centres would avoid the 'mixed messages' problem. If local GPs could initially build up relationships with homeless people in the centres, they could then try to encourage them to continue that relationship within the environment of the general surgery. There would be other advantages. In contrast to the salaried doctors, local GPs would be able to offer greater continuity of care, would in theory be able to provide 24 hour cover, and would not suffer from professional isolation. The argument for using local GPs is particularly strong where the centre is residential; for example, in hostels or detoxification units. Here residents have an address and can be located, and GPs themselves appear to feel that it is easier for them to fulfil their contract to provide 24 hour care to a hostel resident than to someone living on the streets.

The assumption was that some GPs would not be willing to undertake this work unless they were paid. They could become visiting medical officers to a number of centres as indeed they are in other areas. Alternatively they could be paid a fixed sum for each session held at one of the centres and, in addition, they could claim a temporary resident fee for each patient seen. A further option, where a patient was seen regularly, was that the patient could be permanently registered. We were warned that a drawback of this was that it could create problems because the people seen at the centres might already be permanently registered with a GP elsewhere.

There are, therefore, strong arguments for absorbing the general medical services aspect of the schemes into mainstream services, but what about the future of the services offered by the other team members in the two areas? Should they continue to be provided by a special and separate team, or should they too be delivered as part of mainstream provision? The nurses, whether employed by the scheme or not, were very highly regarded by the consumers. Did it matter whether they were actually employed in a special and separate team with one particular doctor or not? The nurse in West London Day Centre was not employed as a member of the team and neither was the nurse in Cable Street Day Centre, but they both provided a very similar service to the nurse who was a team member. Many of the problems homeless people wanted help with could have been dealt with by a nurse, and did not necessarily require a doctor. Clearly nurses do need to work with and have the support of general practitioners for the full range of nursing and medical services to be available to homeless people, but it is debatable whether the advantages of working in a special team with a particular doctor outweigh the potential disadvantages.

What about the alcohol counsellor, social worker and CPN in East London? How far were they part of a 'team'? Did it matter whether or not they had a doctor and nurse as part of their team? The alcohol counsellor working for the East London pilot scheme found that over time her workload evolved to a point where she spent more time providing support, training and back-up to centre staff than working with individual clients. Essentially she developed her role independently of the 'team' although she valued the opportunity of working closely with one doctor who was sympathetic to her aims and way of working.

The social worker became increasingly interested and involved in resettlement work. The extent to which this development was influenced by his membership of the 'team' was difficult to assess, but it appeared that he too used the opportunity offered by membership of the team to develop a more flexible way of working with the homeless than he had hitherto been able to do. In both instances the 'team' facilitated the development of innovative and imaginative work practices by individual workers.

The CPN's experience was quite different. He had previously worked in institutional settings and found it difficult to integrate into a community-based team committed to outreach work. The fact that mental health care services for homeless people were not successfully developed by a CPN in the context of a specialist 'team' setting does not mean that these services were not needed. Our findings show just the reverse.

On balance our findings lead us to recommend relocating within mainstream provision the services currently provided by specialist team members, but this means that consideration needs to be given to ways of promoting and ensuring that these services are actually made available and responsive to homeless people. Two important areas where resources for meeting the needs of homeless people appear to be lacking are mental health care and detoxification facilities. The pattern of use of the schemes also highlighted the need for more counselling, support and health education services. More generally, users gained a good deal of satisfaction from the service offered by the pilot schemes because it was offered on their home ground, and the delivery style was such that trust was developed. This outreach aspect of service delivery is an essential component of any planned service for homeless people and would need to be continued if the services currently offered by the pilot schemes were absorbed into mainstream provision.

One suggestion is that Health Authorities and Social Services Departments in the two project areas (and perhaps other areas where there is a particular problem of homelessness) might appoint specialist resource workers. For example, concerning the district nursing stance, the two Health Authorities might appoint a specialist nurse(s) with community training. These nurses could act as a resource for nursing staff in the health district in order to ensure that a nursing service is provided for homeless people within mainstream provision. Several advantages might follow from this arrangement: a sharing of responsibility among those nurses in the district would help prevent 'burn out'; the general knowledge base of all nurses in relation to homeless people could increase with the help of the specialist resource nurse; and with the appointment of a specialist resource worker there might be a greater likelihood of health service managers taking a greater degree of responsibility for ensuring that an adequately staffed nursing service is provided for this vulnerable group. Some similar sort of arrangement might be made available by the Community Psychiatrict Nursing Service in both areas. The relevant social services departments might also designate a person with specific responsibility for homeless people.

Mainstream commitment to tackling the problem
The pilot schemes have undoubtedly demonstrated that there is a need for special health care services for single homeless people to deal with the high incidence of serious alcohol abuse, mental health problems and other associated problems, not least among which is isolation from society in general and dislocation from family networks and support in particular. But, although we recommend special services, we do recommend that these services are firmly rooted in mainstream provision. There is an enormous danger that special services provided by special teams only serve further to marginalise people who are already operating on the borders of society. However, simply rooting these special services in mainstream provision does not necessarily guarantee a 'good' service. There has to be a commitment to tackling the problem. Single homeless people still have a very low priority in the minds of service planners and there is always the danger that in times of financial stringency services for the homeless will be the first to go.

10 Recommendations

Homeless people do not belong to a homogeneous group for policy-makers to focus on and there is no all-embracing solution to ensure that all homeless people get primary health care when they need it. This study has examined two pilot schemes set up in two areas in London to provide primary health care for homeless people the majority of whom were male and single. It was generally agreed that their contribution was valuable in improving health care provision for the people they saw in the centres, but the evidence presented in the report suggests that their main value lay in the lessons which can be learned from their experience.

I. Homeless people and health care provision

1. In spite of the achievements of the pilot schemes outlined in the report, we do not recommend the continuation of these health care schemes in their present form. Existing mainstream health care services should be made more flexible to meet the main primary health care needs of the majority of single homeless people. At the same time, special health care services should be developed *within* mainstream services and targeted at specific groups of homeless people who have specific health or social problems.

2. The aim should be for local GPs to provide general medical services for the majority of single homeless people, either within their own surgeries or through establishing regular clinics or sessions at day centres, hostels and night shelters. Single homeless people should be encouraged to register with them. Consideration would have to be

267

given to how these GPs should be paid for providing services outside their own surgeries.

3. The use of salaried doctors to deliver services to single homeless people is not recommended, since the disadvantages of lack of 24-hour cover, inability to register patients, and potential marginalisation of an already stigmatised group of people outweigh any advantages. If salaried doctors recommend patients to register with other GPs, they may destroy the trust they are trying to build up with a vulnerable group of patients.

4. Local GPs should take over the clinics already set up in the centres by the project doctors, but the aim should be to provide general medical services in this way only to the small number of people who would never be likely to go to GPs' surgeries.

5. There is a need to educate all GPs about the needs and characteristics of homeless people so that they are more prepared to take them on as patients. A change in GPs' attitudes towards homeless people is essential if general medical services are to be made more flexible for this client group.

6. GPs should be given greater back-up and ancillary staff in order to feel able and willing to take on homeless people as patients. GPs' reluctance to treat single homeless people may be related to practical problems of time, space and facilities.

7. Family practitioner committees should take a stronger lead in securing access by homeless people to a good standard of general medical care:

(i) they should be more flexible about registration where a patient has no fixed address and should make their policy on this clear to GPs;

(ii) they should become better informed about the health care needs of homeless people and should share this knowledge with other practitioners and agencies;

(iii) they should explore the feasibility of setting up local initiatives where necessary to meet the needs of homeless people;

(iv) they should ensure that they take on GPs with the skills and commitment to treat homeless people in areas where their health care needs are not being met.

II. Special needs

9. The services of the health care teams provided by the pilot schemes were available only in day centres, hostels and night shelters. An investigation should be made of the health care needs of homeless people who do not use these centres, such as street dwellers, homeless women and homeless people from ethnic minorities, and urgent consideration should be given to improving ways of reaching them and meeting their needs.

10. Similarly, the services of the health care teams were not used by homeless families, whose need is said to be considerable. Again, urgent consideration should be given to improving ways of providing primary health care to homeless families.

11. It is recommended that a high priority should be given to the development of services specifically to deal with mental health and alcohol-related problems among single homeless people, and that counselling and advice services on a range of health and social issues should be developed. These were seen by local voluntary and professional workers to be the main health care needs of single homeless people which were not being met by mainstream services.

12. All these services should be firmly rooted within mainstream provision, but delivered on an outreach basis where necessary by specialist workers who can share their expertise with others and provide support for the staff of centres used by homeless people.

13. It is recommended that all health care provision for single homeless people should have strong links with local housing initiatives, since there was considerable evidence that their health care needs were thought to be inextricable from their living conditions.

14. There is an urgent need for health promotion and health education programmes to be targeted at single homeless people to encourage them to look after their health, to inform them about their rights to health care and to advise them how to use mainstream services. This should be

provided in places where they congregate and on an outreach basis for those who do not use traditional agencies and centres for homeless people.

III. Special projects

15. It should not be assumed that the setting up of centrally inspired initiatives with central funding is the most appropriate way of tackling difficult social problems at a local level. The experience of the pilot schemes indicates that schemes of this nature, whether locally or centrally initiated, must ensure widespread consultation at a local level before they start. They should be set up with tightly focused and potentially achievable objectives and with a firm management structure and on-going management support. This may be easier to ensure if they arise from a local initiative.

16. In special projects of this kind using multidisciplinary teams careful consideration should be given to the exact composition of the teams and the ways in which they should relate to mainstream services. If team members come from different disciplines with different professional cultures, a clear definition of roles, responsibilities and lines of accountability needs to be laid down from the outset. The team members should be appointed at the same time and all members should be in post before any attempt is made to deliver services.

11 Summary

1. This study evaluated the two pilot schemes of primary health care for homeless people which were set up in 1986 by the Department of Health and Social Security. One scheme was based in East London and was managed by the City and East London Family Practitioner Committee (FPC). The other was located in Camden and was managed by the Camden and Islington FPC. Each scheme was staffed by a multidisciplinary team of workers. The main objectives of the schemes were in the short term to provide a good standard of primary health care to homeless people in the locality of the managing FPC and, in the longer term, wherever possible to secure their admission to the list of a general medical practitioner.

The evaluation
2. The aims of the research were to assess the schemes in the light of their objectives and to comment on the appropriateness of the schemes as models of primary health care provision for homeless people. Our study concentrated on single homeless people because it was this group who used the schemes. Many of the issues we explored have broader relevance to the provision of primary health care to homeless people generally.

3. Over a twelve-month monitoring period (1 January 1987 - 31 December 1987) we collected detailed information about all users of the two pilot schemes. We had worked closely with both teams to establish a medical record system which could be used by them for practical purposes and by us for our research and monitoring purposes.

271

4. We interviewed a total of 190 homeless people about their health care experiences, 50 per cent of whom had used the pilot schemes' services. In both project areas we also interviewed: (i) all team members and their managers; (ii) samples of professionals concerned with the statutory provision of health or social services to homeless people; (iii) representatives of voluntary agencies offering health care, counselling or social services to homeless people; and (iv) the wardens of the day centres, night shelters and hostels where the project doctors had established regular clinics.

The pilot schemes

5. The team in East London comprised a salaried doctor, an alcohol counsellor, a community psychiatric nurse (who left the project in May 1987), a social worker and a project co-ordinator. In Camden the team was made up of a salaried doctor, a nurse and a project co-ordinator.

6. The FPCs employed *salaried doctors* to work for the schemes. The service offered by these salaried doctors was more limited than that offered by local GPs to the general population. They did not provide 24 hour cover, they had no locum cover when they were on holiday and they had no mechanism for registering patients.

7. All team members undertook *outreach* work. They visited day centres, hostels and night shelters where homeless people congregated, instead of expecting users to come to their base.

8. Since both schemes were channelled through particular centres they were available only to people who attended these centres.

9. During the monitoring period the doctor in East London held regular clinics in five centres; these included two day centres, an evening centre, a short-stay hostel and a detoxification unit. In the same time period the doctor in Camden established regular clinics in two day centres and a night shelter.

10. Other team members in both areas established regular sessions, but not necessarily in the same centres as the doctor. They also visited a number of other centres on a more ad hoc basis. Their roles and work patterns evolved during the monitoring period both in response to the needs of clients and staff and according to their own particular interests

and expertise. Team members provided support, advice and training for centre staff as well as a service for homeless people.

11. Team members rarely started from a base-line of no health care provision at the centres they visited, but existing services were usually provided on an ad hoc basis by volunteers and were not part of mainstream provision.

12. The facilities available to both teams in individual centres varied considerably. The majority lacked some of the standard amenities that were necessary for team members, and in particular the doctor, to provide a good standard of service.

13. Team members had to develop outreach services which were attractive to homeless people and also acceptable to centre staff. At the beginning of the projects they also had a considerable amount of administrative work.

14. Many of the lessons to be learned from the pilot schemes concerned their structure and management and the dynamics of multidisciplinary teams. The teams shared a number of common weakness: they suffered from a lack of clear management advice about how they should operate; team members were appointed incrementally and by different authorities; there were no clear lines of accountability and there was no clear definition of responsibility. Both teams struggled to work through the difficulties of group dynamics while at the same time trying to develop an innovative service in a limited time period and under close scrutiny.

Use and users of the schemes

City and East London pilot scheme
15. A total of 885 individuals used the City and East London pilot scheme one or more times during the 12-month monitoring period (1.1.1987 - 31.12.1987). Most of these users were men, reflecting the predominant use of the centres by men. Almost 50 per cent of users were aged between 35 and 54, 28 per cent were younger than 35 and 5 per cent were over retirement age. Just under a third of all users of the scheme were living rough, skippering or squatting. Of the rest around 16 per cent were temporarily housed in short-stay hostels, 17 per cent

were more settled in long-stay hostels and 22 per cent had some form of their own accommodation.

16. Almost half those who had used the scheme during the monitoring period thought that they were registered with a GP, although the registration may have been of little value because the GP was too far away or they were confusing permanent and temporary registration.

17. The 885 individuals who used the East London scheme during the monitoring period made a total of 3,198 consultations. Just over half did so once only during the calendar year and almost three-quarters of these had consulted the doctor. Around 5 per cent of users consulted more than 12 times during the calendar year and these 47 individuals made between them 830 consultations.

18. Fifty-one per cent (1,631) of all consultations made during the monitoring period were with one of the project doctors. Respiratory complaints were the most common presenting problems accounting for 19 per cent of all doctor consultations. Other fairly common categories of presenting problems were 'Dermatology', 'Psychiatric' and 'Trauma'. A quarter of all doctor consultations were recorded as being alcohol or drug-related, and the vast majority of these involved alcohol abuse. Homeless people using the schemes had a variety of social as well as medical problems. Just over half of all consultations with the project doctors resulted in a prescription or repeat prescription. Almost 13 per cent required some kind of dressing and a similar proportion resulted in providing a medical certificate. Fourteen per cent resulted in users being referred to hospital. Sixteen per cent resulted in advice only.

19. Just over a quarter (901) of all the consultations made during the monitoring period occurred with the Health Authority Nurse working at Cable Street Day Centre who was not employed as a member of the team. In over half of all the consultations with her the users sought general advice about a social or medical problem. In 41 per cent of consultations she provided advice only and took no further action. She gave general nursing care, predominantly dressings for wounds or for chronic skin complaints, in just under a third of consultations.

20. Approximately 9 per cent (288) of all the consultations made during the monitoring period occurred with the alcohol counsellor. Many were not alcohol specific; she also provided general advice and counselling for a variety of social problems. Overall, approximately 40 per cent of all consultations with the alcohol counsellor were alcohol, or very occasionally drug, related. Almost two-thirds involved the user making a specific arrangement for a repeat appointment, usually for 'continuation counselling'. The alcohol counsellor did group work as well as individual counselling and held around 60 group sessions during the 12-month monitoring period.

21. Around 11 per cent (359) of all consultations during the monitoring period took place with the social worker. Almost two-thirds of these involved people wanting help with their housing problems. At least 15 per cent concerned requests for help with welfare benefits. Almost half the consultations resulted in advice only. Just over a quarter resulted in referrals to statutory or voluntary agencies dealing with housing and homelessness.

22. Too few consultations occurred with the community psychiatric nurse to warrant analysis.

Camden and Islington pilot scheme
23. A total of 576 individuals used the Camden pilot scheme one or more times during the 12-month monitoring period. Again, the majority of users were men. Around half the users were in the age range 35-54 and about 5 per cent were over retirement age. Users of the Camden scheme were more likely than those in East London to be living rough or skippering, were more frequently housed temporarily in bed and breakfast accommodation, and were less likely to have their own accommodation.

24. Just over one third of those using the Camden scheme claimed they were registered with a GP, compared with almost a half in the East End. This may reflect the greater geographical mobility among homeless people in the Camden area.

25. The 576 people who used the Camden scheme during the monitoring period made a total of 2,022 consultations. The pattern of frequency of use of the scheme was similar to that found in East London.

Around 58 per cent of people who used the scheme did so once only. Approximately 5 per cent had been seen by the project doctor or nurse more than 12 times during the calendar year and between them had made a total of 483 consultations.

26. The consultation statistics in Camden tend to underestimate the amount of contact the nurses had with users and overestimate the action on consultations taken by the doctor. This is because information about consultations was recorded under the doctor's name only, when the doctor shared clinics with the nurses.

27. Fifty-three per cent (1,073) of all consultations during the monitoring period were with the project doctor. Sixteen per cent of all doctor consultations involved a dermatological condition, 13 per cent involved a respiratory complaint, 11 per cent involved a psychiatric problem and in 10 per cent the user had sought some form of general advice. Thirteen per cent were recorded as being alcohol or, more rarely, drug-related. This figure is not comparable with the equivalent figure for the East London project because there were differences between the doctors in recording whether a consultation was alcohol-related. Sixty per cent of consultations with the Camden doctor resulted in a prescription; 15 per cent ended with the doctor giving the patient advice only and no other treatment; and 10 per cent required some kind of dressing. Patients were referred to a local GP or to hospital less frequently in Camden than in East London.

28. Just under a quarter of all consultations made with the Camden team during the monitoring period were with the project nurse. A further quarter of all consultations were made with the nurse on the staff at West London Day Centre who was not a member of the team. They spent a lot of their time talking to users who were seeking advice about a social or medical problem or simply wanted a chat, as well as providing nursing care. Other common complaints were categorised either as 'Dermatology' or 'Trauma'. A third of all the consultations with one or other of the nurses resulted in advice only and no further treatment. Almost a third required general nursing care. Just under a quarter resulted in repeat prescriptions, but as in East London this did not mean that the nurses were able to prescribe drugs; they were only

able to give patients medication such as paracetemol. Their referral activity was not extensive.

29. In both project areas team members recorded at each consultation how acceptable they thought users of the pilot schemes would be in an ordinary GP's surgery, using a simple three-point scale. In City and East London the acceptability of 70 per cent of users was rated as 'good' at the time of their first contact with the pilot scheme. In Camden the equivalent figure was 65 per cent. In both project areas less than 6 per cent of users were rated as 'poor'.

Voice of the consumer

30. We interviewed 190 homeless people, 50 per cent of whom had used the projects' services: 90 of these interviews were at centres in East London where the project doctor had established regular clinics (45 of them users); and 100 interviews at centres in Camden where regular clinics were set up (50 of them users). Ninety per cent of the sample were men and 10 per cent women, reflecting the fact that very few women used the centres where the surgeries were held. The ages of those interviewed ranged from 9 per cent of the sample who were under 25 through to 5 per cent who were 65 or over. This survey of homeless people was done on a quota sampling basis because it was impossible to find a suitable sampling frame which would have enabled us to select a random sample.

31. Almost a quarter of the people included in the sample said they had some form of their own accommodation. They continued to use day centres because they lacked the emotional, practical or financial support necessary to cope on their own.

32. Sixty per cent of the overall sample thought that they were registered with a doctor, but the proportion registered was markedly lower among those interviewed in Camden (51 per cent) than those in East London (70 per cent), and was much lower among those sleeping rough, skippering or living in a squat than among those who were living in hostels or hotels, or who had some form of their own accommodation.

33. Over 80 per cent of those not registered with a GP had not tried to get themselves registered during the previous year. For many homeless people, as for many housed people, registering with a GP was not a

priority, since they could see no good reason for registering with a GP unless and until they were ill. Others thought that registration was a waste of time, given their mobility. They preferred to use a hospital accident or emergency department or to use the services of the project doctor when he visited the centre. For some, lack of motivation to register was tied up with low expectations about their health or their rights to health care.

34. Just over two-thirds of the people we interviewed said that at some point during the previous year they had wanted to see a doctor: 39 per cent had consulted a local GP; 35 per cent had used a doctor visiting the day centre, night shelter or hostel they attended (in most cases this was one of the salaried doctors working for the pilot schemes); 13 per cent had used a hospital doctor, either in out-patients or in an A and E department; and a few had attended Great Chapel Street Medical Centre. Eighty-three per cent of those who had seen a doctor in the previous year were satisfied with the treatment they had received. (One third of these people were talking about their level of satisfaction with the medical services provided under the pilot scheme.) Single homeless people in our sample reported particular difficulties in finding GPs who were sympathetic to alcohol, drugs or mental health problems.

35. Just over half the homeless people we interviewed had been admitted to hospital at some point during the previous five years, mostly with some form of trauma. In 74 per cent of cases a GP had not been involved in the admission to hospital, usually because people had been picked up off the streets and taken to hospital by ambulance. For a tiny minority, getting admitted to hospital had not been easy and a common complaint was that hospitals, like GPs, often treated homeless people as 'morons'. Around two-thirds of those who had been in-patients had been discharged without having talked to staff about where they would go on discharge, but this was not necessarily the fault of hospital staff. Some individuals chose not to discuss their discharge plans.

36. Our sample was designed to ensure that half the people we interviewed had used one or more of the services offered by the pilot schemes. In both areas the convenience of the service was the most common reason for choosing to use the pilot scheme instead of any other source of health care. Many users of the schemes were apparently

already registered with a GP: 43 per cent in Camden, compared to 78 per cent in East London. Those who were already registered tended to use the project doctor only when they had a minor problem, but would go to their own GP for a more serious complaint.

37. Those who had used the schemes said that it was not always or predominantly for general medical services. Mental health problems were common and a high proportion of consultations were alcohol-related. Many wanted advice about a social or medical problem, or simply a chat with someone who they thought understood their circumstances.

38. In both areas the majority of users were highly satisfied with the services offered: they liked seeing the doctor or other team member in the familiar environment of the day centre, hostel or night shelter; access to the project doctor was relatively simple compared to registering with a GP; team members gave them time to talk about their problems and treated them with respect.

39. Consumers were sometimes frustrated about the non-availability of the doctor on certain days at the particular centre they attended. The project doctors visited each centre once, twice or at the most three times a week.

40. Neither users nor non-users expressed an overwhelming preference either for using special health care facilities, or for using a GP: 49 per cent of people said they would prefer to be registered with a local GP and use the surgery; 31 per cent said they would prefer to use the special health care services provided at the centres; 12 per cent had no clear idea about which type of service they wanted; 4 per cent wanted access to both types of provision and a few showed no interest in using any type of health service provision.

41. About one-third of those who had used the schemes said they would have tried a casualty department or gone to their own GP if the schemes had not been available. The rest were less confident about finding an alternative source of care and some simply would not have bothered to look for a doctor.

Views of the providers

42. Team members thought that the National Health Service was not flexible enough to accommodate the needs of homeless people and that GPs were reluctant to take on patients who were homeless. They also thought that homeless people had low health expectations and that, for them, registering with a GP was not a priority.

43. Team members believed that there was a great deal of educative and promotional work to be done, both with GPs and with the homeless, if more homeless people were to use ordinary GP services.

44. The main strengths of the schemes identified by team members were: they provided a service for a client group not well served by mainstream services; the teams were multidisciplinary; team members were committed to the needs of homeless people; they went out to meet homeless people in their own environment; and their approach was flexible. The schemes also raised the profile of the health care needs of homeless people and offered support and training to local voluntary agencies, particularly those centres participating in the schemes.

45. Weaknesses of the schemes identified by team members mainly concerned the structure, organisation and management of the schemes. They also thought that their presence could undermine the uptake of local mainstream services: users who established a relationship with them might be reluctant to register with local GPs; other professionals might off-load onto them their general responsibility for homeless people.

46. In both areas team members judged their schemes to have provided a good standard of care to people who normally had difficulty in obtaining health care. They found it difficult to comment on the extent to which the schemes had actually improved the health status of individuals. Both teams acknowledged that they had been less successful in getting people to use mainstream services.

47. Team members in East London agreed that a specialist care team needed to continue, but individuals had different views about the ideal format of this team and the extent to which team members should be integrated into mainstream services. The Camden team were not in favour of continuing a special and separate service for homeless people.

In both areas there was agreement that the project doctor's job could and should be absorbed into more flexible mainstream provision.

48. The Chairmen and Administrators of the two managing FPCs agreed that existing health care provision for homeless people was inadequate, but disagreed about whether or not special and separate provision was necessary for this client group, or whether resources and effort should be directed at trying to integrate them into mainstream provision.

49. Both FPCs thought that the problem of getting local GPs to take on homeless people was largely one of attitudes and inaccurate stereotyping, but there was also recognition that among the homeless population there were many time-consuming and demanding patients and this presented a problem for over-loaded inner-city GPs. Neither FPC believed that lack of an address automatically precluded registration, but they suspected that a convenient way for GPs to avoid facing up to the problem was to insist on a home address.

50. Both FPCs had found it hard to incorporate managing the one-off schemes into their staffing and administrative structures. In both localities collaboration between a number of different authorities had proved difficult.

51. The major strengths of the schemes identified by the managing FPCs concerned the commitment and expertise of team members and the prominence given to the problems of homelessness and health care. Their major weakness was that they had been under-managed, both strategically and operationally.

52. The FPCs came to the conclusion that if projects like these were to have a chance of success they needed to have tightly focused and potentially achievable goals. Neither FPC recommended continuing the pilot schemes in their present form, although they suggested that the projects and their evaluation might result in transferable ideas. It was thought that health care provision for homeless people needed a many-pronged approach and the pilot project had acted as just one safety-net. A more appropriate way of tackling the problem might be to fund specific sessions by local GPs.

53. The FPCs suggested how all FPCs could take a stronger lead in securing access by homeless people to a good standard of general medical care: FPCs should be more flexible about registration; they should be more imaginative in their procedures and more creative about their use of funds; and they should target their recruitment policy towards problem areas, such as homeless people, and ensure they took on GPs who had the skills and commitment to treat these people.

Views of the wardens

54. The wardens commonly thought that addiction problems, particularly alcoholism and drug abuse, were major health hazards for clients using their centres. They singled out the need for tackling mental health problems as a priority.

55. The wardens knew of few GPs who were willing to provide primary health care to homeless people and attributed this largely to the stereotypical images that GPs, and their receptionists, held about homeless people.

56. Wardens found it difficult to get emergency care for users or residents who came to them with a serious health problem. The most common causes of referral to hospital were drug over-doses and psychiatric problems, along with trauma resulting from accidents or assaults.

57. Wardens liked the schemes because they provided a regular service to homeless people in a familiar environment. They also liked the flexibility and informality of the approach taken by team members. They felt that the schemes had helped to promote the credibility of local day centres and hostels by raising the profile of homeless people and their problems. Individual team members had also provided support and training for centre staff and this was greatly valued.

58. Weaknesses of the schemes identified by wardens included: lack of emergency out-of-hours cover; lack of specialist psychiatric help; lack of integration with mainstream services; lack of support for project team members; lack of clarity surrounding some of the team members' roles; the drawback that the services would not reach homeless people who did not use the centres; the temporary nature of

the schemes and the uncertainty about what would happen when their funding expired.

59. They agreed that the schemes would have achieved some success if they had reached people who had not seen a doctor before, and if they had networked people into local community services. But there was recognition that these indicators were very difficult to turn into reliable outcome measures.

60. There were additional health care services which wardens would have liked to have had provided at their centres: some form of psychiatric care and counselling; a greater emphasis on preventive health care; health education and information on diet and nutrition; chiropody; dental treatment; health care specifically directed to women using the centres; help and advice concerning drug addiction; a delousing facility nearby or on site; an occupational therapist to help people with physical difficulties; and more detoxification facilities, including day beds in hospitals.

61. The majority of the wardens thought that ideally it would be best if homeless people could use ordinary health care services, but most were of the opinion that special and separate health care services were necessary in the short term at least. Integration into mainstream services was seen as a realistic aim for many, but not all, homeless people.

62. There was little optimism among wardens that homeless people would of their own accord make more use of local GPs if the schemes were discontinued, without an effort being made to arrange a handover to local practices.

63. There was a general consensus among the wardens in both areas that the schemes should be continued, either in their current form or with some modifications.

Views of professionals and voluntary workers

64. The overwhelming majority of the 34 GPs interviewed said there was at least one hostel, night shelter or day centre used by homeless people within a one mile radius of their surgery, but none provided regular sessions at any of these centres. Almost half said they had been

called out in the past year to provide emergency services to a user or resident at one of these places.

65. Most GPs interviewed were reluctant to take on homeless people because they were concerned about creating an additional burden to their already heavy caseload and they thought that homeless people would be disruptive and unacceptable in their appearance or behaviour to other patients using their surgery. They also raised the problems of lack of time, facilities and back-up from ancillary staff, particularly for single-handed GPs in smaller practices.

66. The mobility of homeless people was said to give rise to numerous obstacles to continuing care, in particular the difficulty of tracing medical records, and also created a problem with regard to payment for the service.

67. Most GPs said they would be more likely to treat homeless people as temporary residents than to give them permanent registration. They did not necessarily regard people living in hostels as homeless and implied that it was easier to fulfil their contract to provide 24-hour care to a hostel resident than to someone living on the streets. The majority of GPs said that their FPC would not allow them to register a patient who did not have an address.

68. Just under a quarter of GPs thought that the existing provision of primary health care services for homeless people was satisfactory, a similar proportion thought it was generally poor and around half were non-committal.

69. Three-quarters of the GPs interviewed knew about the existence of the pilot schemes while the rest had not heard of them. We found little evidence of referral activity or any other type of interaction between local GPs and the project teams.

70. Some GPs thought the schemes had improved the access of homeless people to primary health care by providing a multidisciplinary approach and specialist expertise. Others thought that they should never have been set up in the first place because existing services were adequate. About half the GPs in both areas considered that the pilot schemes could be transferred successfully to other areas, about a quarter were unsure about this and the rest were strongly against the idea.

71. We interviewed a total of 42 district nurses, community psychiatric nurses and social workers. Only two district nurses and five CPNs said that they provided regular sessions at hostels, night shelters or day centres used by homeless people.

72. Nurses and social workers were more inclined than GPs to think that housing difficulties were at the root of the health care problems experienced by homeless people.

73. The CPNs and social workers were strongly critical of the inadequacy of existing provision of health care services for homeless people, but the district nurses knew little or nothing about the present provision.

74. In East London only one of the district nurses and less than half of the CPNs knew about the scheme in their area, whereas in Camden most of the district nurses and CPNs were at least aware of their local scheme. Like the GPs, the nurses and social workers we interviewed had had minimal interaction with the pilot schemes.

75. The nurses, CPNs and social workers who knew about the schemes identified a number of strengths: the schemes provided a multi-disciplinary team approach to the problem; team members were committed and effective; and they raised the profile of the health care problems and needs of the homeless. They also identified a number of weaknesses: there was insufficient publicity or feedback about the schemes and not enough interaction with local service providers; the teams were small given the extent of the problem; and the continuity of the schemes was uncertain.

76. They suggested several criteria to assess the success of the schemes; a count of attendances to indicate the level of take-up; consumer satisfaction; how far the medical needs of the homeless were met; and how far links were established with hostels and with local service providers. Roughly two-thirds of the nurses, CPNs and social workers who knew about the schemes thought that the model as developed in their locality could be transferred successfully to other areas, so long as it was not followed too rigidly.

77. We also interviewed six junior casualty officers, six nurses and three hospital social workers working in the casualty departments of

two London teaching hospitals. All had experienced difficulties in providing services for homeless people. They referred to the general problems of follow-up and after-care, and specifically mentioned inadequate psychiatric support and lack of social work back-up. They also emphasised that lack of accommodation was the fundamental problem which needed to be tackled.

78. Most of the casualty staff knew little about health care provision outside the hospital setting, but all believed that single homeless people tended to use the A and E department inappropriately: for example, attending casualty for minor complaints and problems that a GP could deal with; presenting with long-term chronic problems; coming in to get prescriptions or wanting help with alcohol or drug-related problems; and simply trying to get a bed or warm place to stay for the night. Homeless people were commonly thought to use accident and emergency departments in preference to a GP because hospitals were seen to be more accessible and treatment was available at all hours.

79. Only three of the hospital staff we interviewed in East London had heard of the pilot scheme in their area. None of the hospital staff we interviewed in West London knew about their local pilot scheme.

80. In each project area we interviewed representatives of the main co-ordinating agency for local organisations concerned with the homeless. We also spoke to representatives of 12 local agencies. These people in the voluntary sector tended to have a more negative view than the health care professionals about the appropriateness of mainstream health care services for homeless people. Particular concern was expressed about the problems encountered by homeless people who were chronically mentally ill.

81. All but two of the organisations we contacted knew about the pilot scheme in their locality. The strengths they attributed to the schemes were similar to those already described by the GPs and other health care professionals. In addition, they emphasised that it was important that the schemes were *statutory* because this indicated that the government was taking the health care problems of homeless people seriously. There was some criticism of what they saw as a top-down solution to the problem by government, and they emphasised the lack of

consultation with local agencies before the projects were introduced. There was also concern that the life of the projects was too short.

82. The voluntary bodies judged that the projects had at the very least reached some people who would otherwise have gone without health care. The clear message was that the experience of the pilot schemes should be shared, even though there was no consensus about whether the approach as developed locally by the pilot schemes could or should be transferred to other areas.

Special and separate provision of primary health care

83. Just over two-thirds of all the GPs, health care professionals and the representatives of voluntary bodies thought that single homeless people in their locality needed special and separate provision of primary health care services. However, many believed this to be the case in the short term, but not in the long term. It was suggested that special projects like the pilot schemes could be used to help change the attitudes of GPs and other health care professionals towards taking on homeless people, and that they could be an entry point into mainstream provision.

84. The main argument made against special provision was that it isolated homeless people even further from society. Another concern was about what would happen when the funding for the special schemes ran out.

85. The diversity of views expressed about the future provision of health care for single homeless people indicated that there was no simple solution to the problem. Some homeless people could be encouraged to use mainstream services, but it was also thought that there was a sizeable minority who would not be able or willing to do so.

12 Postscript

There have been certain changes in the staffing arrangements and activities undertaken by the two pilot schemes since the monitoring period ended in December 1987. This postscript summarises the main changes that have occurred since then and is based on information supplied by the two teams.

City and East London pilot scheme

Management structure and staffing

1. Changes have been made to improve the management structure of the East London scheme. A new management body has been set up which includes the main line managers of the project team members, and representatives from the voluntary sector.

2. A new community psychiatric nurse was appointed in July 1988 and for the first time since the scheme's inception the team were able to operate at full strength with all posts filled. They plan to add a psychologist to the team from March 1989.

3. The alcohol counsellor left the project in July 1988. She was replaced by another alcohol counsellor who was employed to work with the project and also to do some sessions at Inform-AL, the local alcohol counselling agency in Tower Hamlets.

4. A new full-time project administrator was appointed in August 1988.

Activities

5. Several new initiatives were started which were geared towards homeless women. These included:

- a service for women only, provided at the Cable Street project;

- an experimental female GP service at St. Botolph's Crypt for a trial period of five months. Having assessed the service, the team concluded that it would be more appropriate for a nurse practitioner to provide this session, and it will be taken over by the nurse, funded by the Health Authority, who works with the team.

6. The team was involved in co-ordinating a small number of local research projects. These included:

- a patient-held record trial for the chronically mentally ill;

- a psychologist investigating learning difficulties among the single homeless;

- a medical student attached to the team studying the health beliefs and accommodation of chronically mentally ill patients.

7. Voluntary sector provision in the area has changed (for example, centres have closed or changed their objectives). Services provided by the team have changed in response. For example, team members have extended their services to a number of other local day centres and hostels.

8. The team have been active in publicising their activities through presentations to statutory and voluntary agencies, public meetings and teaching commitments.

9. Team members increased their involvement in voluntary sector management through representing the East London scheme on the management committees of various local agencies.

Camden pilot scheme

Management and staffing

1. All the original team members employed by the Camden scheme have moved on to other jobs since the monitoring period finished in December 1987. The project nurse left first, followed by the administrator in June 1988 and the salaried doctor in July 1988.

2. The team has been replaced. A new nursing sister was appointed in July 1988 and a new salaried doctor started in August 1988. The project administrator was recruited in January 1989.

3. The new team continued holding the surgeries which their predecessors had set up at the West London Day Centre and the Simon Community Night Shelter.

4. The clinics at the Arlington Drop-In Centre were not continued because the Centre was closed following a fire. This Centre is due to open again in March 1989 and the team will resume surgeries there.

5. The nursing sister who had worked alongside the original team at the West London Day Centre (but who was employed by the centre and was not actually part of the team) took up an innovative new post with Bloomsbury Health Authority as Nurse Practitioner to the homeless. The new project team hoped to work closely with her.

6. The new team established an advice and referral clinic at Levita House, a huge complex of temporary accommodation owned by Camden Council. Their aim was to offer advice on any health issue, but they were particularly interested in promoting issues central to the health of women and children, for example, childhood immunisation. The Advocacy Service based at the National Temperance Hospital provided the project doctor and nurse with translation services to help them communicate with the large Bengali population at Levita House. The team plan to set up another advice and referral clinic on similar lines in a large drop-in centre for families.

7. The new project doctor established a system of taking referrals from Area 5 Social Services to assist in mental health assessment at Bow Street Magistrates Court.

8. The team were instrumental in acquiring the services of a visiting psychiatrist to the West London Day Centre as a result of their networking with local statutory and voluntary agencies.

References

Bone, M., *Registration with general medical practitioners in Inner London: a survey carried out on behalf of the DHSS*, HMSO, 1984.

DHSS, *Primary health care in Inner London*, Report of a study group commissioned by the London Health Planning Consortium, (Chairman: Sir Donald Acheson), 1981.

DHSS, *Promoting better health: the Government's Programme for improving primary health care*, Cm. 249, HMSO, 1987.

Leighton, J., 'Primary medical care for the homeless and rootless in Liverpool, *Hospital Hlth Serv. Rev.*, August 1976, 72(8), 266-267.

Liverpool Central and Southern District Community Health Council, *Primary medical care and the single homeless in Liverpool*, (undated).

Locker, D. and Dunt, D., 'Theoretical and Methodological Issues in Sociological Studies of Consumer Satisfaction with Medical Care', *Social Science and Medicine*, 1978, Vol.12, pp.283-292.

McCarthy, M. (ed.), *London's health services in the 80's*, King's Fund Project Paper No.25, 1980.

NFA Day Centres Action Research, *Action for a change*, Research report, 1987.

Powell, P.V., 'A "house doctor" scheme for primary health care for the single homeless in Edinburgh', *Journal of the Royal College of General Practitioners*, 1987, 37, pp.444-447.

Shanks, N.J., 'Consistency of data collected from inmates of a common lodging house', *Journal of Epidemiology and Comunity Health*, 1981, 35, pp.133-135.

Shanks, N.J., 'Medical provision for the homeless in Manchester', *Journal of the Royal College of General Practitioners*, 1983, 33, pp.40-43.

Single Homelessness in London Health Sub-Group, *Primary care for homeless single people in London: a strategic approach*, 1987.

Appendix 1   Methodology

(A)   The sampling of homeless people

1. Agreement was reached with the relevant Ethics Committees and Local Medical Committees that we could interview homeless people using the pilot schemes in the two areas. We also got clearance from the wardens of the centres through which the pilot schemes were channelled to interview clients on their premises. We agreed not to interview at any centre at times when the project doctors were holding clinics because of their concern that our interviewing might be directly linked by consumers to the clinic services.

2. For the purposes of this study a homeless person was defined as one who had no fixed address or who was dwelling in a hostel used primarily by homeless people. However, pilot interviewing had shown that a number of people attending the day centres had their own accommodation of some kind, and our sample included some people in this category.

3. We interviewed 190 homeless people, 50 per cent of whom had used the schemes' services: 90 of these interviews were with individuals attending centres in East London with regular clinics (45 of them users); and 100 interviews were with people using the centres in Camden with regular clinics (50 of them users). Half the interviews were conducted in June 1987 and the other half in November 1987 to allow us to explore any seasonal differences concerning the health problems and experiences of respondents, and to note any differences in knowledge and perception about the schemes as they became more established. The reason for the lower number of interviews in East London was that

during the monitoring period the regular medical service provided by the scheme was withdrawn from one of the centres where we were interviewing.

4. Interviews were carried out on the premises of the day centres, night shelters and hostels where the project doctors had established regular clinics. In City and East London we conducted 10 interviews in each of five centres in June and 10 in four centres in November: five users and five non-users of the project team's services. In Camden we conducted 25 interviews in each of two centres in June and repeated this in November to achieve the total of 100 interviews. In June we interviewed 13 users and 12 non-users and in November we interviewed 12 users and 13 non-users of the schemes.

5. A user was someone who had used the services provided by one or more of the project team members at that centre or at one of the other centres visited by the project teams. A non-user was someone attending the day centre, night shelter or hostel who, at the time of interview, had not used the services provided by the project doctor or by any other team member.

6. These interviews were done on a quota sampling basis because it was impossible to find a suitable sampling frame which would have enabled us to select a random sample of interviewees. Many of the homeless people attending the centres through which the services were channelled were highly mobile and some used the centres on a one-off basis. We could not predict who would attend on a specific day.

Contact procedure

7. Each interviewer was allocated a number of centres to visit. The quota controls for numbers of users and non-users were determined in advance. Interviewers were also given a guide to the age and sex of people attending each centre and were asked to try and reflect these proportions in their quota samples. However, the final selection of persons to be interviewed was left to the interviewers. While it was pointless to try and interview someone who was very obviously drunk or exhibiting bizarre behaviour, or who was completely withdrawn, very few people fell within these categories. In Booth House and Providence Row Refuge no-one was considered unapproachable and in

the other centres around 5 per cent of attenders only on any one day were judged to be incapable of being interviewed.

8. The interviewers took the advice of staff about the best place to start looking for interviews. In some instances centre staff also tried to help the interviewers by steering them towards people they knew to be co-operative, but this was avoided as far as possible. In most of the centres a room was made available where interviews could be conducted in private, but the majority of respondents preferred to be interviewed in the part of the centre where they were approached; for example, the day room, canteen or craft workshop.

9. Different zones within the centres attracted different types of clientele. For example, people using the canteen or craft workshop, in centres where these facilities were available, tended to be more articulate and approachable than those who were slumped in seats in the television room. To ensure that the sample included a broad range of types of homeless people attending the centres, interviewers approached people in a variety of locations.

10. Interviewers explained the purpose of the survey and reassured respondents that their response would not in any way affect their use of health care services provided at the centre or anywhere else. A written description of the survey was given to respondents who wanted more information.

11. It was expected that each interview would last approximately 15-20 minutes, depending on how much respondents had to say. Interviews with non-users were sometimes shorter than this. Other interviews took considerably longer, either because respondents were inarticulate, or because they related extracts from their life-story to illustrate their views or their experiences of health care.

Achieving quotas

12. Once interviewers had reached their quota of either users or non-users in a particular centre they stopped interviewing people in that quota and concentrated on achieving their target for the other group.

13. We did not want to interview any individual more than once, so in November the interviewers checked that respondents had not been

interviewed already in June. We did not ask respondents for their names, but we did collect their initials and date of birth which enabled us to check to make sure we had not duplicated any interviews.

Response rate
14. Professionals working with the homeless people had been pessimistic about the potential response rate. In fact there were surprisingly few refusals: of the total number of individuals approached in June, 18 per cent refused to be interviewed (Table A1.1, p.300); and of those approached in November, 20 per cent refused (Table A1.2, p.301). Those who refused generally said they were not interested; some thought that we were wasting our time because the government did not care what homeless people thought; and a few simply shook their heads, told the interviewers to go away or ignored their presence altogether. There was a danger that those who refused would be the most inarticulate and down-trodden among the homeless population using the centres, but the interviewers noted that this did not appear to be so.

Questionnaires and interviewers
15. The questionnaires were structured in that questions were asked in a predetermined sequence and using identical wording for each interview. However, certain questions were only applicable to users of the pilot teams' services. As we wanted to elicit the views and experiences of homeless people a fairly high proportion of the questions were open-ended, requiring the interviewer to record verbatim responses. The team of five interviewers were given extensive oral and written briefing on the questionnaires and the background to the research. There were also in-depth debriefing sessions after both the June and November rounds of interviewing.

(B) The sampling of health care professionals
1. This survey was designed to achieve interviews with 120 health and social service professionals working in the locality of the two pilot projects. It was intended that the sample would comprise: 40 general medical practitioners; 20 district nurses; 20 community psychiatric nurses (CPNs); 20 local authority social workers; and 20 health or social

services staff based in hospitals. These totals were to be divided equally between the two areas.

2.   The relevant Local Medical Committees agreed that we could approach GPs in their areas and Bloomsbury Health Authority and Tower Hamlets Health Authority gave us clearance to interview district nurses and CPNs.   While the Social Services Departments in Tower Hamlets and City of London agreed that we could interview social workers employed by them, the Social Services Departments in Camden and Westminster declined to participate.   The accident and emergency consultants in two large London teaching hospitals facilitated our interviews with a sample of casualty officers (SHOs).

3.   The interviews were carried out in October, November and December 1987.   Some professional groups, particularly the GPs in Camden, were difficult to get interviews with and as we intended to complete our interviewing by the end of the year, we interviewed slightly fewer people than planned.   The breakdown of our actual sample of health care professionals by project location and by profession is shown in Table A1.3 (p.301).

General practitioners
3.   We drew our sample of GPs from those postal districts where the clinics set up by the project doctors were located, using the Medical Lists of the relevant Family Practitioner Committees (FPCs).   These lists contained the names of 'responsible' GPs in contract with those FPCs.

4.   In East London we selected at random 25 GPs from the City and East London Family Practitioner Committee's Medical List. We drew our sample from the 34 GPs listed under the E1 postal district. We achieved interviews with 18 GPs; 6 refused and we failed to make contact with one other.

5.   In Camden we selected at random 25 GPs from a combined total of 44 GPs in the NW1 postal district (from the Camden and Islington FPC list) and the W1 postal district (from the Kensington, Chelsea and Westminster FPC list). We achieved interviews with 12 GPs; 12 refused and we could not make contact with one other. In Camden we also interviewed two GPs in a health centre in NW5 and two in a health

centre in NW8. These health centres were outside the boundaries of the relevant postal districts, but we knew from talking to clients and centre staff that they were often used by homeless people attending the centres.

District nurses

6. In East London 10 district nurses were selected at random from a list of 21 nurses working in three health centres in the vicinity of the scheme. We interviewed all 10 district nurses.

7. In Camden scheme 10 district nurses were selected at random from a list of 50 district nurses (excluding auxiliary nurses) working for Bloomsbury Health Authority in groups 1 and 2, which covered both the Camden and Westminster parts of the Authority. We achieved interviews with 7 district nurses; 2 refused and we could not make contact with one other.

Community psychiatric nurses

8. In East London 10 CPNs were selected from a list of 12 CPNs who were working in teams whose specialisms were relevant to homeless people; namely those dealing with alcohol-related problems, emergency clinics, primary care and tertiary care. We interviewed all 10 CPNs.

9. In Camden 10 CPNS were selected from a list of 14 CPNs who staffed the two teams working in the vicinity of Camden scheme. We interviewed all 10 CPNs.

Local authority social workers

10. In City and East London social workers were selected from staff lists provided by Tower Hamlets Social Services Department and City of London Social Services Department. The sample of social workers was not drawn on a random sample basis. The team in City of London was very small and the Director of Social Services suggested individuals who she thought would be able to make a contribution to the study.

Hospital staff

11. We interviewed 6 junior casualty officers (SHOs), 6 nurses and 3 hospital social workers either working in or, in the case of the social workers, taking referrals from the casualty departments of two large London teaching hospitals. The sample of casualty officers and nurses was divided equally between the two hospitals, but we were not able to interview any social workers in West London because the relevant Social Services Department had declined to participate in the survey. In both project areas the samples of casualty officers were drawn at random from staff lists. It was not possible to draw the sample of nurses on a random basis and those we interviewed were nominated by the accident and emergency department consultant in each hospital; 3 were sisters and 3 were staff nurses. The 3 social workers we interviewed in East London were those who had the most contact with the accident and emergency department.

Questionnaires and interviewers

12. The questionnaires were structured in that for each professional group questions were asked in a predetermined sequence and using identical wording for each interview. Many of the questions were applicable to all professional groups. As in the case of the client interviews a high proportion of the questions were open-ended, requiring the interviewer to record verbatim responses. The interviews were carried out in the respondent's place of work, which was usually a surgery, clinic or hospital. We used the same team of interviewers who had conducted the interviews with the homeless people. All were given extensive oral and written briefing on the questionnaire.

Health care for single homeless people

Table A1.1 Response rate for interviews with homeless people in June 1987

	Total	City and East London pilot scheme centres					Camden pilot scheme centres	
	Sample	Cable St day centre	St Botolphs	Prov. Row	Tower Hamlets Mission	Booth House Detox.	Arlington Drop-In	W. London day centre
Total number of people approached who satisfied quota requirements	126	15	14	10	18	10	32	27
Completed interviews (i.e. quota targets)	100	10	10	10	10	10	25	25
Refused	26	5	4	0	8	0	7	2

Table A1.2   Response rate for interviews with homeless people in November 1987

	Total	City and East London pilot scheme centres					Camden pilot scheme centres	
	Sample	Cable St day centre	St Botolphs	Prov. Row	Tower Hamlets Mission*	Booth House Detox.	Arlington Drop-In	W. London day centre
Total number of people approached who satisfied quota requirements	118	10	13	11	–	11	38	35
Completed interviews (i.e. quota targets)	90	10	10	10	–	10	25	25
Refused	28	0	3	1	–	1	13	10

* No interviews were conducted at Tower Hamlets Mission in November because by then the regular clinics held by the project doctor had been closed down.

Table A1.3   Sample of health care professionals

		Profession				
Project	Total professionals	GPs	Community Nurses	Community Psychiatric Nurses	Social Workers	Hospital accident & emergency staff
City & East London Project	52	18	10	10	5	9
Camden Project	39	16	7	10	–	6
Total	91	34	17	20	5	15

Appendix 2   Staffing Arrangements

Each pilot scheme consisted of a multidisciplinary team of workers who were employed to provide primary health care to homeless people within the locality of their responsible Family Practitioner Committee (FPC). The key difference in the way that general medical services were provided was that the FPCs employed *salaried doctors* to work for the schemes instead of using local GPs. This appendix looks at the implications of this and also summarises the background and experience of each team member employed on the schemes, the responsibilities attached to their posts and to whom they were managerially and professionally accountable.

Salaried doctors

Authority for employing salaried doctors on the schemes derived from the Secretary of State's powers under Section 56 of the 1977 NHS Act to sanction alternative arrangements if he thought that general medical services were not meeting the needs of certain sections of the population. The report on Primary Health Care in Inner London (Acheson Report, DHSS, 1981a) had identified the homeless as a group who were unable or unwilling to register with a GP and had recommended this use of the Secretary of State's powers to set up alternative provision to meet their needs.

The terms and conditions of service for the salaried doctors employed by the schemes were set out in a contract of employment for a salaried medical practitioner, drawn up by the DHSS and authorised by the Secretary of State. This contract was between the Family Practitioner Committee, as the employer, and the individual doctor. It drew on a hospital doctor's contract, modified to take account of the unique status of the project. In particular, it had to incorporate some of the general medical and pharmaceutical regulations.

Under this contract the remuneration arrangement for the project doctors was different from that of an independent contractor. They were paid a salary instead of receiving fees and allowances for services provided. Their rate of pay was set at the level of the Senior Registrar scale, which is a basic hospital grade and is the same grading used for trainee general practitioners.

There was considerable disquiet among the medical profession concerning the level of remuneration for the posts and the fact that it was a *training* grade rate. The General Medical Services Committee, in particular, argued publicly that the pay was too low for a job which carried as much, or more, responsibility than that demanded of a local GP and advised doctors not to take these posts because of the disagreement over the level of pay (*British Medical Journal*, 3 May 1986). Only a minority of GPs were said to be in favour of a salaried service.

Under the salaried medical practitioner's contract the service provided by the project doctors was more limited than that provided by GPs. They did not provide 24-hour cover or continuity of care, they had no locum cover for when they were on holiday and they had no mechanism for registering patients. Although salaried doctors are generally not able to prescribe drugs because they are not on an FPC's list of general medical practitioners, this drawback was overcome in both project sites. The doctor employed by Camden and Islington FPC was already on their list because he had previously worked as a GP in a practice in their area. He stayed on their list while working for the project. In City and East London arrangements were made for the project doctor to be included on the FPC's list, following negotiations between the FPC, the Local Medical Committee and the DHSS.

City and East London pilot scheme: staffing arrangements

Salaried doctor

The job description for the salaried doctor included both the provision of general medical services to any homeless person within the locality of the FPC, and the referral of patients to other professionals or agencies for further care or opinions, with particular emphasis on assisting patients to register with local GPs. The post also included supervision of the primary care team.

The first project doctor was in his early thirties. He had not found an immediate vacancy in general practice locally after completing his GP training so he had taken on a lectureship in the Department of General Practice and Primary Care at St. Bartholomew's Medical College. While in this post he had also been funded for two years from 'Acheson money' (the £9 million or so which, in response to the Acheson Report, the government had set aside to fund a wide range of initiatives for improving primary health care in the inner cities) to research and develop primary care services for homeless people. This funding started in April 1985. However, he had not completed these two years before his funding was re-directed to the pilot scheme. He joined the project as the salaried doctor in March 1986, 10 months before the monitoring period started.

This doctor left the project in March 1987 to go to general practice. His successor was in his late twenties and took up the post in April 1987. He already had some experience of working with homeless people through doing locum work as a GP in Central London and as the visiting medical officer to a day centre in Pimlico. He had also had contact with homeless people as a casualty officer. His GP trainee year had been spent in a practice which had a long-standing commitment to the homeless. It had supplied visiting medical officers to the Camberwell 'spike' since 1947 and covered several hostels, treating users on a temporary resident basis.

Project co-ordinator

The responsibilities of the project co-ordinator were largely those of secretarial support to colleagues and ad hoc office management. The post also included maintaining record systems.

The first project co-ordinator was appointed in November 1985 and remained in post until the end of the monitoring period. He had previously worked in the Registration section at Lambeth, Southwark and Lewisham Family Practitioner Committee. He had not worked with homeless people before.

Alcohol counsellor

The team had already had a change of alcohol counsellor before the monitoring period began in January 1987. The first counsellor had been appointed by the Tower Hamlets Inter-Agency Group for Alcohol Services in May 1986 and had worked with the East London team for six months on a one-day a week basis. He left the project in November 1986, mainly because he was unable to provide the growing time commitment required by the project team because of the demands of his main job.

His successor, a woman in her mid-thirties, joined the team in November 1986. She was employed part-time and had a joint appointment; she worked two days a week for the project team and two days a week for Inform-AL, a co-ordinating agency sponsored by Tower Hamlets Inter-Agency Group for Alcohol Services. She had not worked with homeless people before, but had been with an Alcohol Advisory service, running a local counselling centre.

The first alcohol counsellor had concentrated on development work with the local day centres. It was envisaged that his successor would build on this and move on to do more concrete things: for example, spending more time with other team members and with wardens of the centres, advising them and helping them to gain confidence in dealing with alcohol problems; and running group discussions with clients, as well as offering individual counselling.

Social worker

The person appointed to the social work post was in his late twenties and had qualified as a state registered nurse in 1980. Although he had no professional social work qualification, he had experience of working with homeless people. Before joining the project he had been employed as a social worker at St. Botolph's Crypt, where he had been a key worker to a group of clients, mainly involved in resettlement work. He thought the pilot scheme would offer a certain amount of flexibility in meeting the needs of homeless people which had not been possible in the day centre setting.

He wrote his own job description and he wanted to develop activities such as: visiting centres where homeless people congregated, with a view to providing them with social work services; developing a special interest and expertise in single homelessness; developing links with statutory and non-statutory organisations to provide a more co-ordinated service for people of no fixed abode; providing education, training and support to day centre and hostel staff.

Community psychiatric nurse

The job description for the CPN set out the general aim of providing a psychiatric nursing service to homeless people in Tower Hamlets as part of a project team, and detailed the role and function of the CPN under three main headings: psychiatric nursing intervention and therapy; professional and administrative responsibilities; education, training and supervision.

The CPN who was appointed to the project was in his early thirties. He was qualified both as a registered general nurse and as a psychiatric nurse. He had not worked in a community setting before joining the project and he had also not worked with homeless people before. He wanted a community post and this was one of his main reasons for applying for the job with the project team.

The CPN found it difficult to develop his role within the pilot scheme and eventually left the project in May 1987. He was not replaced until May 1988, five months after the monitoring period had finished.

Team management

Although they were charged with managing the scheme, the FPC were the employing authority for two team members only; the salaried doctor and the project co-ordinator. The DHSS also channelled funding through Tower Hamlets Health Authority, the Local Authority Social Services Department and through Inform-AL, the local umbrella agency for alcohol services.

This assortment of different employers of team members created both the problem of different geograpical responsibilities and the potential for confused lines of accountability:

(i)   The project doctor was employed by the FPC to provide medical care for the unregistered homeless in their locality. He was managerially accountable to the FPC Administrator and professionally accountable to the full Committee.

(ii) The CPN was employed by Tower Hamlets Health Authority to work in their area, which was more limited than the locality of the City and East London FPC. He was directly responsible to the Director of Nursing (Psychiatry) at Tower Hamlets Health Authority and reported to the Senior Nurse in the Community Psychiatric Nursing Service. Negotiations about the future of the CPN, and later about his replacement, were complicated by the fact that the CPN was employed by the Health Authority and not the FPC who were managing the scheme. For him personally this also created a risk of conflict or confusion between two different lines and styles of management and accountability: the project with its particular style of outreach work; and the Community Psychiatric Nursing Team with its broader goals and more traditional way of working.

(iii) The social worker was employed by Tower Hamlets Social Services Department. If he had stuck rigidly to working within their boundaries, this would have excluded him from some of the centres where the project team operated; for example, one of the centres falls within the boundaries of City and Hackney Social Services.

(iv) The alcohol counsellor was not employed by any of these statutory authorities. She was appointed by Inform-AL and accountable to their Steering Group.

Camden and Islington pilot scheme: staffing arrangements

Salaried doctor

The job description for the salaried doctor in Camden identified this person as a key member of the primary care team charged with identifying homeless people, who were not otherwise receiving health care, and providing it directly to them, whilst at the same time looking to their future needs. As in East London, this included referral of patients to other professionals or agencies for further care or opinions, with particular emphasis on assisting patients to register with local GPs. The brief for the salaried doctor in Camden also included leadership of the team and devising a joint approach to the provision of care.

The salaried doctor in Camden first joined the project in June 1986 for six months as a locum. He was appointed to the permanent post in November 1986. He was in his early thirties and had previously been a principal in general practice in Inner London, but had left that position after seven months, partly because he considered that general practice within inner cities was often failing to provide primary care to some of the most needy individuals in society.

By joining the project he thought that he would be able to offer primary care to a client group who were often unable to obtain health care through any of the conventional channels. Through this he hoped to improve the overall health status of homeless people in the locality. He had not worked specifically with homeless people before becoming involved in the pilot scheme, but he had encountered them in general practice and in his training. He had experience of providing medical cover to a women's alcohol centre, but this centre had not catered for homeless women.

Project nurse

The job description for the project nurse set out the nursing and administrative responsibilities attached to the post, but was subject to review in the light of changing service needs.

It was envisaged that the nurse would provide skilled nursing care and advice to patients both in the capacity of working with and under the guidance of the doctor, and through identifying individuals independently of the doctor, but with his support and advice as necessary. The post also included the promotion of positive health care and education by offering advice and assistance to welfare workers and individuals.

The nurse who was appointed to the project in August 1986 was in her mid-twenties. She had been doing agency nursing before joining the pilot scheme and she had worked at a medical centre in Central London set up specifically for the treating the homeless.

Project co-ordinator

The job description for the project co-ordinator in Camden stated that, in addition to co-ordinating the project, the person appointed was also expected to provide administrative and secretarial support to the primary care team, organise the office and maintain information systems.

The project co-ordinator employed by the FPC had qualified both as a state registered nurse and as a registered mental nurse. She had not worked with homeless people before becoming involved in the pilot scheme. She had previously been employed as a manager of a youth and community centre, funded by the GLC.

Team management

As the team was smaller and involved fewer professional disciplines than in East London, the problem of multiple employing authorities was not so marked, but nevertheless it did exist. The FPC was the employing authority for the project co-ordinator and the salaried doctor but not the nurse. The accountability arrangements for the project doctor were the same as in East London; he was managerially accountable to the FPC Administrator and professionally accountable to the full Committee. The project co-ordinator was responsible to the FPC Administrator.

The DHSS funded Bloomsbury Health Authority to employ the nurse. She was accountable to the Director of Community Nursing Services and responsible to the Senior Nurse, District Nursing. In her day-to-day work she was also accountable to the project doctor.

Appendix 3   Centres Visited by the Project Teams

(i)   City and East London Pilot Scheme
The main centres visited by City and East London team members during the monitoring period (1 January 1987 - 31 December 1987) are listed by centre type in Table A3.1 (p.319), along with the approximate date of their first visit at each centre.   It should be noted that their service input at these centres was not necessarily constant over time.

Locations for surgeries held by the project doctor
In this Appendix we give additional information about the five centres described in Chapter 2, where the first project doctor and then his successor held regular surgeries.

(i)   Cable Street Day Centre
This voluntary sector project in the East End provides a service to single people who are in or have experienced housing need.   It receives funding from the London Boroughs Association, various charitable trusts and private donations.   The project has two parts: a day centre and a hostel.

The day centre is open between 12.30 p.m. and 4.00 p.m. Monday to Friday and provides a social meeting place for men and women over the age of 16.   At the time of our interview, the staff complement at the day centre included 2 full-time members, 1 part-time member and 6 volunteers.

There is room for approximately 70 people in the centre. The current drink policy is less exclusive than in the past. Previously users could not drink before coming in to use the centre; now this ruling is more relaxed but users still cannot drink on the premises.

Health care at the centre

The centre had a tradition of medical care provided by a nursing sister who described herself as a 'nurse practitioner'. When her services were closed down the centre asked the project doctor to step in. He began visiting in May 1985.

This centre also acquired the services of a part-time nurse, paid for by the Health Authority, shortly after the project doctor had set up his surgery there. Staff as well as users often confused her with the project team. Also, as she worked alongside the project doctor when he held surgeries there, it became increasingly difficult to distinguish her contribution from that of the pilot scheme. We therefore considered her as a team member for the purposes of collecting information about clients' use of and responses to the service as a whole.

(ii) St. Botolph's Crypt Centre

This centre is located in a Church in East London and has provided services for homeless men and women since 1962. It now operates as a day centre and an evening centre. The day centre is open three days a week between 10 a.m. and 4 p.m. The evening centre is open every weekday between 6 p.m. and 8 p.m. There are 9 full-time members of staff who work on a rota basis and approximately 60 volunteers. The funding for the centre comes from several sources: statutory grants; trusts; and parochial and personal donations.

The project team's services were only available at the evening centre. The number of people using the evening centre is recorded on a daily basis and throughout the calendar year 1985 a little over 27,000 attendances were noted. On any one evening there is room for about 250 people.

A new extension to the centre, along with reconstruction and modernisation of the existing building, was completed during the monitoring period. The bright new building improved the environment for clients and enhanced the facilities offered. It included a new medical room.

Health care at the centre

This centre was offering users some access to health care before the pilot scheme started. A volunteer doctor and a chiropodist visited weekly, and several volunteer nurses worked there on an ad hoc basis. In addition, members of staff were able to provide social work services to users. These services notwithstanding, the centre was said to be in desperate need of medical services and the project doctor started visiting in May 1985.

(iii) Providence Row Refuge

Established in the 1860s, this centre is a short-stay hostel for single homeless men and women. It is situated near Spitalfields market, and is funded by grants from the London Boroughs Grant Unit, rent payments, hostel deficit grant and donations.

The hostel has 45 beds and take-up is high, with a bed occupancy level of 89 per cent in the winter of 1985 and 85 per cent in the summer of 1986. More recent figures are expected to be higher. Residents are usually accommodated for six weeks only, but this can be extended. The average length of stay is between three and four weeks.

Since October 1985 the hostel has been open for 24 hours a day. Before this, residents had to be outside the building between 9 a.m. and 4 p.m. and they had tended to visit other local day centres during this time. The hostel now provides a small day room and kitchenette, but does not intend to compete as a day centre providing day centre activities.

Overall there are 17 full-time members of staff and 16 part-timers. They work on a rota basis and include social workers and care workers. The size of the social work team has increased and this has improved and extended the level of contact with residents. As a result there has been an increase in the services provided and better and more appropriate referral work.

Health care in the centre

In the past the hostel had been covered by a local GP, but for a number of reasons the staff had decided to dispense with his services. They approached the project team for help and the project doctor started a regular weekly surgery at the hostel in March 1986.

Staff at this hostel included social workers and care workers who were able to offer social work services to residents and make appropriate referrals. For a short time during the monitoring period the hostel employed a community psychiatric nurse. She resigned from the post in May 1987, but remained working as a CPN within Tower Hamlets Health Authority.

(iv) Tower Hamlets Mission

This day centre is run by one of the missions operating in the East End. The day centre opened in 1982 but the Mission has a long history of serving the needy and poor in the area, particularly deprived families, and instructing them in Christianity. The landscape of poverty in the area has changed and the Mission is now heavily used by single homeless people. Its sources of funding are Trust investments and some London Boroughs Association money.

The centre can accommodate a maximum of 150 people. Except on Mondays, when it is open between 7.30 a.m. and 3.30 p.m., the day centre is not open all day. On other weekdays it is open for a couple of hours first thing in the morning and again in the early evening. On Sundays it is open between 2.30 p.m. and 4.30 p.m. and on Saturdays it is closed. There is a women-only session on Tuesdays between 11 a.m. and 4 p.m.

The day centre at the Mission is run by 3 full-time members of staff, 3 part-timers and 19 volunteers. There is a part-time social worker on site. The only rules of eligibility for using the centre are that individuals have to be over 18 years of age, and to avoid disruptive behaviour they are not allowed to bring drink into the centre. During the monitoring period the Mission was undergoing fundamental changes; in particular, it was converting an attached property into a residential unit offering detoxification facilities for men.

Health care in the centre

This centre had no history of providing health care for clients, but it did have a qualified social worker on the staff who provided a social work service on site on two days a week. Centre staff had asked for their Mission to be included in the pilot scheme, and the first project doctor started twice-weekly surgeries there in October 1986. These sessions were taken over by his successor in April 1987.

Neither of the project doctors was entirely happy about locating surgeries at this centre. The first project doctor suspected that they would not be well used since the centre had no tradition of health care, whereas Whitechapel Mission nearby had a volunteer doctor who was well known to homeless people. Also, it was thought that the character of the centre was changing with the construction of a residential rehabilitation unit for men wanting detoxification. Both project doctors were aware that more and more people using this day centre were settled with local GPs, and they thought that providing an outreach service to these people was an inappropriate use of their skills.

The surgeries at Tower Hamlets Mission were eventually withdrawn towards the end of 1987 and in March 1988 were re-located at Whitechapel Mission, which by this time had lost the services of the volunteer doctor. People attending the day centre run by this Mission included a group, made up of chronic alcoholic middle-aged men, who tended not to use other day centres and who the team thought could well use their services. A local general practice took on responsibility for providing medical cover for the new residential unit at Tower Hamlets Mission.

(v) Booth House Detoxification Unit

This is a detoxification unit which opened in 1975 and is located in the basement of a large Salvation Army hostel for men in Whitechapel. It provides treatment for male alcoholics. The unit's funding comes from the Salvation Army, the London Boroughs Association and the DHSS.

Detoxification facilities are scarce and places at the unit are in demand. During the period September 1975 - October 1986 there were 3,800 admissions to the unit: 10 per cent were in the age group 18-29; 36 per cent were aged between 30 and 40; and 54 per cent were aged over 40. The majority of these admissions were UK nationals: 40 per cent were English; 33 per cent were Scottish or Welsh. However, 24 per cent were Irish. The remaining 3 per cent came from a broad range of countries.

The unit has ten detoxification beds and also has the use of four dry-wing post-detoxification holding beds in another part of the hostel. Many, but not all, of the men admitted to the unit are homeless.

The unit provides 24-hour provision seven days a week and is open to callers from 9 a.m. to 9 p.m. with certain restrictions. Treatment is normally short-term. There is a seven-day detoxification programme, which may be extended according to requirement to an approximate maximum period of 10-14 days. Residents are required to remain permanently in the unit in night clothing whilst undergoing detoxification. They may leave sooner at their own request following discussion with staff. A total of 9 people work in the unit; 8 full-time and 1 part-time.

Health care at the centre
Residents at this unit already had access to medical care before the pilot scheme began. Two local GPs each provided a weekly service and the unit employed 3 nurses (2 full-time and 1 part-time) who worked on a rota basis.

One of the GPs stopped visiting because his caseload became too heavy and when the unit started looking around for his replacement he recommended the project doctor. The first project doctor started a regular weekly surgery at the unit in October 1986. The services of the other local GP who had been holding a weekly surgery at the unit before the pilot scheme began continued, as did the nursing services.

Camden and Islington pilot scheme
The main centres visited by the doctor or nurse working for the Camden and Islington pilot scheme are listed by centre type in Table A3.2 (p.320), along with the approximate date of their first visit at each centre.

Locations for surgeries held by the project doctor
In this Appendix we give additional information about the three centres described in Chapter 2, where the project doctor held regular clinics.

(i)   The Arlington Drop-In Centre

This is a day centre in Camden funded jointly by Camden Social Services Department and Bloomsbury Health Authority. It was set up in April 1982. The centre caters for homeless men and women. It is open between 9 a.m. and 4.30 p.m. on weekdays and is closed at the weekend. It has room for about 45 people, but often admits more.

The centre provides a place where people can meet, obtain free tea, coffee and soup, and use the recreational facilities. There is a TV room, equipment for playing snooker, and also an art room. There is only one full-time member of staff. He is assisted by one part-timer and 4 volunteers.

Health care at the centre

The team approached this centre to discuss the health needs of their clients and whether they were being met through existing services. At that time the centre provided no medical cover for clients and was keen to use the resources offered by the pilot scheme. Two months later, in November 1986, the project doctor started to hold surgeries there twice a week. The project nurse attended during these surgeries and also held two further clinics a week on her own. Subsequently a consultant psychiatrist started visiting the centre for a two-hour session on a fortnightly basis.

Both the project team and centre staff agreed that facilities for providing a health service at this centre were poor and they were frustrated at the lack of response they had from the relevant authorities in trying to improve these conditions. There was a room where the doctor and nurse could see patients, but this did not have a sink with running water and there was no couch for examinations. There was also a lack of privacy for patients waiting to use the service. Inadequate facilities also prevented the centre from taking advantage of a chiropody service offered by Bloomsbury Health Authority on a sessional basis. The chiropodists were willing to come only if certain improvements were made, and these were still outstanding at the end of the monitoring period.

(ii) West London Day Centre

This day centre in West London opened in 1975 and operates under the auspices of the Methodist Church. It receives funding from the Methodist Church, the Westminster City Council, and from various grants and donations.

The day centre is open seven days a week to men and women over 25 years of age, but the opening times vary. It offers a wide range of services and facilities, including meals at basic cost, and on an average weekday the centre is used by between 100 and 180 people. There are 12 full-time members of staff, 2 part-timers and 3 residential volunteers. One member of staff is a housing advice and resettlement worker who provides help and advice to those seeking permanent accommodation.

Health care at the centre

This day centre had a history of providing health care for its users and offered excellent facilities for delivering a health service, the only drawback being that the surgery was up several flights of steep stairs. The Camden team needed to find locations for their outreach clinical work and when the project doctor learned that the local GP who provided a weekly surgery at this centre wanted to give it up he took it on, even though the centre was outside the boundaries of his managing FPC. He established twice-weekly surgeries there in September 1986.

Since at least 1979 this centre had employed a nurse who was part-funded by Bloomsbury Health Authority. She had provided nursing cover on her own as well as working with the local GP during the weekly surgery. When the project doctor took over from the local GP and started holding regular surgeries at the centre she worked with him. The project nurse only visited this centre if their own nurse was away on one of the surgery days.

(iii) The Simon Community

This night shelter moved to its current premises near St. Pancras and King's Cross Stations in mid-1987. It is run by a voluntary organisation which also has a number of residential group homes and does outreach work on the streets at night.

The shelter has certain founding principles: it does not aim to be a hostel; and there are only three house rules - no drink, no drugs and no violence. It receives no money from central government and the workers regard this as an important way of retaining their independence. Most of their funding comes from public donations and a newsletter which they produce quarterly.

The night shelter has 22 beds for homeless men and women. It is open between 7 p.m. and midday in the summer when on an average day about 18 of the beds are likely to be occupied. In the winter the shelter opens an hour earlier and most of the beds are occupied. Most of the people using the shelter are overnight guests, some of whom come one night a week on a regular basis. The maximum length of stay is usually two weeks, but if workers think that a person's needs cannot be met elsewhere then they can sometimes stay longer.

The number of workers changes periodically because they move between the night shelter and the group homes. At the time of our visit in January 1988 there were 7 full-time workers.

Health care at the centre
Regular sessions by the project doctor and nurse at this centre did not start until November 1987, shortly after the night shelter had moved to new premises. The team had been in contact long before this, but had held back from visiting the shelter at its old premises because they had not wanted to damage the relationship it had built up with a local health centre. The change of premises had disrupted this link because it was located further away from the health centre and the shelter had turned to the team for help.

The doctor set up regular surgeries on two mornings a week. The project nurse worked with him at one of these surgeries and in addition visited the shelter twice a week on her own. The shelter was able to provide a separate room which could be used as a medical room, but it had no couch or running water. There was, however, a sink and a toilet suitable for the disabled just around the corner. A major problem was that the room was also freezing cold in the winter.

**Table A3.1 Main centre visited by the City and East London project team
with approximate date of first visit**

	Team member				
	First project doctor (left project March 1987)	Second project doctor	Alcohol counsellor	CPN (left project May 87)	Social worker
Booth House (detoxification unit)	Oct '86	April '87	—	—	—
St Botolphs Crypt (evening centre)	May '85	April '87	Jan '87	—	—
Cable Street Day Centre[1] (day centre)	May '85	April '87	Jan '87	Jan '87	July '87
Providence Row Refuge[2] (short stay hostel)	March '86	April '87	Jan '87	May '86	—
Tower Hamlet Mission (day centre)	Oct '86	April '87	Jan '87	—	April '87
Whitechapel Mission (day centre)	—	March '88	Dec '86	—	April '87
Caplin House (hostel)	—	—	Dec '86	—	—
Tower House (hostel)	—	—	—	—	June '87

(1) Cable Street Day Centre had the half-time services of a Health Authority nurse. For the purposes of our evaluation she was considered as a team member, with the proviso that she was an 'extra' resource which could not be counted elsewhere.

(2) The American doctor who joined the project team during his sabbatical in England took over the clinic at this centre for the six-month period, September 1987-March 1988.

Health care for single homeless people

Table A3.2 Main centres visited by the Camden and Islington project team with approximate date of first visit

Centre	Team member	
	Project doctor	Project nurse
Arlington Drop-in Centre (day centre)	Nov '86	Nov '86
Simon Community Night Shelter (night shelter)	Nov '87	Nov '87
West London Day Centre[1] (day centre)	Sept '86	—
Parker Street Hostel (hostel)	—	July '87
St Mungos Hostel (Argyle Street) (hostel)	—	Jan '87

(1) West London Day Centre employs a district nurse, part funded by Bloomsbury Health Authority, who for the purposes of our evaluation was considered as a team member; with the proviso that she was an 'extra' resource which could not be counted on elsewhere.

A Review of the Literature on Primary Health Care for Single Homeless People

Marie-Anne Doggett

Introduction

In 1987 an International Year of Shelter for the Homeless was called by the United Nations in a 'worldwide attempt to reduce homelessness wherever it is found' (Miller, 1987). In Britain, the first task was to increase awareness of the crisis and the government announced major research efforts into various aspects of homelessness (Hansard, 1 April 1987).

This review has been completed as a background paper to the Policy Studies Institute study of two pilot primary health care schemes in London, which were set up and funded by the DHSS for a limited period. For the purposes of this study a homeless person was defined as one of no fixed abode, or dwelling in a hostel used primarily by other homeless people.

From a vast literature on both homelessness and primary care services in Inner London, it has been necessary to select material specifically on the provision of primary health care to the single homeless – a field which in itself has not been well researched. As the bibliography shows, a great deal of the material surveyed is of an 'unofficial' or 'semi-published' nature, much of it produced by voluntary organisations and non-statutory bodies of various types. In addition, the changing landscape of homelessness in the 1980s, brought about by demographic trends, changing aspirations, increasing unemployment and government interventions (SHIL, 1986) has meant that much of the research from earlier days can no longer be applied to present-day conditions.

Homelessness: problems and characteristics

A definition of homelessness is no easy task, either as a matter of law or a matter of policy (Arden, 1986). The definitions provided by the legislation are not sufficient to comprehend the true nature of homelessness, since major groups such as young single people or childless couples are often excluded (Greve et al., 1986), even though they may experience some of the worst conditions of any social problem in Britain today (Barrett et al., 1984).

In the early 1980s, a government-funded research report defined as homeless any single people 'with no home of their own' and concluded that the single homeless were 'a heterogeneous and ill-defined target population' (Drake et al., 1982). More recently, homeless young people have been observed 'from all walks of life' (Saunders, 1986), while patients of a medical centre for the homeless have been described as 'as varied as those seen in any general practice' (Toon et al., 1987). In fact, homelessness is affecting increasing numbers of people and a wide cross-section of the community (SHIL, 1986).

Who are the homeless?

Drake et al. (1982) reported that the homeless included women as well as men, the under 20s as well as the over 65s, the employed as well as the unemployed, and those with job skills and higher education as well as the unskilled and poorly educated. They also commented on the disproportionately high numbers of young people in their sample.

Concern for the plight of homeless young people has been growing, since many of them have no rights to public or private housing (Housing Rights Campaign, 1987), much of which, in any case, is irrelevant to their needs (SHIL Sub-Group, 1987). Attitudes are said to be inconsistent, since society seems to expect young people to show initiative, but then criticises them when they fail and find themselves in difficulties (Saunders, 1986). Government benefit systems increasingly enforce mobility on young people (SHIL Sub-Group, 1987), the results of which are frequently seen as increased physical and emotional turmoil (Stein, 1987). Especial concern has been expressed for those under 18, since few local authorities grant tenancies at this age, even though young people can legally leave home at 16 (Saunders, 1986). In addition, the Children's Society have estimated that some 75,000 children under 17 run away from home each year (Hansard, 10 February, 1987), and the pattern of young people's lives after leaving care is often disturbing, with frequent moves and dissatisfaction with accommodation resulting from a lack of preparation for independent living (Stein, 1987; Saunders, 1986).

Alongside the very young, elderly homeless people are also regarded as highly vulnerable, whether as a result of high mobility (DHSS, 1981a), poor living conditions (McKechnie and Wilson) or concentration in unsuitable lodging houses and hostels (SHIL Sub-Group, 1987). The majority of elderly single homeless people are thought to come from broken marriages, mental hospitals, local authority care, the Armed Forces or prison (Channel 4 TV, 1987). In order to be able to live successfully outside an institution the elderly need higher levels of support and care than are currently funded (SHIL, 1986) and improved accommodation more suited to their needs (DHSS, 1981).

Meaningful observations on homelessness faced by ethnic minorities are often hampered by lack of data (Greve et al., 1986). Language problems create obvious barriers (DHSS, 1981a), overcrowding is thought to be particularly severe amongst ethnic minority communities (Tower Hamlets, 1987) and access to voluntary and statutory agencies may be limited, or there may be suggestions of racism in housing management practices (Saunders, 1986).

Although single blacks and Asians may avoid institutions such as lodging houses, hostels or resettlement units, their needs are no less urgent (SHIL Sub-Group, 1987). Men may lose their jobs if they cannot live near to traditional areas of employment (Tower Hamlets, 1987) and the problems faced by girls and women from ethnic minorities are even more severe, and their needs sadly under-researched (Saunders, 1986).

Indeed, women in general suffer from a lack of provision of services, with fewer hostel beds and fewer organisations to help (City and Hackney CHC). Although homeless men may outnumber women by as many as 3:1 (Drake et al., 1982) there are fears that the true proportion of women may be hidden by this very lack of provision and by the fact that they are considered more likely to try to help themselves through friends (Saunders, 1986).

According to the Channel 4 television programme in 1987, most local authorities now report that over 50 per cent of their total applicants for housing are single, but many still feel that their main responsibility is to homeless families. Cutbacks in housing finance, the decline in council housing and in the private rental sector, and the priority and points allocation systems have all favoured families over the single homeless (Stein, 1987). Vigorous support campaigns have ensured that the problems of homeless families in temporary accommodation are well documented (Howarth, 1987; Bayswater Hotel, 1987) and there is a growing literature on their needs, particularly those of children and travelling families (Drennan and Stearn, 1986; Lawrie, 1983; Streetly, 1987). By contrast, very little is known about the needs of the single homeless, although at least one writer has commented that if society has accepted a moral and social obligation to help dependency groups such as the elderly and handicapped, then it should likewise support single homeless people as much as those with children (Maitra, 1982). Any services provided today should be based on the recognition that homelessness is a fact of life for the young, the elderly, ethnic minorities and women as well as white men (SHIL Sub-Group, 1987).

Myths and stereotypes

The term 'homeless single person' was first used in a National Assistance Board survey of hostels and lodging houses in 1966 (Powell, 1987). In the conditions then prevailing, the single homeless were widely perceived as vagrants, dossers or tramps, and research had reinforced this view of a specific group with severe problems in addition to homelessness (Drake et al., 1982). By the mid 1970s, there was a growing awareness that there is no 'typical' single homeless person, that the term can mean different things to different people and that the only factor which may unite the group as a whole is lack of accommodation. There is increasing evidence that the single homeless may be ordinary people in circumstances in which anyone could find themselves (Saunders, 1986), but stereotypes change slowly. In one recent report, even the homeless themselves were applying the label 'dosser' in a self-denigrating way which implied that sleeping rough defined a person's whole being (Central London Outreach Team, 1984).

Social services and housing departments still often regard the single homeless as 'deviant' (Channel 4 TV). They are considered to have personality 'inadequacies' which lead them into homelessness, but many such difficulties may result from the deprivation which comes from lack of accommodation, rather than cause it (Davies, 1974). People who lead a 'nomadic' life are likewise often considered deviant and are therefore unpopular, both with the general public and with institutions which serve them (Holden, 1975). For too long public policy has hidden behind such stereotypes and 'in the absence of an accurate assessment, stereotypes are considered to be self-evident truths' (Saunders, 1986).

Popular images include the dirty old alcoholic sleeping rough in parks and under railway arches, the young drug addict frequenting Central London and the middle-aged mentally ill woman (Drake et al., 1982). Although such characters undoubtedly still exist, the problem should be reviewed in the light of research evidence. Most young single homeless people are 'ordinary youngsters with everyday desires' (Channel 4 TV), whose homelessness tends to be a condition of 'constantly having to move on ... and make do' (Mariasy, 1987). The myth of the 'gold-paved London streets' is no longer so strong as it once was (Hodgkin, 1987) and it is not always the youngest people in metropolitan areas who are the heaviest drug users (Drake et al., 1982).

Although there are no statistics, large-scale migration amongst young people does not appear to be a serious problem and voluntary agencies are receiving increasing numbers of requests from Londoners in London and other locals in their own cities (Saunders, 1986). Contrary to popular belief, hostel residents are not necessarily transient - 84 per cent had been at Arlington House in Camden for over 5 years during a recent survey (Green, 1985). SHIL believes that an assumption of high mobility amongst the single homeless is unwarranted and that homeless people are no more mobile than 'yuppies', professionals or executives (SHIL Sub-Group, 1987). Homeless does not necessarily mean rootless (Stearn, 1987).

One problem which arises from all these stereotypes is a sense of discrimination and stigmatisation (Davies, 1974). In those sleeping rough, a sense of worthlessness and a low level of self-esteem were prevalent, even though only a small proportion had serious personal problems (Central London Outreach Team, 1984). It is thought that any service which can help break down the segregation will also help break down the damaging myths (SHIL Sub-Group, 1987).

Why are people homeless?

The stereotyping outlined above has often resulted in the 'personal pathology' theory of homelessness, which regards the condition as an inherent quality within certain individuals. Although vigorous efforts are now being made to understand homelessness in terms of the factors which precipitate it, there is no doubt that, once homeless, a 'vicious downward spiral' tends to come into play, so that a loss of dignity, a socially unacceptable appearance and an 'unbalanced' state of mind all make it nearly impossible to find a home (City and Hackney CHC).

In general terms, homelessness results from the overall shortage of accommodation in this country and the lack of appropriate accommodation for different groups, especially young people (Saunders, 1986). In 1975 local councils and housing associations were building 175,000 new houses; this figure fell to only 40,000 in 1985 and at the same time the private rented sector fell from 24 per cent of all housing stock in 1961 to only 8 per cent today (Mariasy, 1987). In London demand for accommodation has been further increased by the plans to close 30 large psychiatric institutions by 1995 and the reduction of direct access hostel bed spaces from 6,100 in 1981 to 5,300 in 1985 (Livingstone, 1985).

About 40 per cent of people accepted as homeless give the reason that friends or relatives no longer feel able to house them (Hansard, 1 April 1987), and this family breakdown is one of the most common reasons why young people make use of voluntary agencies (Saunders, 1986). In addition, marriage break-up was cited as the main cause of homelessness by around 20 per cent of those accepted in 1986, while a further 20 per cent had been evicted from private rented accommodation (Hansard, 10 February, 1987).

Of course, authorities must take into account the differences between voluntary and involuntary homelessness. Young people who choose to leave home will probably exhibit rather different coping mechanisms from those who are forced out (Saunders, 1986) and temporary homelessness can sometimes be a part of the lifestyle associated with different jobs for single people (Drake et al., 1982).

Who takes responsibility?

The Housing (Homeless Persons) Act 1977 gave local authorities a statutory duty to house the homeless, even people they had not previously regarded as priorities, such as pregnant women, those involved in family disputes and those with mental handicap (DHSS, 1980). This Act continues to apply in Scotland, but in England and Wales has been replaced by the Housing Act, 1985 - Part III: Housing the Homeless (Arden, 1986). Local authorities must offer advice and assistance to anyone who is unintentionally homeless or threatened with homelessness according to certain priorities, which include single people vulnerable through old age, mental illness or handicap, physical disability or other special reasons, such as young people at risk of sexual or financial exploitation (Saunders, 1986). In reality the Act is open to widely differing interpretations, often influenced more by available housing stock than by other considerations, especially in London (Greve et al., 1986). The legislation appears to give housing authorities powers, but not duties, so minimum standards are not easily enforceable (Hansard, 10 February, 1987), and many single people in need fall through the net.

Local authorities still need take no responsibility for single people from outside their areas who have no connection with them. This has led to an active role for various voluntary agencies who try to plug the gaps (Saunders, 1986) and the voluntary sector seems to be shifting its support towards helping homeless people run their own campaigns and building access to mainstream services, not simply providing alternatives to them (Barrett et al., 1984).

Where do homeless people go?

Overall it is claimed that some 50 per cent of all those accepted as homeless go immediately into permanent accommodation (Hansard, 10

327

February, 1987), but this masks considerable differences in individual areas. For example, Camden gave permanent accommodation to only 151 households in 1986-7, compared with 1,710 who were offered temporary accommodation; in Tower Hamlets the corresponding figures were 526 and 1,221 (CIPFA, 1987).

The Department of the Environment does not collect information on the numbers of households placed in temporary accommodation (Hansard, 3 March 1987), but the Chartered Institute of Public Finance and Accountancy does (CIPFA, 1987). Throughout England and Wales in 1986, 213,200 households claimed homelessness, of which 51,912 were given temporary accommodation by local authorities *(New Society*, 22 January 1988). By the end of 1987, 19,000 households were in temporary accommodation in London, of which 8,500 households (i.e. 30-40,000 people) were in bed and breakfast hotels, 1,600 in hostels and refuges, 4,000 in short-life accommodation, 1,200 in accommodation leased temporarily from private landlords and 4,000 individuals at home with relatives (London Housing Unit, 1987). It was estimated that it would cost £163 million to keep them there. For comparison, the average cost of keeping a family in a B&B hotel was thought to be £30 per day, or £12,000 per year, whereas the average cost, allowing for all debt charges, management and maintenance, of building or acquiring a new council house in Greater London was estimated at £5,500-£7,000 (Hansard, 10 February, 1987).

Latest statistics show that 51 per cent of accepted households were placed in B&B accommodation in London with 12 per cent assigned to hostels, 5 per cent to women's refuges, 11 per cent to short-life dwellings and 21 per cent to 'other' accommodation (CIPFA, 1987). Concern is expressed that fewer than one-third of the households in B&B have actually been placed there by local authorities and the remainder form part of the 'hidden homeless', many living in grossly inadequate conditions (Greve et al., 1986).

In addition, short-term hostels are increasingly being used to offer long-term solutions for which they were never intended (Saunders, 1986). Although there has been progress in improving or closing some of the old-style, larger hostels, and an increase in smaller, better-standard, non-specialist provision, there has been little development of new direct-access provision or special provision for young people, women and ethnic minorities (SHIL, 1986).

Finally, there are estimated to be 15,000 people who may be sleeping rough in London, with a national figure of around 500,000 (Matthews, 1986). According to one survey, over half of those who constantly sleep rough may prefer to do so because they dislike the available alternative accommodation (Central London Outreach Team, 1984). More worryingly, recent estimates for the numbers of single homeless people in London include up to 30,000 who may be squatting, and point out two disturbing trends: skippering in completely empty property for short periods and overnight use of trains for temporary shelter (London Housing Unit, 1987).

The size of the problem

The question of exactly how many people are truly homeless in this country is difficult to answer mainly because of the lack of adequate statistics (Channel 4 TV) especially in Inner London where the Homeless Persons Units are heavily pressurised (Greve et al., 1986). Information relating to the number of persons currently homeless is not collected centrally (Hansard, 2 April 1987) and neither the DoE nor the DHSS have comprehensive data (Saunders, 1986). Much evidence is anecdotal and/or incomplete - the result of informed opinion rather than statistical analysis (Davies, 1974).

Official statistics which are available usually relate to the number of households accepted as homeless by local authorities, though this may be less than half of all those who apply (Greve et al., 1986), and usually concern families. Such acceptances have risen from 53,000 in 1978 to 103,700 in 1986, though the actual numbers of those who regard themselves as homeless has probably now reached a quarter of a million. In 1986, 44 per cent of all households accepted were in the Greater London area (Hansard, 10 February, 1987).

Because single homeless people are not guaranteed provision under the Housing Act Part III (HMSO, 1985), and are not therefore often included among households accepted as homeless, estimates of their true numbers vary widely – from 64,500 in London (London Housing Unit, 1987) to 2,000,000 nationwide (CHAR advertisement, 1988). For young people the position is equally uncertain. The government states that their numbers are increasing (DHSS letter, 1976) and organisations like the Piccadilly Advice Centre and Centrepoint report large increases in requests for temporary accommodation (Saunders, 1986). Again estimates are often only 'guesstimates' and range from 80,000 in 1985 (Campling, 1987) to almost 300,000 who may be staying with others while awaiting a place of their own in London (Mariasy, 1987). When all age groups are taken into account this figure could rise to as many as 915,000 Londoners (London Housing Unit, 1987).

Whichever figures are most accurate, the fact of the 'hidden homeless' remains – single people without homes or family support, dependent on the housing market and consigned to life in low-standard, high-cost establishments (Saunders, 1986).

Changes over time

Some of the main social and policy changes of recent years have had marked effects on the problem of homelessness. For example, the decision to close Resettlement Units and replace larger hostels and lodging houses with small-scale group homes or cluster housing has meant that bedspaces have been lost. The older premises have increasingly taken on the function of resident nursing homes for chronically physically and mentally ill people, especially the elderly, while younger people have been forced into B & B hotels, squats or onto the streets (SHIL Sub-Group 1987). Short-term pressures of demand and the slow development of alternative provision have forced some modification of the original plans in some instances (Greve et al., 1986), where full closure would mean that the level of welfare services, sheltered housing and other community resources would be 'embarrassingly exposed' (Green, 1985).

A further area of concern is the growing evidence that adequate provision is not being made for the community care of ex-psychiatric patients. Research suggests that this policy will generate an annual flow of over 2,000 single people in London alone, who will require housing and support (Greve et al., 1986). Community care cannot work without a proper home, appropriate primary care services and community support, so that the need for suitable accommodation for mentally ill single people can only become of greater priority (City and Hackney CHC).

Perhaps one of the most controversial decisions of recent times was the April 1985 amendment of the board and lodgings Regulations. This was seen as evidence of hardening government attitudes and attempts to make financial savings without consideration of the wider policy implications (Saunders, 1986). The financial limits allowed for B&B were said to force young people into overcrowded accommodation. The restrictions on the length of time they could claim the allowance and the six-month ban on return to the same area meant that they could not be resident in one place long enough to qualify for council accommodation, and that their links with local labour markets would also be lost (Saunders, 1986). Such compulsory 'nomadism' also meant that they would lose contact with social, family and medical support systems (Channel 4 TV) and some observers were convinced that 'the misery, the desperation, the hopelessness we have seen is the exacerbation of what was already an appalling situation' (Piccadilly Advice Centre, 1985). Others estimated that as many as 64,000 young people were affected by the new Regulations within the first three months of their introduction (Mariasy, 1987). Many believed that the assumptions underlying the legislation were, quite simply, wrong, that the young people affected had no other choice open to them but to be in the type of accommodation they were in, and that the only result of the changes would be reinforced poverty (Robertson and Matheson, 1986).

In spite of a considerable amount of monitoring work, few of the important underlying questions about what has happened to people affected by the changes can be answered. One author could only suggest, tentatively, that there was 'not enough evidence about what happened to claimants to conclude that little hardship has been caused' (Berthoud, 1986).

Further difficulties were foreseen as a result of the introduction of the new Social Security Act, changes to the Housing Benefit system and the Housing Bill in 1988 and the transfer of board and lodgings to Housing Benefits in 1989. It was feared that the proposed changes might represent 'financial disaster' for many, with the likelihood of increased rents and reduced benefits for all single, childless under 25 year olds (Lunn, 1987; London Housing Unit, 1987).

Camden and Tower Hamlets

The most up-to-date picture of homelessness in these two boroughs can be gained from the CIPFA Homelessness Statistics (1986-1987 Actuals). In addition, Jarman (1981) produced some tables of characteristics of both East and West End zones of London, though these are now somewhat dated.

Camden is an area of high population density and many disadvantaged groups. A highly mobile population includes many tourists and visitors as well as students and large numbers of single, non-pensioner households. There are many multi-occupancy rooming houses, with over the national mean of private rented houses and bedsitters. Overcrowding is a serious problem and there is a great lack of amenities and a high crime rate. Employment is mainly in service and non-manufacturing industries, especially catering and office work (DHSS, 1981; Drake et al., 1982). Camden is having to bring its old hostels back into use to cope with its current homelessness crisis and almost all potential rehousing resources are going to the homeless rather than waiting list tenants. Its emergency programme now includes a tough new 'one offer only' allocation policy (Platt, 1987).

Tower Hamlets has also recently removed the limits on the type of offer which can be made, although there are many empty houses and the housing budget is frequently underspent. Homeless tenants represent only 10 per cent of council lettings and although single people and childless couples constitute half the waiting list, only about a quarter of the housing stock is suitable for them. Altogether the council owns about 82 per cent of the housing, with only 8.4 per cent in the private rental sector. Once again overcrowding is a serious problem, especially amongst the ethnic minority communities, mainly Bengalis (Tower Hamlets, 1987). Overall the population is more stable than in Camden, but social, economic and environmental conditions are also very poor, with high unemployment (Rhodes et al., 1986). The area has above the national mean of pensioners, single-parent families, single, non-pensioner households, and students, with a high proportion of elderly and long-term homeless (Drake et al., 1982). The main provision for the single homeless in the past was in large hostels, but bedspaces have been reduced from around 2,000 in 1981 to around 1,000 in 1987 (NFA Day Centres, 1987).

Primary health care in Inner London

In recent years there has been a multiplicity of reports on primary health care, such as the Government's Green and White Papers (DHSS 1986a and 1987), the report from the Social Services Committee (1987), the Cumberlege report (DHSS, 1986b) and an earlier survey of London for the RCGP (Jarman, 1981). Many of these have virtually ignored the problem of homelessness, so that homeless people are frequently left out of service design altogether (SHIL Sub-Group, 1987). Perhaps the document which has attracted the most comment is the Acheson report (DHSS, 1981a), which concentrated on Inner London and produced a comprehensive survey of the problems, together with some 115 recommendations to help alleviate them. Shortly afterwards, a representative of the Health Visitors Association was moved to make a plea for 'no more reports on primary care until the recommendations of the current one have been implemented' (King's Fund Centre, 1981). Her wishes were not granted. Members of the Social Services Committee (1987) were 'disturbed to be told by other witnesses that many of the recommendations in the Acheson report have been ignored', and a survey of primary health care in the inner cities after Acheson concluded that 'neither at national nor local level has a major shift in priorities or resources towards primary health care taken place in practice' (Rhodes et al., 1986). Some additional financial resources were made available nationally, but they did not cover many of the important areas identified by Acheson and were inadequate to provide a sustained shift in priorities. Nevertheless, many of Acheson's ideas have become part of the 'conventional wisdom', even though implementing them has proved painfully slow.

Social deprivation and environmental factors

As long ago as 1979, the Royal Commission on the NHS was pointing out the direct links between social, environmental and cultural factors in the declining inner city areas and various medical problems (Royal Commission, 1979). One year later, the Black report concluded that 'much of the evidence on social inequalities in health can be adequately understood in terms of specific features of the socio-economic environment ... which are strongly class-related in Britain and also have clear causal significance' (DHSS, 1980). Health and illness must be regarded in terms of the social and environmental factors which affect people's lives (SHIL Sub-Group, 1987) and many feel that there is a limit to the improvements which can take place in primary health care as long as the underlying social and environmental problems remain (King's Fund Centre, 1981). In 1986 the government reaffirmed its 'general commitment to the problems of multiple deprivation' (DHSS, 1986a) but the Green Paper contained no mention of homeless people as a particularly deprived group.

Others have spoken of the single homeless as 'a socially deprived group with evidence of increased health care needs' (Powell, 1987). Their environment 'has a debilitating effect on health and encourages apathy as regards health care' (Liverpool CHC). Not only can social deprivation increase levels of clinical morbidity, but there is evidence that deprived groups do not use health services effectively (McCarthy, 1980). For example, poor housing conditions can lead to longer hospital stays, while lack of education and social skills can result in low uptake or inappropriate use of services. In addition, social isolation can be exacerbated by difficulties of access to services, with greater distances to travel, poorer public transport and the possibility of violent attack (DHSS, 1981a). In areas of multiple social deprivation there is a strong need for co-ordination between all branches of the NHS and other local authority and welfare services (Liverpool CHC), as people tend to blur the boundaries between the responsibilities of the various authorities (Tower Hamlets, 1987).

There is no doubt that Inner London is a very deprived area (McCarthy, 1980). Individual Londoners are frequently more isolated than people elsewhere, family unity and support are undermined by depopulation and housing development, and high mobility results in a lack of social cohesion. When the economically successful move away, they are often replaced by more vulnerable groups, such as single young people living alone. Housing stock is often very poor, with much overcrowding, but extensive rebuilding can also break up communities and lead to even more isolation (DHSS, 1981a). Some boroughs, such as Tower Hamlets, have been singled out as areas of particular deprivation, with severe environmental problems detrimental to health, such as lack of open spaces, traffic congestion, water pollution, animal pests and damp housing with increased rubbish (Tower Hamlets, 1987). Unfortunately, many of the areas with the worst social and environmental problems also suffer from the least suitable primary care services (Jarman, 1981).

General practitioner services.

Although based on data obtained over 10 years ago, Jarman's survey of primary care in London remains one of the most comprehensive sources of information on GP services in Inner London (Jarman, 1981). More recent work has confirmed his view that differences among general practices were less marked for the East End than for the West End of London (Smith and Stiff, 1984). Other studies from which the following observations were drawn include the Acheson report (DHSS, 1981a); Heath and Sims, 1984; Tower Hamlets Health Inquiry, 1987; Rhodes et al., 1986.

GPs in Inner London tend to be older than elsewhere. Only 15 per cent of Heath and Sims' sample were under 40, compared with a national figure of 32 per cent, while Acheson reported that 18 per cent were over 65, compared with 6 per cent nationally. According to the Tower Hamlets Health Inquiry, 9 per cent of GPs in that borough are over 70 years of age, whereas in the rest of England and Wales the figure is only 2 per cent. At a time when London's clientele, such as the single homeless, are making extraordinary demands on the health and social services, the need would appear to be for young and enthusiastic GPs with new ideas and approaches (McCarthy, 1980). In practice, the older doctors may prove reluctant to change and resistant to the more modern theories (DHSS, 1981a).

There is general agreement that the introduction of an agreed retirement age for all GPs is a matter of urgency and could bring about immediate improvements (Heath and Sims, 1984; Jarman, 1986). The government hopes that its proposed changes in retirement policy will help replace older, single-handed doctors by younger, group-practising, team-orientated ones (DHSS, 1986a).

Acheson found that 47 per cent of Inner London GPs were born outside the UK, compared with 25 per cent in England and Wales, and Jarman (1981) found that this was a characteristic particularly of East End practice. As long ago as 1974, Davies was calling for more emphasis on care for the homeless in medical school teaching, but Acheson reported that relatively few young, enthusiastic vocationally-trained GPs were being recruited some years later (DHSS, 1981a), and others have since confirmed that postgraduate education among London GPs can often be inappropriate (Heath and Sims, 1984). On the other hand, Smith and Stiff (1984) observed that there was little variation in qualifications and training between doctors in inner city and suburban areas, with similar proportions having received some specific training in general practice.

Although Heath and Sims (1984) commented that there was little income from private practice in their sample, Smith and Stiff (1984) found that more inner city than suburban doctors spent time on private work and on teaching, though similar proportions held hospital appointments.

Acheson concluded that practice organisation was 'probably not the most appropriate to cope with the particular need and problems of Inner London' (DHSS, 1981a). There were fewer group practices and primary health care teams there than elsewhere. Heath and Sims (1984) found that a high proportion of their doctors were still in single-handed practice and of those in groups, the majority were only with one other, despite the DHSS's recommended optimum of 5-6 doctors. Similarly, Smith and Stiff (1984) found fewer doctors receiving the group-practice allowance in the inner city. Recent figures from the Tower Hamlets Health Inquiry (1987) suggest that 21 per cent of GPs are still single-handed there, 31 per cent work with one other doctor and only 16 per cent with four or more, compared with national figures of 13 per cent, 18 per cent and 25 per cent respectively.

Acheson recommended that list size should be at least 1,500 to qualify for full NHS support (DHSS, 1981a). Many doctors kept small lists because of the level of fixed allowances, the ready availability of non-NHS work, or because they were elderly and semi-retired, but it was considered that small lists made the organisation of primary health care services and the relationships between GPs and other health professionals more difficult. Both Heath and Sims (1984) and Smith and Stiff (1984) found list sizes well below the average of 2,000, but many GPs considered their workload to be much greater than colleagues elsewhere, because of the high proportions of immigrant and elderly patients, the poor housing and the multiple deprivation in their areas, and consequently felt that an ideal list size should be below 2,000.

One of the most pressing problems facing primary health care in Inner London remains that of inadequate practice premises (Heath and Sims, 1984). Acheson reported that only one quarter fell within recommended standards and went on to present a lengthy list of basic recommendations, including minimum standards, teams of co-ordinators, review and financial assistance from health authorities and many others (DHSS, 1981a). Rhodes et al. (1986) were able to report several initiatives around the question of GP premises, but the government still acknowledges that there are too many doctors in cramped accommodation, which precludes adequate support staff (DHSS, 1986a). In the recent White Paper (DHSS, 1987) there are plans to give Family Practitioner Committees new responsibilities for drawing up priority programmes and to increase funds for improvement grants and the cost-rent scheme. However, many GPs consider the latter unhelpful, since only average building costs are allowed, whereas costs in Inner London are extremely high (Tower Hamlets, 1987). In Tower Hamlets, two thirds of practice premises are rented from the local authority and their structural framework and maintenance are often poor. Whereas 36 per cent of borough GPs are reported fairly satisfied with their premises, almost half are not satisfied and complain of small rooms, inadequate waiting space, poor toilet facilities, lack of storage for records, lack of accommodation for attached staff, absence of treatment rooms and major structural problems. This reflects the increased dissatisfaction with premises expressed by inner city GPs in Smith and Stiff's earlier study (1984), which also found that they considered that they had adequate access to diagnostic facilities, but not enough direct access to hospital beds where they could retain responsibility for their patients.

The same source revealed that inner city GPs were less likely than others to have good relations with other professionals, particularly with colleagues socially and with hospital staff over patient admissions.

However, their finding that inner city doctors were more likely to describe their local social services as 'good' is contradicted by Heath and Sims (1984), who reported very little satisfaction with the personal social services, mainly because social workers were considered too young and inexperienced, were not available at night and often made contact with GPs too late in the day. Acheson observed that disadvantaged people require the provision of services by a number of health and other agencies, with whom the first point of contact should be a GP group practice working closely with social services and community nurses (DHSS, 1981a). Nurses (see below) are often used as receptionists in Inner London, which is perhaps less surprising when one considers that over 40 per cent of practices may be without any ancillary staff at all (Heath and Sims, 1984). Tower Hamlets is reported to have the lowest proportion of receptionists, practice managers and other ancillary workers in England and Wales (Tower Hamlets, 1987).

Community nursing services

In an ideal world, all community health workers should have an extended brief which would take in issues such as the problems of the single homeless (SHIL Sub-Group, 1987). The value of nurses in special schemes for the homeless is said to be beyond question (Liverpool CHC) and they are thought to represent a greater source of available professional time than other professionals such as GPs (Wootton, 1985). In reality, both the attachment and employment of community and practice nurses in Inner London were less than half of the national rate during the Acheson survey, and he recommended more reliable and sensitive establishment guidelines, which should be at least 20 per cent higher immediately (DHSS, 1981a). Although nurse training has been the area where 'post-Acheson money' has perhaps had the most effect (Rhodes et al., 1986), the professional and economic pressures of living and working in London still contribute to a recruitment and retention problem in the inner city areas (Tower Hamlets, 1987). Community nurses in Inner London tend to be younger, newly-qualified, inexperienced and with heavier caseloads (DHSS, 1981a). They soon move on, especially if they have no commitments, and do not spend as much time in post as colleagues elsewhere (Jarman, 1981). Meanwhile, a lack of integrated community nursing services is believed to be highly significantly correlated with increased hospitalisation rates in general (Jarman, 1981) and increased use of Accident and Emergency Departments in particular (Tower Hamlets, 1987).

The government ordered a Community Nursing Review, chaired by Julia Cumberlege, who recommended that community nursing services should be planned, organised and delivered on a neighbourhood basis of between 10,000 and 25,000 people (DHSS, 1986b). In a later article (Jarman and Cumberlege, 1987), she pointed out that health care and social services are currently provided by many agencies, whose boundaries overlap considerably, and suggested that there would be considerable benefit if common boundaries could be defined. The government has agreed that neighbourhood nursing teams might rationalise the way primary health care teams operate (DHSS, 1986a) and that this may be especially appropriate in inner cities, where there is a traditional pattern of small, overlapping practice areas (DHSS, 1987). However, the White Paper only affirms the need for 'nursing services to be organised flexibly, whether geographically or on a practice basis'.

The debate over the relative merits of attached community nurses and employed practice nurses has been intense. The Black report (DHSS, 1980) called unequivocally for 'an above average number of community nurses to be attached to family practice' in areas where there is a high prevalence of ill health, poor social conditions and few GPs. Acheson (DHSS, 1981a) found that only 25 per cent of community nurses were in attachment schemes in Inner London, compared with 68 per cent nationally, and that practice nurses were employed by 11 per cent of GPs in Inner London, compared with 24 per cent nationally. He did not consider any recommendations necessary 'to disturb the present balance between community and practice nurses', pointing out that attachment could be 'inefficient' in areas of high mobility, high non-registration and high overlap of practices. In one case, fifteen to twenty different GPs were involved in a single block of flats, and many nurse managers have actually 'detached' staff, especially health visitors, in urban areas where GP lists do not cover identifiable geographical areas because they felt that consideration of the integrated needs of the whole community was being impeded.

Individual types of nurses have also received considerable attention in the context of provision of health care services to homeless people. Health visitors play a prominent role with homeless families (Boyer, 1986; Drennan and Stearn, 1986; Lovell, 1986; Lawrie, 1983). As far as single homeless people are concerned, the spotlight often falls on community psychiatric nurses, whose services are keenly sought (Wootton, 1985).

Co-operation and teamwork

An underlying theme of most of the recent official and unofficial reports so far considered, and an inextricable strand in any consideration of general practitioner and community nursing services, is the concept of the primary health care team (DHSS, 1981b). Acheson took pains to emphasise that attachment is not synonymous with teamwork, the aims of which must be integrated and co-ordinated care which is appropriate to the consumer, improved communications, the avoidance of unnecessary duplication and the arrangement of other appropriate services (DHSS, 1981a). There is increasing recognition of the key role of primary health teams in carrying out all the functions of primary health care, whether preventive, diagnostic, therapeutic or caring (SHIL Sub-Group, 1987). Offering a range of services under one roof benefits both patients and staff alike (Jarman and Cumberlege, 1987).

Areas with multiple problems demand greater co-ordination between health and other services (DHSS, 1981a). The 1986 Green Paper calls on all statutory and voluntary agencies to 'maximise resources in the interests of patient care' - and quotes the provision of health care for single homeless people as an example (DHSS, 1986a). A decade earlier, a surgery in a Liverpool Day Centre had improved co-operation within the health services and also between the health and local authority social services (Liverpool CHC). Some years later, the lack of any co-ordinated approach by the authorities in Manchester was partly blamed for diminishing the impact of certain individuals who were working hard to overcome the barriers for single homeless people (Shanks, 1983). The value of such schemes depends in part on their impact on the thinking of service providers (SHIL Sub-Group, 1987), and joint planning is vital if lack of liaison is not to affect public perceptions of accessibility to primary care services (Tower Hamlets, 1987).

Outside London, many health authority services can be provided in the context of the primary care team (DHSS, 1981a) but within the capital such teams are scarcer than elsewhere (Heath and Sims, 1984). Older doctors may be unwilling to accept the concept and many premises are totally inadequate for viable teamwork, or even for staff meetings. Community health workers are often not allowed to cross health district or local authority boundaries straddled by many GP practice areas and the whole impression is one of fragmentation rather than co-ordination (Jarman, 1981; DHSS, 1981a). However, many changes have been proposed in a relatively short space of time. Planners and policy-makers must recognise that the formation of primary care teams cannot take place overnight, particularly with scarce resources (Rhodes et al., 1986).

Camden and Tower Hamlets
Ever since Tower Hamlets was identified in the Black report (DHSS, 1980) as an area in need of special health and social development, there has been considerable concentration on its problems in the literature, culminating in the Tower Hamlets Health Inquiry (1987). As yet nothing similar has been produced for Camden. In Tower Hamlets the Health Authority still considers the general health status of the population to be 'very poor', with an overall standardised mortality rate (SMR) of 114, compared with an average of 97 for other London authorities. For those under 65 years old, the SMR is 31 per cent above average. The high proportion of social classes IV and V in the borough results in more work for primary care staff, with higher than average GP consultation rates, both in and out of hours. There is said to be a great division between the prestigious teaching hospital and the underdeveloped primary care services and a great sense of inequality in the distribution of health care services to local people in the community, which they feel powerless to improve. Lack of consultation and democratic planning results in a 'chaotic mismatch of action and need' and the CHC concludes that 'what we see in this borough is the most acute end of the problem spectrum of primary care in inner cities compared to England and Wales as a whole'.

Primary health care for the single homeless

The nature and extent of health needs and unmet needs

'Need' is notoriously difficult to define and measure (Crombie and Fleming, 1986) and some feel that producing adequate measures of need may be one of London's 'intractable' problems (McCarthy, 1980). Even MPs recognise that 'demands and needs are not the same' (Hansard, 10 February, 1987) but researchers can only conclude that 'current approaches to the measurement of needs in the population for health care services are inadequate to the task' and cannot give enough information on 'what type of health care is indicated or what mix of health care resources might be required (Leavey, 1985). Others are sometimes 'struck by the lack of objectivity' in the way definitions of user need are arrived at (NFA Day Centres, 1987). On a more positive note, SHIL feels that needs and health profiles can be built up through 'community approaches to homeless people', involving overviews from both local authority and non-statutory agencies, pressure and community groups (SHIL Sub-Group, 1987), and the government agrees that there is scope for giving greater emphasis to local information about both medical and social needs (DHSS, 1987). At the same time, information technology must be more fully exploited to link up health indices, social factors and services, so that the correspondence between provision and need can be monitored (Jarman and Cumberlege, 1987).

Since the early 1970s, there has been a growing awareness that the problem of homelessness incorporates a wider number of people and a greater range of needs than was previously considered, when individual problems of illness and disadvantage held sway (Drake et al., 1982). Housing need, i.e. access to decent, affordable accommodation (Saunders, 1986), is now considered paramount and the main feature which homeless people have in common, with only a minority experiencing the multiple personal and social problems which call for formal or informal support networks (Greve et al., 1986). In spite of the Black report's insistence that all local authorities should fulfil their responsibilities in providing for 'all types of housing need which arises' (DHSS, 1980), cutbacks in housing finance have resulted in a decline in both council housing and the private rental sector, which has only made the situation much worse (Stein, 1987). There is growing recognition that social conditions and environment affect both the need for and provision of health care (DHSS, 1981a) and that the areas with greatest need are often those with the poorest medical services (Liverpool CHC). Most public research into the health needs of single homeless people has focused almost exclusively on reception centres, hostels and lodging houses. This has built up a good picture of the functions and ethos of these institutions, but not necessarily of the needs of their inhabitants (SHIL Sub-Group, 1987). It has been suggested that there should be more emphasis on the type of project which examines aspects of the health needs of and services available to the single homeless in the context of both medical and social problems, such as was attempted by the Central London Outreach Team (1984). This will help identify the variety of their disadvantages and the range of health and other support services required to help them (Drake et al., 1982).

Perhaps the most vocal campaigners against the marginalisation of the health needs of single homeless people are members of the Single Homelessness in London Working Party (SHIL). They argue that concentration on the problems of a small section of the population tends to perpetuate stereotypes and traditional images which retain a grip over public policy. Special schemes for providing primary care for the single homeless are often not 'plugged in' to local housing and social services and tend to emphasise 'medical' rather than 'health' requirements. The widespread implications of the fact that homelessness can result in loss of access to health care services tend to be overlooked (SHIL Sub-Group, 1987).

Similarly, an overemphasis on the morbidity characteristics associated with single homelessness is common to many studies which try to assess need. The related concept, that those in greatest need are often those who use services less effectively (McCarthy, 1980), is only recently receiving the attention due to it. SHIL also argues that consideration of access to services, including registration difficulties and the attitude of staff, is imperative if single homeless people are not to be discouraged from taking up available primary care services.

Morbidity and the single homeless
The main message to emerge from recent publications is that homelessness is associated with a high risk of illness, which may take

different forms at different stages (SHIL Sub-Group, 1987). It is notoriously difficult to disentangle cause and effect between homelessness and a range of social and medical problems (Drake et al., 1982). Lack of co-ordination between housing and caring services can sometimes result in disabled people becoming homeless because they can no longer support themselves unaided (SHIL, 1986). Discharged psychiatric patients are often without suitable accommodation when they leave hospital (Davies, 1974) and City and Hackney CHC asks whether the increased mental disorder amongst the homeless is a cause or a result of their homelessness. A recent television documentary was convinced that if people drink or have behavioural problems, this is generally a result of their situation, not the cause of it – as one of their interviewees retorted, 'You'd have to be drunk to sleep in one of these places' (Channel 4 TV). There is other evidence that the homeless lifestyle can lead to drinking as a relief from reality, in which a vicious circle of 'drinking to forget about drinking' becomes established (Central London Outreach Team, 1984).

Overall, homeless people tend to experience a higher incidence of chronic, debilitating illness than others (Powell, 1987), while minor acute illnesses can present particular problems for them when they lack the facilities to look after themselves properly (Toon et al., 1987).

a) Sociodemographic factors
The incidence of problems has been related partly to age and partly to the length of time spent homeless (Drake et al., 1982). Very young people may suffer from more foot and skin problems, indeterminate stomach pains and tension resulting from anxiety (Saunders, 1986). In some instances both anorexia and pregnancy may be the result of exploitation in the search for affection (Channel 4 TV), and single young people living alone may be particularly susceptible to stress, mental illness and drug abuse (DHSS, 1981a). Intermediate age groups (ie. 30-49) seem most prone to a mixture of physical and mental illnesses, especially alcoholism, while those over 50 suffer most from physical disabilities (Drake et al., 1982). The same source reveals that all medical and social problems, together with the use of medical facilities, tend to increase with the length of time spent homeless, although this seems to apply mainly to the younger age groups. This

may be either because late middle-aged and elderly people are picked up more by the caring services and are technically no longer homeless, or, or course, they may simply die. Drake et al. (1982) also found only marginal differences in the problems experienced between the two sexes: women seemed to drink less and men tended to have more multiple problems. The least educated appeared to have the most problems.

More evidence has been accumulated regarding the influence of the type of accommodation on morbidity patterns. The Royal Commission on the NHS (1979) acknowledged that medical problems can be directly connected to poor housing and the Black report underlined the fact that security in housing has health benefits (DHSS, 1980). In spite of this, some councils remain unwilling to recognise the links between poor housing and health (Tower Hamlets, 1987) and little attention is paid to the subject in many areas where the majority of single homeless live in hostels and lodging houses (Liverpool CHC). In general, those with the 'direst accommodation difficulties' tend to experience the most problems (Drake et al., 1982). Hostels are also singled out as examples of concentrated suffering, where incidence of chronic physical and mental disease is high (SHIL Sub-Group, 1987), in spite of the opinions of wardens who may take a more positive view of their residents' health than do local GPs (Wootton, 1985).

b) Types of pathology
Around 50 per cent of single homeless people questioned about their health claim to have no disability at all (Central London Outreach Team, 1984; Drake et al., 1982) and about one half to two thirds are thought not to have any serious problems. However, the remaining sizeable minority suffer from a variety of illnesses and as many as one in twenty may have four or more problems at the same time.

c) Physical illness and handicap
Jarman (1981) found little significant variation in physical illness between the London boroughs, and other surveys show that between 30 and 50 per cent of disabilities are thought to have a physical cause (Digby, 1976; Drake et al., 1982). Of these, pulmonary disorders give rise to grave concern because of their persistence (Channel 4 TV).

Tuberculosis still represents a real problem for some health authorities, such as Tower Hamlets (DHSS, 1980). Throughout Inner London there is a high rate of TB per 100,000 population (DHSS, 1981a) and amongst single homeless vagrants and those in hostels the rate is estimated at 10-15 per cent (Morrell, 1967; Tandon, 1986) or a fifty times increased risk (Stearn, 1987). Despite fears of a public health hazard and suggestions that X-ray screening should be the most appropriate means of identifying sufferers (DHSS, 1976), mass radiography services no longer visit many hostels (Wootton, 1985).

Other respiratory disorders have a high prevalence amongst the single homeless (Tandon, 1986) and may represent the type of disorder on which most time is spent (Liverpool CHC). Incidence of bronchitis has been reported as 10 per cent (Morrell, 1967) and 17 per cent (Shanks, 1983) and the risk of lung cancer estimated as a seven times increase for hostel dwellers (Stearn, 1987). Upper respiratory tract infections are common (Holden, 1975) and may well became chronic if neglected, while insanitary conditions may contribute to the spread of other infections and parasitic infestations (City and Hackney CHC).

Skin complaints and disorders of the legs and feet are traditionally associated with those who sleep rough, in shelters or hostels (Dickinson and Dickinson, 1987; City and Hackney CHC; Liverpool CHC). However, in a more recent study Toon et al. (1987) note that 58 per cent of their sample had good foot hygiene, with a further 38 per cent considered average and only 4 per cent poor. Most problems arose from ill-fitting and worn footwear and 21 per cent had severe foot problems, especially ulceration and blistering.

Epilepsy is also considered 'fairly common' (City and Hackney CHC) and hostel dwellers may be nine times more likely to suffer from it than others (Stearn, 1987). In some quarters, gastrointestinal disorders were reportedly high (Tandon, 1986) with 11 per cent of one recent sample suffering from peptic ulcer (Toon et al., 1987).

One area where the single homeless seem particularly prone to problems is that of accidental trauma. Incidence statistics vary between 2 and 16 per cent (Central London Outreach Team, 1984; Digby, 1976; Morrell, 1967; Toon et al., 1987).

Of those single homeless who had been hospitalised in these surveys, about 50 per cent may have been so for physical reasons and a further 15 per cent for accidents (Digby, 1976). Many may be afraid of going into hospital, for fear of dying or losing their hostel place (Davies, 1974). Toon et al. (1987) observed that a high proportion of their consultations (14.7 per cent) were referred to hospital, but that many of these did not receive appropriate treatment, for various reasons.

d) Mental illness and handicap

Mental illness rates in Inner London are higher than in Outer London or the rest of England and Wales (Jarman, 1981). Among the single homeless, estimates of the incidence of psychiatric illness vary from around 10 per cent in a mixed population (Drake et al., 1982) to over 80 per cent in a reception centre where ex-psychiatric patients had failed to find suitable community accommodation (Liverpool CHC). Between 30 and 40 per cent of hostel dwellers may have had mental illnesses in the past or present, though for women this figure may be over 50 per cent (Digby, 1976), and between 8 and 17 per cent of cases may have been serious enough for hospitalisation (Drake et al., 1982; NFA Day Centres, 1987). Those in hostels may be up to 57 times more likely to suffer from mental illness than others (Stearn, 1987).

Disruptive behaviour associated with psychiatric illness can be a very real problem, both to hostel wardens who are not trained in psychiatric care (Wootton, 1985) and to health care staff in hospital out-patient and other areas, where such patients engender antipathy and treatment of physical illness becomes problematic as a result (Morrell, 1967).

As one might expect, anxiety and depression associated with the strain and insecurity of homelessness are common (McKechnie and Wilson, 1986), especially among young people (Saunders, 1986). Problems with unemployment (Digby, 1976; Drake et al., 1982) compound with those of accommodation, which is especially limited for violent young people (Saunders, 1986), those with drug and alcohol problems (Drake et al., 1982; SHIL, 1986) and those individuals who prefer to sleep rough rather than go to unsuitable accommodation (Central London Outreach Team, 1984).

Of gravest concern is the lack of comprehensive community care for ex-psychiatric in-patients. In 1976 health authorities were asked to take into account the needs of homeless single clients with high levels of mental disorder and alcoholism when discussing joint care planning (DHSS, 1976). Ten years later there was still a 'serious shortfall of accommodation available and only a very small number of new units, despite community care initiatives' (SHIL, 1986). One South London psychiatric hospital is reported to have discharged five patients to hostel accommodation and 26 to no fixed address between June 1985 and June 1986 (Stearn, 1987).

e)   Alcoholism
Both alcohol and drug abuse are thought to be disproportionately high in Inner London (DHSS, 1981). Estimates of incidence of alcoholism among the single homeless range from 10 to over 30 per cent, according to the population surveyed (Drake et al., 1982; Liverpool CHC; Morrell, 1976; Toon et al., 1987; NFA Day Centres, 1987). Amongst those sleeping rough the problem is considered more prominent than any other area of need, excepting poverty and homelessness itself (Central London Outreach Team, 1984). Those who live in hostels may be 177 times more prone to alcoholism than others – by far the greatest increased risk of all health conditions (Stearn, 1987).

Problem drinkers often experience poorer health (NFA Day Centres, 1987). Associated problems include duodenal ulcers, malnutrition, peripheral neuritis, weak legs, blackouts and injuries. Aggressive behaviour can give rise to isolation and guilt, but can also lead to arrest, loss of employment and barring from health provision (Central London Outreach Team, 1984), especially from GPs (Davies, 1974).

Provision for single homeless people with alcohol problems is poor. Some boroughs do not have any statutory provision at all, and even good voluntary schemes are usually restricted to men (City and Hackney CHC).

f)   Drug abuse
Although drug abuse often occurs in conjunction with alcoholism, it is less visible and most of the drugs abused may not be perceived as powerful or potentially harmful if they are prescribed by doctors or casualty departments (Central London Outreach Team, 1984). Estimates of incidence are usually below 10 per cent (Drake et al., 1982;

NFA Day Centres, 1987) and relatively small numbers may experience accommodation problems as a result of drug addiction – only 3 per cent in Drake et al.'s sample (1982). Nevertheless, the numbers of single homeless people who present at hospital A&E departments with problems associated with drug or alcohol abuse serve to highlight the lack of suitable provision (Liverpool CHC).

g) Mortality
Premature ageing and death are held to be more frequent amongst the homeless (Channel 4 TV) and there is a reported significant excess mortality among lodging house dwellers (Shanks, 1983). Poorer social conditions tend to be linked with higher standardised mortality ratios and in Inner London suicide is around 50 per cent more likely than elsewhere (DHSS, 1981a).

Social problems and the single homeless
Recognition that social and medical problems are inextricably linked is widespread. Holden (1975) remarked that 'it is not easy to separate the medical from the social aspects of the house and its residents', referring to an experimental scheme in North London for homeless young people. Health problems are embedded in social conditions and people with social problems are more likely to visit a doctor than any other social service (SHIL Sub-Group, 1987). Drake et al. (1982) found that 8 per cent of their sample could be considered to have 'social' problems and that many of these were young people, mainly with accommodation difficulties. The Central London Outreach Team (1984) also noted that about half of the requests they received for advice from people sleeping rough were for temporary or permanent accommodation. They also commented on the very apparent problem of loneliness among their sample – the single homeless may have many acquaintances, but few friends.

Health of the single homeless and the general population
The nature and definitions of morbidity can vary from study to study and meaningful comparisons are not always possible. The Third National Study on Morbidity Statistics from General Practice, 1981-82, is the most up-to-date source of information on the nation's health in

general, though this was not published until 1986 (RCGP, 1986). A consensus view remains that single homeless people have worse general health than the rest of the population (SHIL, 1986), that they suffer from more physical illness, psychiatric disorder and alcoholism (Leighton, 1976) and that they require more than average medical care (Shanks, 1983) as a result of their environment and lifestyle (Liverpool CHC) and behaviour (Davies, 1974).

Powell (1987) confidently asserts that both registration with GPs and utilisation of health care services is low among the single homeless compared with the general population. Evidence for the access which single homeless people have to primary health care services, based on their registration with GPs, attitudes towards them, use and misuse of hospital casualty departments and awareness of services, is far less extensive than for some of the other areas reviewed so far, thus making comparisons with the general population even more uncertain.

Access to primary health care for single homeless people
For many, the crucial factor involved in the provision of primary health care to the single homeless is not so much the availability of services as their delivery (Shanks, 1983), and these commentators have identified the main problem as one of access to primary care facilities (SHIL Sub-Group, 1987). Difficulties in gaining access to medical services can affect the expression of demand for them in a group which already tends to express less effective demand, despite greater need (Liverpool CHC).

The study of access to GPs now requires consideration of relative need, class inequality, practice organisation, spatial accessibility and the nature of the doctor-patient relationship (Leavey, 1985). In addition, a lack of liaison between primary care, hospital and social services staff can result in public perceptions of inaccessibility (Tower Hamlets, 1987).

a)   Registration with GPs
Amongst surveys of single homeless people, rates of registration with a GP have ranged from 26 to 84 per cent in different parts of the country (SHIL Sub-Group, 1987). The DHSS claims that only 1 per cent of the whole population is not registered with a GP (DHSS, 1987) but alarm

bells sounded when the Acheson report suggested that this figure might be as high as 30 per cent in Inner London (DHSS, 1981a). Subsequent investigation by Bone (1984) revealed that the situation was 'less disturbing' than feared, although it must be pointed out that her figures do not include any 'vagrants'. She found no evidence that the situation was much worse in Inner London as a whole than in the country generally, and concluded that only 3 per cent of the population there had registration problems. Of those not permanently registered (i.e. around 5 per cent), about four-fifths were so 'from choice or inertia' and only about 1 per cent remained unregistered because of actual or expected difficulties. On the other hand, there was some evidence that those in greatest need were the most likely to be rejected, for example the elderly, those with chronic illness limiting their activity and those with psychiatric problems.

Figures for Tower Hamlets and Camden revealed that around three-quarters of all unregistered people lived in Camden, Kensington, Chelsea and Westminster, areas with higher levels of preference for private doctors and increased numbers of highly mobile young people and foreign visitors. In Camden, 66 per cent lived under one mile from their doctor, 22 per cent lived more than one mile away and 12 per cent were not permanently registered. In Tower Hamlets, equivalent figures were 73 per cent, 25 per cent and 2 per cent. Failures to register at the first attempt were also clustered in Camden (15 per cent) whereas in Tower Hamlets the figure was 7 per cent (Bone, 1984).

The reasons for non-registration of single homeless people have been manifold but fall essentially into two camps - patient inability or unwillingness and GP reluctance, of which the latter is considered more significant (Liverpool CHC; City and Hackney CHC) and is dealt with more fully below.

Many single homeless people feel they have no need of medical care (NFA Day Centres, 1987); they may have low expectations for their health, be embarrassed about their appearance or suspicious as a result of previous unhappy experiences with primary care (Liverpool CHC); they may view registration as severing the link with an area identified as home if they are in temporary accommodation, thus heightening their sense of rootlessness (SHIL Sub-Group, 1987). For Acheson (DHSS, 1981a) high mobility was one of the main causes of non-registration and Bone (1984) confirmed that higher rates of non-registration did occur in young, unattached adults, as they did in social classes I and II, people recently arrived at their current address, foreigners and Old Commonwealth citizens. For many, an inability to 'negotiate the system' seems to be behind their non-registration, either because they do not know how, especially ethnic minorities (DHSS, 1981a) or because they find the world of medical cards, appointment systems and waiting rooms totally alien to their way of life (Leighton, 1976; City and Hackney CHC; Holden, 1975). Although Family Practitioner Committees have powers to allocate any patients who are experiencing difficulties in registration to a given doctor's list (DHSS, 1986a) there is concern that only a minority of people know about this possibility (Bone, 1984) and that more publicity should be given to the FPCs' role here (DHSS, 1981a).

There are those who claim that the process of temporary registration provides a financial incentive for GPs, who thereby receive a capitation fee several times per year (Stearn, 1987). People who do not intend to stay in one place for more than three months are not entitled to register with a doctor unless they are in need of treatment and cannot therefore register in advance of actual illness; in some cases, people of no fixed address find it impossible to register even temporarily (DHSS, 1981a). However, according to SHIL (SHIL Sub-Group, 1987) this assumption of high mobility is unwarranted amongst many hostel and lodging house dwellers. Earlier, the DoE survey had reported that 63 per cent of single homeless people had lived more than one year in their current county and more than 40 per cent in their current district or borough (Drake et al., 1982).

The implications of non-registration are twofold. First, there is evidence that difficulties in obtaining primary care itself are experienced by many (Drake et al., 1982). Secondly, without a GP, there are problems involved in admission to hospital care and, on discharge, with on-going after care – in other words 'a missing link in the chain of treatment' (Davies, 1974). One of the government's main objectives in its Green Paper (DHSS, 1986a) is to raise the general quality of services, including simplification of the ways in which patients can select and change their doctors. It recognises that the continuity of care which GPs provide for people on their lists and their ability to arrange for patients to receive the most appropriate form of specialist treatment are 'hallmarks of our system'. In addition, as suggested by Heath and Sims (1984), many people in Inner London view their GP as a first point of reference in any crisis, not just for health services, and therefore rely on him to maintain good contacts with hospital and other services, many of which may seem rather fragmented (Jarman, 1981).

b) Attitudes of GPs towards the single homeless
Perhaps second only to the problems raised by not having a doctor at all, are those associated with 'authoritarian, unsympathetic or uninterested' doctors (Davies, 1974). Reluctant GPs are often cited as the main reason behind difficulties of access to primary care for the single homeless (Liverpool CHC) and there are complaints of lack of understanding (Wootton, 1985), resistance to requests from the homeless for medical care (Shanks, 1983) and 'not wanting to know' (Digby, 1976). In the 1970s there was 'a less than even' chance of succeeding in attracting the services of a local GP to projects in hostels and day centres (Davies, 1974), and Digby (1976) reported that 8 per cent of all hostels, especially those which did not cater for specialist groups such as alcoholics or drug-abusers, had no access at all to any kind of medical advice. At the same time, many local GPs were aware that they were not giving a good medical service to the homeless and experienced sensations of frustration as a result (Holden, 1975).

The reasons given by GPs to explain their reluctance include fears of abuse, disruption and unreliability (Leighton, 1976), hostility from other patients (City and Hackney CHC), excessive workload (DHSS, 1981) and transience (Bone, 1984). In other words, most are highly influenced by the stereotypes of homelessness which we considered earlier. In one hostel in the former Victoria Health Authority, the warden considered that 10 per cent of the residents had problems affecting their social acceptability, whereas the GP thought that the figure was 80 per cent (Wootton, 1985). The views of some doctors are obviously coloured by their experiences with their more problematic patients, but negative attitudes from the medical profession are said to foster negative attitudes amongst the single homeless (Liverpool CHC), who then became suspicious of conventional channels (Shanks, 1983).

Whatever their reasons, most doctors seem to reject the single homeless by claiming that their lists are full – 68 per cent in Bone's sample (1984) and still the most commonly mentioned response in a more recent analysis (NFA Day Centres, 1987). We have already seen why some doctors in Inner London maintain smaller lists than elsewhere in the country but there have been various suggestions for incentives to encourage more registration. Many of Acheson's (DHSS, 1981a) recommendations on this point appear to have been ignored (Rhodes et al., 1986); for example, there is still no London weighting for GPs, in spite of the burdens of higher living costs in the capital (Tower Hamlets, 1987). Jarman (1986) has recently recommended the payment of an additional registration fee for fully registering all new patients and others have put forward the idea of extra financial allowances for GPs with a special interest in homelessness (Wootton, 1985). The government's Green Paper (DHSS, 1986a) speaks of 'adequate incentives to doctors to practise in ways which encourage people to join their lists', while the subsequent White Paper (DHSS, 1987) confirms that a new allowance will be made for those working in deprived areas. The exact mechanisms by which such incentives will be put into practice remain the subject of heated debate.

SHIL has recommended that all GPs throughout the country should be salaried (Stearn, 1987) but most London GPs do not wish to lose their independent contractor status (Smith and Stiff, 1984). Several experiments with salaried family doctors are already taking place (DHSS, 1987), including, of course, the two pilot schemes for providing primary care for the homeless in Camden and Tower Hamlets whose evaluation lies behind this review. To some, however, the provision of such special salaried doctors is detrimental to any hope of integrating services for the homeless into the main stream of primary care provision and may actually remove some single homeless people from the lists of GPs with whom they were previously registered (Stearn, 1987). Others point out that such schemes place a heavy burden on one service to maintain the 24-hour commitment necessary and may give rise to the undesirable practice of uncontrolled multiple consultations and prescriptions (Powell, 1987).

c)   Information on rights and services

Advisory services are well developed in London, where some, such as the Piccadilly Advice Centre, act as an information source for others (Saunders, 1986). However, there is a danger that much of the available information is somewhat fragmented, and may remain in the hands of individual advice workers or projects, without wider dissemination. There is a great need for information leaflets and posters to be displayed in places used by homeless people, such as post offices, bus stops, DHSS offices, shops and day centres, and for these to be available in different languages (SHIL Sub-Group, 1987).

The government is concerned that both CHCs and FPCs should produce more comprehensive information about local services (DHSS, 1987). It regards the availability to individuals of information about local practices as part of its quality of care commitment and wants to see the involvement of local consumer groups and local media in disseminating practice information. This would help patients choose the sort of practice they want, raise public awareness of doctors and their services, and encourage people newly moving into an area to register with a GP rather than leave it until a time when they might have to use a hospital casualty department (DHSS, 1986a).

d)   Use of Accident and Emergency Departments

Acheson commented on the unacknowledged use of hospital A&E Departments by mobile young people, vagrants, hostel dwellers, commuters and tourists (DHSS, 1981a). Statistical evidence is confusing, ranging from Bone's assertion (1984) that there is no evidence that Inner London residents make disproportionate demands on hospitals nor that they are especially liable to use them as primary care services, through SHIL's contention that, contrary to general impressions, the use made of A&E Departments by the single homeless is only 'occasional' (SHIL Sub-Group, 1987), to Powell's crude attendance rates of 37:100 single homeless at risk per annum, compared with 8:100 patients at risk per annum in Edinburgh (Powell, 1987). In some cases, half of all presentations by single homeless people at A&E Departments are seen as 'misuse of services', mainly as a result of the 'breakdown of primary health care systems' (Liverpool CHC); in others just over one quarter of all people who used an A&E Department might not have done so if the general practice system was working perfectly (Bone, 1984). As many as 95.4 per cent of regular attenders may be single homeless people (Powell, 1987) or homeless men may represent only 2.5 per cent of all attendances (Leighton, 1976). There would appear to be some consensus that around 50 per cent of attendances at A & E Departments in Inner London may not be true emergencies (DHSS, 1981a; Davison et al., 1983), but little agreement as to the proportions who were not registered with a nearby GP, ranging from less than 1 per cent (Bone, 1984), to 23-25 per cent (DHSS, 1981a) to 40 per cent (Leighton, 1976).

Whatever the truth of the figures, it may well be that even statistically small numbers of 'problem' patients create a false impression of larger numbers if they are difficult to manage and spend a long time in the department (Davison et al., 1983). Staff attitudes may range from suspicion (Davies, 1974) based on lack of training in dealing with social problems (Leighton, 1976) to discrimination based on irritation or fear of verbal or physical abuse (City and Hackney CHC).

One of the most worrying reasons for the use of A&E Departments appears to be the non-availability of GPs, especially during weekends or at night (Heath and Sims, 1984). There may be a wide variation in surgery hours – from 10 hours to 48 hours per week in a recent survey in Tower Hamlets, where 36 per cent of people who used the local A&E Department did so because their local surgery was closed (Tower Hamlets, 1987). Deputising services are a cause of great concern, especially among single-handed doctors, and though there is little information on their use, there is a fear that patient confusion may result in increased use of A&E Departments, especially by parents anxious for their children's health (DHSS, 1981a). The government has recognised that answering machines and systems which intercept or redirect telephone calls can be 'a substantial impediment to sick and anxious people, especially when there are language and cultural difficulties' and has called for 'difficulties in gaining access by telephone' to be tackled (DHSS, 1986a).

The question of the appropriateness of A&E Departments to the needs of single homeless people is two-sided. There are those who advocate that they should take on a primary health care role and accept that they are part of a network of community provision (SHIL

Sub-Group, 1987), but in many cases A&E doctors have no experience of general practice and there are many fears that their recommended treatments would therefore be 'inappropriate' (DHSS, 1981a). Secondly, there is the vexed question of whether or not single homeless people make 'appropriate' use of A&E services – that is, for accidents and emergencies rather than for basic primary care. Powell (1987) calculated that, where a primary care scheme for hostel dwellers existed, 57 per cent of A&E attendances were deemed appropriate and 43 per cent were considered more appropriate to primary care, compared with 29 per cent and 71 per cent for attendances from single homeless outside those hostels. Single homeless people are considered 'more likely' to attend for conditions which a GP could treat (Maitra, 1982), but these may be the 'complications' brought on by lack of previous primary care, or 'preventable' emergencies (Leighton, 1976). Presentations relating to drug and alcohol abuse or psychiatric illness may highlight the general lack of suitable treatment or after-care facilities (Liverpool CHC). Those attending for non-medical reasons, in search of food, money, warmth and shelter, for example, should not be assumed to have only a social problem, since psychiatric problems are often not recognised as such and referral to an inappropriate social worker, and hence to inadequate or inappropriate accommodation, might only increase the problem (City and Hackney CHC).

Responses to the health needs of the single homeless
Historically, the medical care of the homeless has been 'at best perfunctory' and has relied largely on the efforts of sympathetic individuals (Shanks, 1983). Over thirty years ago it was reported that the main gap in welfare legislation was in the lack of facilities for dealing with illness in elderly lodging house men (Sargaison, 1954). In the 1970s there were still difficulties in obtaining medical care for such people (Davies, 1974) and the DHSS felt obliged to remind health authorities of their responsibilities (DHSS, 1975 and 1976). Throughout this period, and into the 1980s, there has been some concentration on the health and medical needs of the residents in hostels, lodging houses and resettlement units, and, more recently, investigation into the particular problems experienced by homeless families in bed and breakfast hotels. However, organisations like SHIL

are convinced that 'traditional images of single homelessness retain a grip over thinking', whereas in reality there is a 'new landscape' of homeless people who are young, often female and often black (SHIL Sub-Group, 1987).

What is needed therefore is a response which challenges the sterotypes and myths of homelessness and provides a range of services, in line with Green Paper thinking (DHSS, 1986a). Perhaps some of the most important ingredients in providing medical care for the homeless are time and compassion (Holden, 1975; Wootton, 1985) and an informal approach is of the essence (Liverpool CHC). Those schemes which have been set up, many on an experimental basis, reflect the variety of approaches to the problem which have been adopted. After all, as Edwina Currie emphasised, 'The Department does not issue guidance centrally to health and local authorities on services specifically for the single homeless. Authorities are expected to plan according to local needs and circumstances' (Hansard, 25 February 1987).

a) Separate services
These typically take the form of open access clinics, such as Great Chapel Street, London (El-Kabir, 1982), Luther Street, Oxford (Stearn, 1987) and Bridge Centre, Newcastle upon Tyne (Maitra, 1982), or medical input into hostels, lodging houses, resettlement units or day centres, such as the Edinburgh house doctor scheme (Powell, 1987), various experiments in Liverpool (Liverpool CHC) and services provided at Arlington House, Camden and Tower House, Tower Hamlets (SHIL Sub-Group, 1987).

Open access clinics try to create the 'right atmosphere' and to develop appropriate responses to anti-social behaviour (Saunders, 1986) but there are suggestions that their success may be due more to the tenacious vision of a few key individuals than to the nature of the schemes themselves (SHIL Sub-Group, 1987). Access is usually very easy, without an appointment or the 'barrier' of a hostile receptionist, and anonymity can be preserved. On the other hand, clients need to 'accept their subculture' in order to make their way there and this may then prove more difficult to break out of. Clinic workers are more likely to be able to provide flexible teamwork, be good listeners, introduce innovatory practices and provide some specialisation, but they may not be well placed to deal with non-medical needs and may not be able to draw on wider community resources. This may tend to confirm the segregation of their client group from others and promote an emphasis on personal pathology. Record keeping is usually much simplified, but, where patients are not permanently registered, there may be difficulties about 24-hour coverage and full medical histories may not be available when needed. Perhaps one of the most serious indictments of open access clinics stems from their very 'success', when local GPs tend to refer all their single homeless patients to them and do not make any efforts at all to improve their own service (Stearn, 1987).

More than 10 years ago Digby expressed the view that there was a 'great need for clinic facilities in some of the larger hostels and lodging houses' (Digby, 1976). The Acheson report (DHSS, 1981a) subsequently called on all health authorities to arrange for medical and nursing services for hostels and there are now several schemes in existence. In many cases, there is a considerable input from the non-NHS or voluntary sector (Wootton, 1985) and staff get a great deal of personal satisfaction from caring for residents. However, this short-term advantage must be set against the longer-term disadvantage of eroding the motivation to replace these institutions altogether and ensure that all single homeless people, whatever their age, are in suitable accommodation or receiving appropriate care (SHIL Sub-Group, 1987). Those in favour of on-site provision in hostels argue that their size and isolation militate against their integration into the normal primary health care services (Tandon, 1986), that they are easy of access and informal (Liverpool CHC) and that special links can be built up with appropriate hospital specialists when necessary (Shanks, 1983). Other advantages may include the preventive care possibilities that are opened up through personal knowledge and long-term relationships with residents and the holistic approach that is facilitated by being able to address social and environmental, as well as medical, problems (SHIL Sub-Group, 1987). On the other hand, accommodation for the services may be less than adequate and lack of full medical notes a major problem (Powell, 1987). In addition, institutionalised relationships may distort personal development, lower expectations of health and 'label' inmates in ways they find impossible to challenge (SHIL Sub-Group, 1987).

Overall, separate health care provision for the single homeless would appear to have the support of only a minority of people. Some have pointed out the advantages of having staff both trained in primary care skills and with specialist knowledge of homelessness: 'Growth of expertise and knowledge among those providing health care for the homeless may be an important way of changing attitudes, just as the hospice movement has changed attitudes to the terminally ill' (Toon et al., 1987). They have also argued that to worry about the stigmatisation of the single homeless is unrealistic when so many find it difficult to deal with health service bureaucracy, are suspicious of authority and live 'disorganised' lives which militate against using the normal facilities and complying with treatment offered there. However, for the most part the advantages of sympathetic, easy-access services seem outweighed by the disadvantages of not addressing the central problem of the majority of single homeless people, especially young people, women and ethnic minorities. Such services are very limited in number and cannot cover the needs of the single homeless for 24-hours-a-day cover, 7 days a week, yet where they do exist they may be absolving local GPs from a sense of responsibility or denying patients their right to choose another GP (Stearn, 1987). Special clinics may also be more vulnerable to cuts in times of financial restraint (City and Hackney CHC); their work can all too easily be marginalised, since they are not linked into any framework for social policy planning (SHIL Sub-Group, 1987).

b) Fully integrated services

Spearheaded by SHIL, several groups are campaigning for single homeless people to be fully integrated into revitalised primary care facilities 'while accepting that this will not always be possible' (Toon et al., 1987). Separate services and special schemes may act as disincentives to full access and cannot be totally comprehensive, whereas integrated services can deliver co-ordinated, multi-service responses, adopting a holistic approach and involving consumer participation. Special services are often based on the 'old stereotypes' rather than 'current reality'; fully integrated primary health care services can be part of a pattern of local networks, cultures and support systems, part of a wider effort to develop conditions in which physical and mental health can flourish and part of a community approach to health care, involving community workers, action groups and the single homeless themselves (SHIL Sub-Group, 1987).

Those who may find this view 'utopian' should take heart from the increasing number of GPs who are 'seeing the homeless as ordinary patients' as stereotypical images of homelessness are revised (Stearn, 1987). In Edinburgh, after experimenting with a 'workmen-in-camp' scheme of house doctors in hostels, the recommendation was made that future provision should 'involve re-integrating the single homeless into normal health service provision through their registration with general practitioners' (Powell, 1987).

c) Special services to assist access
Faced with such differing ideologies, the inevitable compromise has taken place and several schemes now incorporate the dual function of improving access to general services on an integrated basis, while providing direct primary care services for a limited time. In the long term this may prove rather confusing for clients, there may be continuity difficulties and such schemes may still be marginalised within the NHS (SHIL Sub-Group, 1987). For the moment most are still in their infancy, awaiting full evaluation. They include the Leeds Health Care for Homeless People Project and the Manchester and Salford Health Care for Homeless People Project. The two London-based schemes – the East London Homeless Health Project and the Camden and Islington Health Care Project – are the subject of the Policy Studies Institute evaluation, of which this review of the literature is an integral part.

References
Arden, A. *Homeless persons - the Housing Act 1985 Part III*. Legal Action Group, 1986.

Barrett, H. et al. *Homelessness and the voluntary sector*. ARVAC, 1984.
Bayswater Hotel Homelessness Project. *Speaking for ourselves: families in Bayswater B&B*, 1987.

Berthoud, R. *Supplementary benefit Board and Lodgings payments: the effects of time and price limits.* PSI, 1986.

Bone, M. *Registration with general medical practitioners in Inner London: a survey carried out on behalf of the DHSS.* HMSO, 1984.

Boyer, J. 'Homelessness from a health visitor's viewpoint'. *Health Vis.* November 1986, *59*(11), 332-3.

Campling, J. 'Shelter for the homeless'. *Soc. Work Today*, 12 January 1987, 22.

Central London Outreach Team. *Sleeping out in Central London.* GLC, 1984.

Channel 4 Television. *Homeless*, three-part documentary broadcast on 30 March, 6 April, 13 April 1987.

CHAR advertisement, *New Society*, 15 January 1988, 12.

Chartered Institute of Public Finance and Accountancy. *Homelessness statistics 1986-87 actuals.* CIPFA, 1987.

City and Hackney Community Health Council. *Homeless and healthless: health care for single homeless people in an inner city health district*, (undated).

Crombie, D.L. and Fleming, D.M. 'The third national study of morbidity statistics from general practice'. *J.Roy. Coll. Gen. Pract.* February 1986, *36*(283), 51-2.

Davies, A. *The provision of medical care for the homeless and rootless.* CHAR, 1974.

Davison, A.G. et al. 'Use and misuse of an accident and emergency department in the East End of London'. *J.Roy, Soc. Med.* 1983. *76*, 37-40.

DHSS. Letter: Provision of medical care for the vagrant population. DC59/75. DHSS, 1975.

DHSS. Letter: Health care for homeless, rootless people, 1976.

DHSS. *Inequalities in health. Report of a Research Working Group.* (Chairman: Sir Douglas Black.) DHSS, 1980.

DHSS. *Primary health care in Inner London.* Report of a study group commissioned by the London Health Planning Consortium. (Chairman: Sir Donald Acheson.) 1981a.

DHSS. *The primary health care team.* Report by a Joint Working Group of the SMAC and the SNMAC. HMSO, 1981b.

DHSS. *Primary health care: an agenda for discussion.* Cmnd. 9771. HMSO, 1986a.

DHSS. *Neighbourhood nursing: a focus for care.* Report of the Community Nursing Review (Chairman: Julia Cumberlege.) HMSO, 1986b.

DHSS. *Promoting better health: the government's programme for improving primary health care.* Cm.249. HMSO, 1987.

Dickinson, E.J. and Dickinson, R. 'Medical care for the homeless'. *Lancet,* 25 April 1987, *1*(8539), 980-981.

Digby, P. Wingfield. *Hostels and lodgings for single people.* HMSO, 1976.

Drake, M. et al. *Single and homeless.* HMSO, 1982.

Drennan, V. and Stearn, J. 'Health visitors and homeless families'. *Health Vis.* November 1986. *59*(11), 340-2.

El Kabir, D.J. 'Great Chapel Street Medical Centre'. *BMJ,* 13 February 1982, *284,* 480-1.

Green, J. 'The resettlement process from Arlington House': report from a HCT seminar, 22 January 1985. *Housing Rev.* May-June 1985, *34*(3), 97-8.

Greve, J. et al. *Homelessness in London*: a statement and recommendations by the research team. Submitted to the GLC, 1986.

Hansard, 10 February 1987, Housing and homelessness debate, col. 175-262.

Hansard, 1 April 1987, col. 1090-1.

Hansard, 2 April 1987, col. 597.

Heath, M. and Sims, P. 'The GP in the inner city: a survey of a London health district'. *J.Roy. Coll. Gen. Pract.* 1984, *34,* 199-204.

Hodgkin, J. 'Living loose'. *New Society,* 8 September 1987, 14-16.

Holden, H.M. 'Medical care of homeless and rootless young people'. *BMJ,* 22 November 1975, *4,* 446-8.

Housing Act 1985. Part III: Housing the homeless. HMSO, 1985.

Housing Rights Campaign. *Housing is a right for all.* (Information Pack, 1987, p.2).

Howarth, V. *A survey of families in bed and breakfast hotels:* report to the governors of the Thomas Coram Foundation for Children, 1987.

Jarman, B. 'A survey of primary care in London'. *RCGP. Occasional Paper,* No. 16, 1981.

Jarman, B. 'Quality in general practice: a focus on inner cities'. *J.Roy. Coll. Gen. Pract.* 1986, *36,* 395-6.

Jarman, B. and Cumberlege, J. 'Developing primary health care'. *BMJ,* 18 April 1987, *294,* 1005-8.

King's Fund Centre. *Primary health care in Inner London.* A report of a conference held at the King's Fund Centre on 22 September 1981.

Lawrie, B. 'Travelling families in East London: adapting health visiting methods to a minority group'. *Health Vis.* 1983, *56*(1), 26-8.

Leavey, R. *Access to GPs: a fair share for all?* A report prepared for the DHSS. Univ. of Manchester Dept. of General practice, DHSS Research Unit, 1985.

Leighton, J. 'Primary medical care for the homeless and rootless in Liverpool'. *Hosp. Hlth Serv. Rev.* August 1976, *72*(8), 266-7.

Liverpool Central and Southern District Community Health Council. *Primary medical care and the single homeless in Liverpool,* (undated).

Livingstone, K. *Homelessness in London:* a report by the leader of the GLC. GLC, 1985.

London Housing Unit. *New Year 1988: another disastrous year for London's homeless.* The Unit, 1987.

Lovell, B. 'Health visiting homeless families'. *Health Vis.* November 1986, *59*(11), 334-7.

Lunn, T. 'Trapped by the age barrier ...'. *Soc. Serv. Insight,* 30 January 1987, 8-9.

McCarthy, M. (ed.) *London's health services in the 80s.* King's Fund Project Paper No. 25, 1980.

McKechnie, S. and Wilson, D. *Homes above all. Housing in Britain: the facts, the failures, the future.* Shelter, (undated).

Maitra, A.K. 'Dealing with the disadvantaged - single homeless, are we doing enough?'. *Pub. Hlth Lond.* 1982, *96*, 141-4.

Mariasy, J. 'Young people and homelessness'. *Everywoman*, November 1987, 12.

Matthews, P. 'Doctors for the homeless and rootless'. *BMJ*, 21 June 1986, *292*, 1672.

Miller, K. 'Homeless year aims for all party commitment'. *Loc. Gov. Chron.* 9 January 1987, 9.

Morrell, D.C. 'The Edinburgh common lodging house: a challenge in medical care'. *Scot. Med. J.* May 1967, *12*(5), 171-7.

NFA Day Centres Action Research. *Action for a change.* Research report, 1987.

New Society, 'Homelessness costs double'. 22 January 1988, 7.

Piccadilly Advice Centre. *Bored with lodging?* A report on the effects of the new board and lodging regulations, 1985.

Platt, S. 'London homeless: the crisis erupts'. *New Society*, 4 December 1987, 9-11.

Powell, P.V. 'A "house doctor" scheme for primary health care for the single homeless in Edinburgh'. *J.Roy Coll. Gen. Pract.* October 1987, *37*, 444-7.

Powell, P.V. 'Use of an accident and emergency department by the single homeless'. *Health Bull. (Edin.)* 1987, *45*(5), 255-62.

Rhodes, G. et al. *Primary health care in the inner cities after Acheson.* PSI, 1986.

Robertson, S. and Matheson, C. *Enforcing vagrancy.* West End Co-ordinated Voluntary Services, 1986.

Royal College of General Practitioners, Office of Population Censuses and Surveys and DHSS. *Morbidity statistics from general practice, 1981-82: third national study.* HMSO, 1986.

Royal Commission on the National Health Service. Report. (Chairman: Sir Alec Merrison). HMSO, 1979.

Sargaison, E.M. *Growing old in common lodgings.* Nuffield Provincial Hospitals Trust, 1954.

Saunders, B. *Homeless young people in Britain: the contribution of the voluntary sector.* NCVO, 1986.

Shanks, N.J. 'Medical provision for the homeless in Manchester'. *J.Roy. Coll. Gen. Pract.* January 1983, *33*, 40-3.

Single Homelessness in London Working Party. *Single homelessness in London*, 1986.

Single Homelessness in London Health Sub-Group. *Primary health care for homeless single people in London: a strategic approach*, 1987.

Smith, C. and Stiff, C. 'Problems of inner city general practice in North East London'. *J.Roy. Coll. Gen. Pract.* 1984, *35*, 71-6.

Social Services Committee. *Primary health care.* Vol. 1: Report together with the proceedings of the Committee. Session 1986-87: First report. HMSO, 1987.

Stearn, J. 'No home, no health care?'. *Roof*, May-June, 1987, 16-19.

Stein, M. 'Young, single and homeless'. *Soc. Serv. Insight*, 19 June 1987, 18-20.

Streetly, A. 'Health care for travellers: one year's experience'. *BMJ*, 21 February 1987, *294*, 492-4.

Tandon, P.K. 'Health care for the homeless'. *J.Roy. Coll. Gen. Pract.* June 1986, *36*, 292.

Toon, P.D. et al. 'Audit of work at a medical centre for the homeless over one year'. *J.Roy. Coll. Gen. Pract.* March 1987, *37*, 120-2.

Tower Hamlets Health Inquiry. Report, 1987.

Wootton, H. 'A new year - but little cheer for the single homeless'. *Hlth Soc. Serv. J.* 12 December 1985, 1564-5.

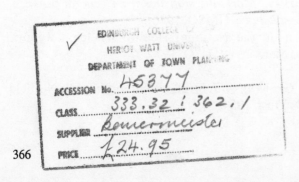